Textbook of
Endocrine Physiology

W9-BPK-850

Textbook of Endocrine Physiology

Fourth Edition

Edited by

JAMES E. GRIFFIN, M.D.

Professor of Internal Medicine
University of Texas Southwestern Medical Center at Dallas

SERGIO R. OJEDA, D.V.M.

Head, Division of Neuroscience
Oregon Regional Primate Research Center

OXFORD
UNIVERSITY PRESS

2000

Oxford   New York
Athens   Auckland   Bangkok   Bogotá   Buenos Aires   Calcutta
Cape Town   Chennai   Dar es Salaam   Delhi   Florence   Hong Kong   Istanbul
Karachi   Kuala Lumpur   Madrid   Melbourne   Mexico City   Mumbai
Nairobi   Paris   São Paulo   Singapore   Taipei   Tokyo   Toronto   Warsaw

and associated companies in
Berlin   Ibadan

Copyright © 2000 by Oxford University Press, Inc.

Published by Oxford University Press, Inc.,
198 Madison Avenue, New York, New York, 10016
http://www.oup-usa.org
1-800-334-4249

Library of Congress Cataloging-in-Publication Data
Textbook of endocrine physiology /
edited by James E. Griffin, Sergio R. Ojeda.—4th ed.
p. cm.   Includes bibliographical references and index.
ISBN 0-19-513540-7 (cloth)—ISBN 0-19-513541-5 (pbk.)
1. Endocrine glands—Physiology. 2. Endocrinology.
I. Griffin, James E. (James Emmett), 1944–
II. Ojeda, Sergio R.
QP187.T43 2000   612.4—dc21   99-057918

9 8 7 6 5 4 3 2 1

Printed in the United States of America
on acid-free paper

Preface

During the past 12 years this textbook of endocrinology has been used by graduate and medical students as they learn physiology, anatomy, biochemistry, and cell biology. The book is intended to provide a solid, clear, and succinct account of basic endocrine function, emphasizing the impact that advances in the biological sciences have on our understanding of physiological processes. The text addresses clinical disorders only as a means of illustrating divergence from normal physiology and normal regulation of endocrine function. The book offers basic insights into endocrinology that should lead to a better understanding of the complex array of endocrine disorders that medical students will encounter in later years. It should also provide a framework for those, who, planning to pursue a career in research, are seeking to identify critical subjects of investigation.

The contributors are well-recognized authorities in the respective fields of research. The first five chapters of the book consider general aspects of endocrine physiology: the organization of the endocrine system, genetic control of hormone synthesis, mechanisms of hormone action, immune-endocrine interactions, and assessment of endocrine function. The next two chapters deal with the neuroendocrinology of the hypothalamus and its relationship to the pituitary gland. Subsequent chapters are devoted to reproductive physiology (sexual differentiation, female reproductive function, male reproductive function, endocrinology of pregnancy), somatic growth and development, thyroid gland physiology, and the adrenal glands. The last two chapters review the multihormonal control of calcium homeostasis and of glucose, lipid, and protein metabolism. Selected clinical examples of altered endocrine physiology are provided throughout the book, without clinical jargon. We have tried to keep the level of discussion in each chapter appropriate for students who are just beginning their medical and graduate education. Despite this necessary simplicity, the book presents the latest advances in the fields of energy metabolism, obesity and control of appetite, discusses novel interactions between the immune and endocrine systems and their implication for tumor growth, and reports on the discovery of new hypothalamic peptides involved in the regulation of pituitary function. Moreover, it discusses in a simple, but accurate manner the recent advances in the fields of fluid and electrolyte balance, hormones of the heart and brain, and offers an account of the discovery of a series of new factors recently identified as critically involved in the regulation of gonadal, adrenal, and thyroid development and function.

For this fourth edition, there are new authors for Chapters 2 and 8. Perrin White has written a new Chapter 2 on "Genes and Hormones," providing a concise description of the techniques used in molecular endocrinology. Keith Parker has written a new Chapter 8 on "Sexual Differentiation," including an expanded section on emerging concepts of the mechanisms of gonadal differentiation. Overall, this edition has 23 new and 13 revised figures. We would like to express our special appreciation to the contributors. We also thank Samia Burns for secretarial assistance and Marty Burgin for preparation of the illustrations.

Dallas, TX   J.E.G.
Beaverton, OR   S.R.O.
2000

Contents

Contributors

NEIL A. BRESLAU, M.D.
Clinical Professor of Internal Medicine
University of Texas Southwestern Medical Center

BRUCE R. CARR, M.D.
Professor of Obstetrics and Gynecology
University of Texas Southwestern Medical Center

M. LINETTE CASEY, M.D.
Associate Professor of Biochemistry
University of Texas Southwestern Medical Center

PINCHAS COHEN, M.D.
Professor of Pediatrics
University of California Los Angeles

DANIEL W. FOSTER, M.D.
Professor and Chairman of Internal Medicine
University of Texas Southwestern Medical Center

JAMES E. GRIFFIN, M.D.
Professor of Internal Medicine
University of Texas Southwestern Medical Center

NORMAN M. KAPLAN, M.D.
Professor of Internal Medicine
University of Texas Southwestern Medical Center

SAMUEL M. MCCANN, M.D.
United Companies Distinguished Professor of Biomedical Science
Pennington Biomedial Research Center

J. DENIS MCGARRY, M.D.
Professor Internal Medicine and Biochemistry
University of Texas Southwestern Medical Center

CAROLE R. MENDELSON, PH.D.
Professor of Biochemistry and Obstetrics and Gynecology
University of Texas Southwestern Medical Center

SERGIO R. OJEDA, D.V.M.
Head, Division of Neuroscience
Oregon Regional Primate Research Center

KEITH L. PARKER, M.D.
Professor of Internal Medicine
University of Texas Southwestern Medical Center

RON G. ROSENFELD, M.D.
Professor and Chairman of Pediatrics
Oregon Health Sciences University

WILLIS K. SAMSON, PH.D.
Professor of Pharmacological and Physiological Sciences
St. Louis University School of Medicine

PERRIN C. WHITE, M.D.
Professor of Pediatrics
University of Texas Southwestern Medical Center

Textbook of
Endocrine Physiology

Organization of the Endocrine System

SERGIO R. OJEDA
JAMES E. GRIFFIN

The evolutionary appearance of multicellular organisms dictated the necessity of establishing coordinating systems to regulate and integrate the function of the different cells. Two basic regulatory mechanisms developed to perform this delicate function: the nervous system and the endocrine system. Whereas the former employs electrochemical signals to send commands to peripheral organs and to receive information from them, the latter performs its regulatory function by producing chemical agents that, in general, are transported by the bloodstream to the target organs.

The two systems are, nevertheless, closely linked. The best-known connection is that of the hypothalamus and the pituitary gland. Hypothalamic neurosecretory cells produce substances that are delivered to the portal blood vessels (see Chapter 6) and transported to the anterior pituitary where they regulate the secretion of adenohypophyseal hormones. Other hypothalamic neurons send their axons to the posterior pituitary where they end in close proximity to the vascular bed of the gland and release their neurosecretory products directly into the bloodstream. The nervous and endocrine systems are further related by the innervation of endocrine glands. Most, if not all, endocrine glands, including the gonads, the thyroid, and the adrenals, receive nerves that appear to control both their blood flow and their secretory activity. In turn, the endocrine system regulates the function of the nervous system. For example, the gonadal and adrenocortical steroids act directly on the central nervous system either to inhibit or stimulate the secretory activity of those neurons that produce releasing hormones involved in the control of the pituitary–gonadal and pituitary–adrenal axis, respectively (i.e., luteinizing hormone-releasing hormone [LHRH] and corticotropin-releasing hormone [CRH]; see Chapter 6).

Although conventional definitions of the nervous and endocrine systems clearly delineate their differences, an absolute distinction between the two systems cannot be made. For instance, the nervous system produces substances that do not act across synapses, but rather are released into the bloodstream and travel to distant target cells. Among these substances of neural origin are the hypothalamic-releasing factors that control the secretion of anterior pituitary hormones; epinephrine of adrenomedullary origin, which upon release into the bloodstream can affect the function of various organs, such as the liver and muscle; and oxytocin and vasopressin, which are secreted by hypothalamic neurons and act on the mammary gland and uterus (oxytocin) to stimulate the activity of contractile tissue and on the kidney (vasopressin) to regulate extracellular fluid volume. Conversely, several peptides originally discovered in the gastrointestinal tract where they exert hormonal actions are now known to be produced in neurons of both the central and peripheral nervous systems where they appear to act as neurotransmitters or neuromodulators. Examples of these hormones are gastrin, secretin, and vasoactive intestinal peptide.

Because of their interrelationships, endocrine glands and the components of the nervous system that regulate endocrine function are referred to as the neuroendocrine system. The discipline devoted to the study of this system is called *neuroendocrinology* (see Chapter 6). It is now clear that the neuroendocrine system does not operate alone; instead, it is subjected to regulatory input from an unexpected source, the immune system (see Chapter 4). The relationship between the neuroendocrine system and the immune system is reciprocal: hormones influence the immune system, and cytokines (the secretory products of the immune system) affect neuroendocrine functions. Most remarkably, immunologically reactive cells have been found to secrete certain hormones such as adrenocorticotropin (ACTH), β-endorphin, prolactin, and LHRH, which until recently were thought to be produced only in the brain and/or pituitary gland.

Perhaps the best characterized neuroendocrine–immune system relationship is that of the immune–hypothalamic–pituitary–adrenal axis. Cytokines, particularly interleukin-1 (produced by antigenically challenged macrophages), act on the hypothalamus to stimulate the secretion of CRH, which, in turn, stimulates the pituitary gland to secrete ACTH. This hormone acts on the adrenal cortex to elicit glucocorticoid secretion. Glucocorticoids then promote the formation of neutrophils in the bone marrow, decrease the formation of monocytes/macrophages and lymphocytes, and inhibit both cytokine and antibody production.

The immune system also affects the secretion of other pituitary hormones via the hypothalamus. Thus, in addition to the stimulatory effect of interleukin-1 on CRH release, cytokines have been shown to depress thyrotropin-releasing hormone (TRH) and LHRH production. In turn, several pituitary hormones and neuroendocrine peptides, including somatostatin, thyroid-stimulating hormone (TSH), and growth hormone (GH), are able to affect specific immunological functions (such as immunoglobulin synthesis, which is enhanced by TSH, and lymphocyte production, which is increased by GH).

The ovary provides another example of the interrelationships between the endocrine and the immune systems. Cytokines directly regulate certain ovarian functions and, as in the case of the neuroendocrine system, ovarian hormones have the ability to affect the immune system. For instance, interleukin-1 synthesis increases in the ovary during the hours preceding ovulation, resulting in a greater production of progesterone and prostaglandins, which in turn have a stimulatory effect on ovulation. Conversely, low doses of progesterone enhance the expression of the interleukin-1 gene in macrophages.

In their definition of a hormone, Baylis and Starling specified that for a substance to be considered a hormone, it should meet the requirement of being produced by an organ in small amounts, released into the bloodstream, and transported to a distant organ to exert its specific actions. This definition indeed applies to most of the "classical hormones" produced by the endocrine glands. It is now apparent, however, that hormones can act on contiguous cells, performing a *paracrine* function, and that they can modify the secretory activity of the same cells that produce them, performing an *autocrine* function. In acting locally, hormones do not need to be transported in the bloodstream, but they still can exert their action in a manner commensurate with their hormonal nature, that is, through binding to specific receptors.

Still, other "nonclassical hormones" such as growth factors of the epidermal growth factor (EGF) family of trophic polypeptides can affect cellular function in a nondiffusible, "juxtacrine" manner. This mode of communication is established when a membrane-anchored growth factor on one cell interacts with its membrane-bound receptor located on an adjacent cell.

ENDOCRINE GLANDS AND HORMONES

The endocrine system is composed of several glands located in different areas of the body that produce hormones with different functions. The major morphological feature of endocrine glands is that they are ductless, that is, they release their secretory products directly into the bloodstream and not into a duct system. Because they are richly vascularized, each secreting cell can deliver its products efficiently into the circulation.

The classical endocrine glands and their known secretory products are listed in Table 1-1. In recent years, the traditional view of the endocrine system's glan-

Table 1-1 Classical Endocrine Glands and Their Hormones

Gland		Hormone
Pituitary	Anterior lobe	Luteinizing hormone (LH), follicle-stimulating hormone (FSH), prolactin (PRL), growth hormone (GH), adrenocorticotropin (ACTH), β-lipotropin, β-endorphin, thyroid-stimulating hormone (TSH)
	Intermediate lobe	Melanocyte-stimulating hormone (MSH), β-endorphin
	Posterior lobe	Vasopressin (AVP) or antidiuretic hormone (ADH), oxytocin
Thyroid		Thyroxine (T_4), 3,5,3'-triiodothyronine (T_3), calcitonin
Parathyroid		Parathyroid hormone (PTH)
Adrenal	Cortex	Cortisol, aldosterone, dehydroepiandrosterone, androstenedione
	Medulla	Epinephrine, norepinephrine
Gonads	Testis	Testosterone, estradiol, androstenedione, inhibin, activin, müllerian-inhibiting substance
	Ovary	Estradiol, progesterone, testosterone, androstenedione, inhibin, activin, FSH-releasing peptide, relaxin, follistatin
Placenta		Human chorionic gonadotropin (hCG), human placental lactogen (hPL), progesterone, estrogen
Pancreas		Insulin, glucagon, somatostatin, pancreatic polypeptide, gastrin, vasoactive intestinal peptide (VIP)
Pineal		Melatonin, biogenic amines, several peptides

Table 1-2 Nonclassical "Endocrine Organs" and Their Hormones

Organ	Hormone
Brain (especially hypothalamus)	Corticotropin-releasing hormone (CRH), thyrotropin-releasing hormone (TRH), luteinizing hormone-releasing hormone (LHRH), growth hormone-releasing hormone (GHRH), somatostatin, growth factors[a] (fibroblast growth factors, transforming growth factor-α (TGF-α), transforming growth factor-β (TGF-β), insulin-like growth factor I (IGF-I)
Heart	Atrial natriuretic peptides
Kidney	Erythropoietin, renin, 1,25-dihydroxyvitamin D
Liver, other organs, fibroblasts	IGF-I
Adipose tissue	Leptin
Gastrointestinal tract	Cholecystokinin (CCK), gastrin, secretin, vasoactive intestinal peptide (VIP), enteroglucagon, gastrin-releasing peptide
Platelets	Platelet-derived growth factor (PDGF), TGF-β
Macrophages, lymphocytes	Cytokines, TGF-β, proopiomelanocortin (POMC)-derived peptides
Various sites	Epidermal growth factor (EGF), TGF-α, neuregulins, neurotrophins

[a]Not considered to be hormones, but they can act as such.

dular nature has been broadened to include production of recognized hormones in organs whose primary function is not endocrine. Perhaps the earliest example of this was the recognition that hormones are produced by cells scattered along the mucosa of the stomach and small intestine. The brain, heart, kidney, liver, and certain blood elements also produce peptides or form active steroid metabolites from circulating precursors that deserve the designation of hormones (Table 1-2). Not all of these hormones will be considered in this volume.

CHEMICAL NATURE OF HORMONES

Chemically, the hormones fall into three general categories. The first comprises hormones derived from single amino acids. They are the *amines,* such as norepinephrine, epinephrine, and dopamine, which derive from the amino acid tyrosine, and the thyroid hormones, 3,5,3'-triiodothyronine (T_3) and 3,5,3',5'-tetraiodothyronine (thyroxine, T_4), which derive from the combination of two iodinated tyrosine amino acid residues.

The second category is composed of *peptides* and *proteins.* These can be as small as thryotropin-releasing hormone (three amino acids) and as large and complex as growth hormone and follicle-stimulating hormone, which have about 200 amino acid residues and molecular weights in the range of 25,000–30,000.

The third category comprises the *steroid hormones,* which are derivatives of cholesterol and can be grouped into two types: (*1*) those with an intact steroid nucleus such as the gonadal and adrenal steroids and (*2*) those with a broken steroid

Amines

OH
|
HO — CH — CH₂ — NH₂
HO (Norepinephrine)

Thyroid Hormones

$$HO—\bigcirc—O—\bigcirc—CH_2—CH—COOH$$

(3,5,3'-triiodothyronine, T₃)

Polypeptides

(Oxytocin)

Proteins

(Growth hormone)

Steroids

CH₂OH
|
C=O
OH

HO

(Cortisol)

(Vitamin D3)

Fig. 1-1 Examples of different categories of hormones. In the case of the protein hormone, each circle represents an amino acid, as shown for the polypeptide hormone.

nucleus (the B ring) such as vitamin D and its metabolites. Figure 1-1 provides examples of these three categories of hormones.

FUNCTION OF HORMONES

Regardless of their chemical nature, hormones are present in the bloodstream in very low concentrations (10^{-7} to 10^{-12} M). Thus, it is not surprising that a prerequisite for any hormone to exert its actions is that it must first bind to specific, high-affinity cellular receptors. These receptors may be located at the cell membrane, as in the case of protein hormones and amines, or in the nucleus, as with thyroid and steroid hormones (see Chapter 3). Another characteristic feature of hormones is that a single hormone can exert various effects in different tissues; conversely, a single function can be regulated by several hormones. Estradiol exemplifies the versatility of some hormones. It is produced by the ovary and can act on the ovarian follicles themselves to promote granulosa cell differentiation, on the uterus to stimulate its growth and maintain the cyclic change of the uterine mucosa, on the mammary gland to simulate ductal growth, on bone to promote linear growth and closure of the epiphysial plates, on the hypothalamic–pituitary system to regulate the secretion of gonadotropins and prolactin, and on general metabolic processes to affect adipose tissue distribution, volume of extracellular fluid, etc. In each case estradiol acts through the same common mechanism, namely binding to high-affinity, specific nuclear receptors followed by attachment of the receptor–steroid complex to DNA regions of genes that are expressed in a tissue-specific manner.

An example of a single function regulated by more than one hormone is the release of fatty acids (lipolysis) from adipose tissue stores. A variety of hormones including catecholamines, glucagon, secretin, prolactin, and β-lipotropin stimulate lipolysis within minutes by activating, via cyclic AMP, a rate-limiting triglyceride hydrolase known as *hormone-sensitive lipase*. Growth hormone and glucocorticoids also stimulate lipolysis, but only after a time lag of 2 hours because they induce the synthesis of hormone-sensitive lipase rather than activate the hydrolase. Other hormones such as insulin, insulin-like growth factors (IGFs) or somatomedins, oxytocin, and gastric-inhibitory polypeptide inhibit lipolysis.

An example of a complex function regulated by different hormones is the development of the mammary gland, which is under the primary influence of prolactin, estradiol, and progesterone and the permissive influence of glucocorticoids, thyroid hormones, and insulin. The effect of these latter hormones is considered permissive because, by themselves, they have little effect, but when they are present the actions of prolactin, estrogen, and progesterone become fully manifested.

Hormones exert their functions in four broad physiological areas. These are reproduction, growth and development, maintenance of the internal environment, and the regulation of energy balance.

Reproduction

Hormones produced by the gonads (androgens, estrogen, progestogens) and the anterior pituitary gland (luteinizing hormone [LH], follicle-stimulating hormone [FSH], growth hormone [GH], and prolactin) interact to regulate the growth and structural integrity of the reproductive organs, the production of gametes, the patterns of sexual behavior, the phenotypic difference between the sexes, and the continuation of the species (through their effects on ovulation, spermatogenesis, pregnancy, and lactation).

Several examples of these interactions can be provided. For instance, estradiol induces hypertrophy and hyperplasia of both the muscular and endothelial layers of the uterine wall; in turn, the secretion of estradiol from the ovary is under the control of the pituitary gonadotropins. Testosterone, which in males is under the control of LH, exerts tropic effects on sex accessory glands such as the prostate and seminal vesicles. Both estradiol in females and testosterone in males play fundamental roles in determining the female and male external appearance at puberty. Testosterone promotes the growth of the testes, scrotum, and penis, and stimulates muscle development, particularly that of the pectoral region and shoulders. Estradiol promotes the development of the female external genitalia and the redistribution of adipose tissue, which localizes more noticeably in the thighs, hips, and breasts (see Chapter 9). Although in humans gonadal steroids do not induce a stereotyped pattern of sexual behavior as in animals, there is no doubt that they are important in maintaining the libido.

Both ovulation and spermatogenesis are processes tightly controlled by the pituitary gonadotropins LH and FSH, which act either directly on the gonads to promote follicular development (ovary) and formation of sperm (testis) or indirectly through their stimulatory effects on estrogen and testosterone secretion. During pregnancy various hormones of placental origin including estradiol, progesterone, chorionic gonadotropin, placental lactogen, and several others (see Chapter 11) contribute to maintaining the normal progression of pregnancy. After delivery another group of hormones, most noticeably prolactin (see above), maintains the structure and function of the lactating breast.

Growth and Development

Various hormones play primary and permissive roles in the timing and progression of growth both for overall body size and for individual tissues. In many cases the local production of growth factors is a result of hormone action. In other instances the production of a growth factor may be hormone independent, but the growth factor interacts with hormones to promote or reduce growth.

The classical hormones involved in the process of growth are GH, thyroid hormones, insulin, glucocorticoids, androgens, and estrogens. Although the stimulatory effect of GH on bodily growth is mediated by a family of peptides known collectively as *insulin-like growth factors* (see Chapter 12), it is unclear to what extent these growth factors are involved in mediating the stimulatory effect of androgens and estrogens on linear growth and acquisition of muscle mass. An example of a hormone that plays both permissive and primary roles in growth is thyroxine. In its absence, GH fails to stimulate skeletal growth, a phenomenon that appears to be related to a reduced ability of the tissue to respond to IGFs. In the central nervous system, however, thyroxine plays a primary role in inducing growth and cellular differentiation. Some of its actions in the brain appear to be mediated by the production of a issue-specific growth factor, nerve growth factor (NGF). Experimental evidence indicates that the synthesis of some peptide growth factors such as the IGFs, NGF, and the epidermal growth factor (EGF) is induced by specific hormones (GH, thyroxine, and androgens, respectively). It is not known whether other peptide growth factors such as fibroblast growth factor (FGF) and platelet-derived growth factor (PDGF) are hormonally regulated. A more detailed discussion of the hormones and peptide growth factors involved in regulating growth is presented in Chapter 12.

Maintenance of Internal Environment

The maintenance of the internal environment involves the control of extracellular fluid volume and blood pressure, the electrolyte composition of bodily fluids, the regulation of plasma and tissue levels of calcium and phosphate ions, and the maintenance of bone, muscle, and body stores of fat.

A multitude of hormones participates in the regulation of these processes. For example, vasopressin or antidiuretic hormone, which is synthesized in the hypothalamus and released from the posterior pituitary, acts on the kidney to induce water reabsorption; aldosterone produced in the adrenal cortex stimulates sodium reabsorption and potassium excretion in the kidney. Thus, both hormones contribute to regulating blood pressure, extracellular fluid volume, and electrolyte composition of bodily fluids.

Plasma levels of calcium and phosphate ions are controlled by parathyroid hormone (PTH) from the parathyroid glands (see Chapter 15). The PTH increases serum calcium concentration mainly through its stimulatory actions on calcium transport in bone and kidney, but also by enhancing intestinal calcium absorption through its stimulatory influence on the renal formation of 1,25-dihydroxyvitamin D. Also, PTH acts on the kidney to increase phosphate excretion.

The functions of the bone, muscle, and adipose tissue are regulated by hormones as diverse as PTH, estrogens, androgens, and GH (bone), and catecholamines, insulin, glucagon, and glucocorticoids (muscle and adipose tissue). Pertinent details are given in Chapters 14, 15, and 16.

Regulation of Energy Balance

For an organism to survive, it must be able to convert the calories contained in food into energy, to store part of that energy for subsequent use, and to mobilize it when necessary. Maintenance of energy homeostasis is of paramount importance for the proper regulation of body weight, which requires a balance between food consumption and energy expenditure. The hypothalamus plays a central role in this process by integrating a variety of afferent sensory, visual, biochemical, and hormonal signals reflecting the nutritional status of the organism. Processing of these signals results in the activation of efferent signals that regulate both feeding behavior and energy expenditure. The latter is regulated via mechanisms controlling the metabolic rate, such as those influenced by the sympathetic and parasympathetic nervous systems, and by insulin, glucagon, and thyroid hormones.

Until recently, the identity of the afferent signals controlling energy balance was unknown. This situation changed dramatically with the identification of leptin as a hormone produced by white adipose tissue that acts on the brain to decrease food intake and increase energy expenditure. Leptin acts through specific receptors, which are particularly abundant in hypothalamic nuclei, such as the ventromedial nucleus and the arcuate nucleus, known to be involved in the control of feeding behavior. Thus, leptin serves as a "lipostat" or "adipostat" that—acting via its strategically located receptors—informs the brain of the status of energy storage in adipose tissue, and modifies the efferent wing of energy homeostasis. One target of leptin action are the neurons of the arcuate nucleus of the hypothalamus that produce neuropeptide Y (NPY), an appetite-stimulating neuropeptide. An increase in plasma leptin levels leads to decreased production of NPY and a corresponding decrease in food intake.

In addition to leptin, recent studies have identified at least three centrally originated peptides that suppress feeding behavior: melanocortinergic neurons of the arcuate nucleus acting via a melanocyte-stimulating hormone receptor known as

MC4-R; a corticotropin-releasing-factor–related peptide known as *urocortin,* produced in the lateral hypothalamus; and an orphan receptor known as *bombesin receptor type-3.* It is possible that at least part of the suppressive effects of leptin on feeding behavior is mediated by one or more of these systems. Accordingly, they should be considered as part of the efferent mechanisms controlling energy balance.

Even more recently, two novel neuropeptides termed *orexin A* and *B* and their receptors have been identified by molecular cloning, found to be produced in neurons of the lateral hypothalamus, and shown to stimulate feeding behavior. Their presence in the hypothalamus and the potency of their actions suggest that orexins represent the homeostatic counterpart of the afferent leptin regulatory system. It is thus clear that the long-held mystery of the mechanisms underlying the regulation of energy balance are being unraveled at an ever increasingly fast pace.

SYNTHESIS AND RELEASE OF HORMONES

Peptide and protein hormones are synthesized in the rough endoplasmic reticulum. As with all proteins, the amino acid sequence of protein hormones is determined by specific messenger RNAs that are synthesized in the nucleus and have a nucleotide sequence dictated by a specific gene. We shall see in Chapter 2 that translation of the specific messenger RNA sequence results in the ribosomal synthesis of a protein larger than the mature hormone. This precursor form may be either a *prohormone* or a *preprohormone.* Prohormones are extended at their amino termini by a hydrophobic amino acid sequence called *leader* or *signal* peptide. Preprohormones are also extended by a signal peptide, but in addition contain internal cleavage sites that upon enzymatic action yield different bioactive peptides. In some instances, preprohormones contain peptide sequences that may not have a known biological activity. These sequences are called *cryptic* peptides. In other instances these peptides may act as "spacers" between two bioactive peptides.

Because of its hydrophobic nature, the *leader* peptide sequence of both preprohormones and prohormones permits the newly synthesized protein to move across the membrane of the endoplasmic reticulum to be transported to the Golgi apparatus. The leader peptide is removed from the hormone before the synthesis of the polypeptide chain is ended and this permits the protein to assume its secondary structure during its transport to the Golgi apparatus. Once it arrives at this organelle, the hormone may be further processed by proteolytic enzymes, which cleave the prohormone generating one or more mature hormones, and/or by other enzymes that add nonprotein residues such as carbohydrates. Whatever the case, the hormone is always stored in granules that fuse with the cell membrane during the release process and allow their contents to be extruded into the extracellular perivascular space. This process is called *exocytosis* and involves the participation of microtubules and the mobilization of calcium across the cell membrane. During release, not only the hormone but also the cleaving enzymes and peptides associated with the prohormone are discharged from the granule.

Amine and steroid hormones are synthesized in a manner much different from proteins. They originate from a precursor molecule (tyrosine and cholesterol, respectively) that is either totally (tyrosine) or partially (cholesterol) transported to the cell of synthesis via the bloodstream. Once inside the cell, these precursor mole-cules are subjected to the sequential action of several enzymes resulting in the for-mation of various intermediate products that themselves may be hormones. Like proteins, amines are packed into granules and are released by a similar process of exocytosis. In contrast to protein hormones, thyroid hormones and steroids, once produced, can freely cross the cell membrane without having to be packed in gran-ules and actively exocytosed.

Although we have discussed mechanisms involved in the formation of hor-mones at their site of origin, well-documented examples exist of hormones that are produced at sites other than those in which their precursor is formed, using these same mechanisms (i.e., proteolytic cleavage of peptide hormone precursors and en-zymatic modification of steroid hormones). In some instances, a hormone with lit-tle activity is converted into an active or more active form by the action of enzymes in the circulation or other tissues. For example, angiotensin II is formed in the cir-culation through the sequential action of the enzyme renin, produced in the kidney to convert angiotensinogen to angiotensin I, and a converting enzyme produced in the lungs that cleaves two amino acids from angiotensin I to form angiotensin II. The androgen androstenedione (produced by both the gonads and adrenal glands) can be metabolized to the estrogen estrone in adipose tissue, and testosterone is con-verted into the more potent androgen dihydrotestosterone in androgen target tissues such as the prostate.

Although protein, amine, and steroid hormones differ in their mechanisms of synthesis and release, a feature they all share is the variability of their blood levels. As we shall see next, fluctuating plasma hormone levels are the consequence of the episodic nature of a hormone secretion.

PATTERNS OF HORMONE SECRETION

The concentration of hormones in the circulation is generally regulated by control loops or feedback mechanisms to allow response to physiologic needs (see below). In addition, the basal secretion of most hormones is not a continuous process but rather has a pulsatile nature. When hormone release is induced by a secretagogue the pattern of response is episodic. Conversely, inhibition of hormone secretion by other hormones always results in suppression of the episodic increases in hormone levels. The pulsatile pattern of hormone secretion is characterized by episodes of release that can be as frequent as every 5–10 minutes; each episode is followed by a quiescent period during which plasma levels of the hormone fall toward basal values. Another discharge then occurs and the cycle repeats itself, often varying in both amplitude and frequency of the pulses. In the case of hormones subjected to negative feedback control (see below), removal of the inhibitory feedback signal results in a marked enhancement of the amplitude and frequency of the episodes of secretion.

Secretory episodes may occur with different periodicities. For example, the most prominent episodes of release may occur with a frequency of about an hour. This mode of release is called *circhoral*. If the episodes of release occur at inter-vals longer than an hour but less than 24 hours the rhythm is called *ultradian*, if the periodicity is of about a day the rhythm is called *circadian,* and if it recurs every day it is called *quotidian.* Release patterns of the latter type are usually referred to as *diurnal* because the increase in secretory activity becomes expressed at defined periods of the day. For example, ACTH has a characteristic diurnal pattern of release with plasma levels rising sharply during the early morning hours.

The release pattern of a hormone may have a much less frequent periodicity. For example, the monthly preovulatory discharge of gonadotropins recurs approximately every 30 days, a pattern of release that has been called *circatrigintan.* Other hormones such as thyroxine exhibit changes in plasma levels that occur over months. If the changes take place on a yearly basis the rhythm is called *circannual* or *seasonal,* as it occurs in relation to the seasonal phases of the year.

Although it is clear that these low periodicity rhythms of hormone release are dictated by either environmental or hormonal cues, the mechanisms underlying the pulsatile release of hormones are unknown. It does appear, however, that secretory cells, including neurosecretory neurons, have the intrinsic ability to secrete their products in a discontinuous, episodic manner. Superimposed on this basic mode of release, the amount of hormone produced, and the frequency of the secretory episodes are modulated by specific negative and positive feedback mechanisms (see below).

The physiological importance of pulsatile hormone release has been best demonstrated in humans and nonhuman primates treated with LHRH, the hypothalamic peptide that stimulates the secretion of gonadotropins from the anterior pituitary (see Chapter 6). Only when LHRH is given in a pulsatile fashion at a frequency of about one pulse per hour is gonadotropin secretion and gonadal function maintained normally; a slower frequency fails to maintain gonadotropin secretion at a level sufficient to support normal gonadal production of steroids and gametes; a faster frequency or continuous administration of LHRH inhibits the secretion of gonadotropins and prevents normal gonadal function. This latter phenomenon, which results from a reduced sensitivity of the pituitary to a frequent or continuous LHRH stimulation, has been applied to the treatment of precocious puberty and to attempts at fertility control using long-acting LHRH analogs (see Chapters 9 and 10).

TRANSPORT AND METABOLISM OF HORMONES

Once a hormone is released into the bloodstream it may circulate freely, if it is water soluble, or it may be bound to a carrier protein. In general, amines, peptides, and proteins circulate in free form, whereas steroids and thyroid hormones are bound to transport proteins. A well-known exception to this rule is provided by the insulin-like growth factors, which, despite being polypeptides, circulate tightly attached to specific binding proteins. Some plasma proteins such as albumin and prealbumin have the capacity to transport nonselectively a variety of low-molecular weight hormones. In contrast, specific transport proteins that are globulins have saturable, high-affinity binding sites for the hormones they carry. These proteins include thyroid hormone-binding globulin (TBG), testosterone-binding globulin (TeBG), and cortisol-binding globulin (CBG).

Binding of hormones to carrier proteins has a profound impact on the hormone clearance rate from the circulation. The greater the binding capacity of the specific protein carrier, the slower the clearance rate of the hormone. Thus, hormones that circulate mostly in bound form, such as thyroxine, have a much slower disappearance rate from the plasma than do hormones that circulate either in free form or only weakly bound. In general, changes in the plasma levels of binding proteins are rapidly followed by adjustments in the secretion rate of the corresponding hormone, so that the fraction of hormone readily available for tissue delivery remains constant and endocrine function remains normal. One well-known example of this is the increase in CBG concentration that occurs during pregnancy as a consequence of estradiol stimulation. While the total plasma cortisol rises as a result of the increased CBG levels, the cortisol available to the tissues remains normal. This is because as the concentration of CBG increases there is a temporary decrease in the cortisol available to target tissues as more is bound to CBG. This results in a temporary increase in ACTH by activation of feedback mechanisms (see below) and increased cortisol secretion to bring the total plasma concentration of cortisol to a higher level and return tissue delivery of cortisol to normal. Thus, in the steady state with intact control mechanisms, alterations in hormone-binding proteins do not affect endocrine status.

The metabolic clearance rate (MCR) of a hormone defines quantitatively its removal from plasma. Under steady-state conditions, the MCR represents the volume of plasma cleared of the hormone per unit of time; usually the units employed are milliliters per minute. If a radioactive hormone is infused into the bloodstream until a constant level is reached and the infusion is then stopped, the disappearance rate of the labeled hormone from the plasma can be determined and the plasma half-life of the hormone calculated. The plasma half-life of a hormone is inversely related to its MCR. Table 1-3 lists the half-lives of several hormones.

Only a small portion of the circulating hormones is removed from the circulation by most target tissues. The bulk of hormone clearance is done by the liver and the kidneys. This process includes degradation by a variety of enzymatic mechanisms such as hydrolysis, oxidation, hydroxylation, methylation, decarboxylation, sulfation, and glucuronidation. In general, only a small fraction ($<1\%$) of any hormone is excreted intact in the urine or feces.

The interaction of hormones with their target tissues is apparently followed by intracellular degradation of the hormone. In the case of protein hormones and amines, degradation occurs after their binding to membrane receptors, internalization of the hormone–receptor complex, and the dissociation of this complex into its two com-

Table 1-3 Half-life of Protein, Amine, and Steroid Hormones in Plasma

Hormone	Half-life
Amines	2–3 min
Thyroid hormones T_4	6.7 days
T_3	0.75 days
Polypeptides	4–40 min
Proteins	15–170 min
Steroids	4–120 min

ponents (see Chapter 3). In the case of steroid or thyroid hormones, degradation may occur after binding of the hormone–receptor complex to nuclear chromatin.

FEEDBACK MECHANISMS

The secretion of most, if not all, hormones is regulated by closed-loop systems known as *feedback mechanisms*. Indeed, the endocrine system as a whole is organized in a hierarchy of closed-loop systems that not only operate between cells but also constitute an essential feature of intracellular regulation. Feedback mechanisms are of two types: *negative feedback* and *positive feedback*. Negative feedback is the prevailing control mechanism regulating endocrine function; in its simplest form it is a closed loop in which hormone A stimulates the production of hormone B, which in turn acts on the cells producing hormone A to decrease its rate of secretion. An example of this type of feedback can be found in the stimulation of adrenal cortisol secretion by the adenohypophyseal hormone ACTH (hormone A), and the resulting inhibition of ACTH release by the increased plasma cortisol (hormone B) levels (Fig. 1-2). In the less common positive feedback mechanisms, hormone B further stimulates the production of hormone A instead of diminishing it (Fig. 1-2). A typical example of a positive feedback loop is that which exists between LH and estradiol. During the menstrual cycle a gradual increase in plasma LH levels stimulates the production of estradiol by the ovary; after reaching a certain level, estradiol induces an abrupt increase in LH secretion, known as the preovulatory surge of LH, because it induces ovulation. Upon reaching maximal levels, plasma LH declines despite the presence of still elevated estrogen concentrations. This latter phenomenon exemplifies the self-limiting nature of positive feedback systems. The secretion of hormone A declines rapidly after its initial activation because the secretory cell has a limited capacity to produce the hormone and because there are always additional negative feedback loops that limit the magnitude of the response.

Endocrine control systems also have *feed-forward loops* directing the flow of hormonal information. These feed-forward loops can be negative or positive. They are intrinsically unstable because they do not function as closed-loop systems. Because feed-forward loops always form part of a large, more complex feedback circuit their performance is closely regulated by subserving closed-loop mechanisms. This concept is diagrammed in Figure 1-3, which shows a feed-forward loop that accelerates the conversion of product 2 into product 3. The latter results in a product 4 that then inhibits the formation of product 2.

Fig. 1-2   Schematic representation of a negative (*a*) and a positive (*b*) feedback loop. The arrows represent stimulation. The blunt-ended lines represent inhibition. EC, endocrine cells; TEC, target endocrine cell; A, hormone A; B, hormone B.

Fig. 1-3   Schematic representation of a feed-forward loop (broken line) that activates the progression of reaction in a hypothetical metabolic pathway. The loop, however, operates within a system tightly controlled by negative feedback systems (blunt-ended line). (Adapted from Rasmussen H: In: *Textbook of Endocrinology,* 5th ed., RH Williams, ed., Saunders, Philadelphia, p. 2, 1974, with permission.)

A well-recognized example of a feed-forward loop is the release of insulin by the β-cells of the islets of Langerhans in response to an increase in plasma glucose concentration. Upon stimulation of its secretion by the elevated glucose levels, insulin acts on the liver to enhance the uptake of glucose. When plasma glucose levels fall to basal levels, insulin mobilization decreases, and glucose uptake is reduced.

As one would suspect, different levels of complexity exist in the organization of endocrine control systems. The simplest is that of a single negative feedback loop. Much more complex is the situation in which one hormone controls the production of another hormone from a different cell type, which, in turn, controls a third secretory cell that produces a hormone(s) that both feeds back upon the first and/or second component of the system and regulates the function of still another cell type. An example of such a system is the hypothalamic control of gonadotropin secretion from the anterior pituitary (Fig. 1-4). While the hypothalamus stimulates the secretion of gonadotropins through the delivery of LHRH to the pituitary gland, the gonadotropins control the secretion of ovarian steroids, which in turn feed back on the

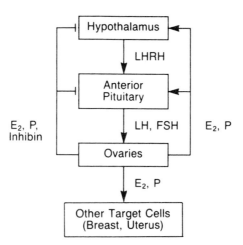

Fig. 1-4   The hypothalamic–pituitary–gonadal axis as an example of a complex endocrine control system. Arrows indicate stimulation and blunt-ended lines represent inhibition. E_2, estradiol; P, progesterone; LH, luteinizing hormone; FSH, follicle-stimulating hormone; LHRH, luteinizing hormone-releasing hormone.

hypothalamus and anterior pituitary to regulate the secretion of LHRH and go-nadotropins, respectively.

MECHANISMS OF ENDOCRINE DISEASE

Endocrine disorders can result from hormone deficiency, hormone excess, or hormone resistance. With some notable exceptions (e.g., calcitonin), hormone deficiency always causes disease. Hormone deficiency is usually the result of a destructive process occurring in the gland in which the hormone is produced. Thus, infection by viruses or bacteria, infarction due to impaired blood supply, physical compression by tumor growth, or attack by cellular or humoral immune mechanisms all may lead to impaired hormone production in most endocrine glands. Alternatively, hormone deficiency states can result from genetic defects in hormone formation such as gene deletion or mutation, failure to cleave a peptide hormone precursor to the active hormone, or a specific enzymatic defect in the formation of thyroid or steroid hormones. Recently, inactivating mutations in cell surface receptors for hormones that stimulate endocrine glands have been shown to cause hormone deficiency (LHRH in the anterior pituitary, LH in the testes, and TSH in the thyroid).

Hormone excess usually results in disease. The hormone may be overproduced by the gland that normally secretes it or by a tissue that is not normally an endocrine organ. Malignancies are often involved in each of these types of hormone excess. Some tumors of endocrine glands (e.g., pituitary, adrenal) are functional and secrete the appropriate hormone for the gland but in an unregulated manner. In some instances, activating mutations in cell surface receptors for stimulating hormones have been found (LH, TSH). In the malignant transformation occurring in nonendocrine tissues (e.g., lung cancer), dedifferentiation may lead to the production of certain peptide hormones. Other mechanisms of hormone excess include the effects of antireceptor antibodies stimulating a receptor instead of blocking its activation, as in the common form of hyperthyroidism, and the ingestion of exogenous hormones, as in the glucocorticoid excess resulting from its therapeutic use.

Hormone resistance as a mechanism of disease has now been described for almost all hormones. In these disorders the hormone is present in normal or increased amounts, but the expected actions of the hormones do not occur. In some cases, because of a mutation, a structurally abnormal peptide hormone is present, causing the resistance (e.g., insulin, PTH). In other instances there are antibodies to the hormone or hormone receptor (e.g., insulin and its receptor). Finally, hormone resistance may also occur as the result of primary receptor defects (e.g., androgen and vitamin D receptors) or defects in the postreceptor mechanisms of hormone action (e.g., insulin, PTH).

SUGGESTED READING

Besedovsky HO, and Del Rey A: Immune-neuro-endocrine interactions: Facts and hypotheses. Endocr Rev 17:64–102, 1996.

Cahill GF: Origin, evolution, and role of hormones. In: *Endocrinology,* 2nd ed., LJ Degroot, ed., Saunders, Philadelphia, pp. 3–5, 1989.

Flier JS: Leptin expression and action: New experimental paradigms. Proc Natl Acad Sci USA 94:4242–4245, 1997.

Kalra SP, Dube MG, Pu S, Xu B, Horvath TL, and Kalra PS: Interacting appetite-regulating pathways in the hypothalamic regulation of body weight. Endocr Rev 20:68–100, 1999.

Merriam GR, and Wachter KW: Analysis of the temporal coincidence of hormonal pulses. In: *Pulsatility in Neuroendocrine Systems* (*Methods in Neuroscience,* Vol. 20), J Levine, ed, Academic Press, San Diego, pp. 326–335, 1994.

Pardridge WM: Transport of protein-bound hormones into tissues *in vivo*. Endocr Rev 2:102–123, 1981.

Rasmussen H: Organization and control of endocrine systems. In: *Textbook of Endocrinology,* 5th ed., RH Williams, eds., Saunders, Philadelphia, pp. 2–30, 1974.

Turek FW, and Van Cauter E: Rhythms in reproduction. In: *The Physiology of Reproduction,* 2nd ed., E Knobil and JD Neill, eds., Raven Press, New York, pp. 487–540, 1994.

2

Genes and Hormones

PERRIN C. WHITE

Much of the knowledge presented in the following chapters has been gained using molecular genetic techniques to analyze the structure, synthesis, regulation, and effects of hormones. This chapter provides an overview of some of the relevant techniques and associated concepts.

GENE EXPRESSION

Deoxyribonucleic acid (DNA) and *ribonucleic acid* (RNA) consist of *nucleotides.* A nucleotide consists of a *base,* a sugar moiety (either deoxyribose or ribose), and a phosphate group. The sugars and phosphates alternate in the backbone of a nucleic acid strand. In general, there are four possible bases. In DNA, these are *adenine (A), cytosine (C), guanine (G),* and *thymine (T).* Adenine and guanine are *purines,* whereas cytosine and thymine are *pyrimidines.* The corresponding nucleotides are *adenosine, cytidine, guanosine,* and *thymidine.* In RNA, *uracil (uridine)* is substituted for thymine (thymidine).

The DNA molecule is double stranded. Each strand has a direction because the deoxyribose molecules forming the backbone are asymmetrical, with the phosphate bonds linking each two sugar molecules going from the 3′ position of one to the 5′ position of the next. Thus, the 5′ position of a sugar molecule is free at one end (the 5′ end) of the strand, and the 3′ position is free at the other. The two strands of a DNA molecule run in opposite directions, so that the 5′ end of one strand is opposed to the 3′ end of the complementary strand.

The DNA strands interact with each other through *complementary (Watson-Crick) base pairing,* in which A and T, or C and G, are paired through hydrogen bonds. Thus, the sequence of one DNA strand unambiguously determines the sequence of the complementary strand during DNA replication.

The length of a DNA segment is typically given in bases or nucleotides (nt) or, if double stranded, *base pairs* (bp). A longer segment is measured in thousands of bases (kilobases, kb) or millions of bases (megabases, mb).

A *gene* may be defined as a segment of DNA within a chromosome that can be *transcribed* to yield RNA that serves a particular function. Many transcripts are *messenger RNAs* (mRNA) that are *translated* into proteins. Others function directly as RNA, including ribosomal RNA and transfer RNA, which are required for protein synthesis, and small nuclear RNAs required for splicing introns out of primary mRNA transcripts (see below).

Genes encoding proteins consist of several components (Fig. 2-1). *Exons* are regions that are retained in mRNA. These are usually interspersed with *introns,* sequences spliced out of the primary transcript before it leaves the nucleus. Exons consist of coding sequences that are translated into protein, and untranslated regions at both ends of the gene. Transcriptional regulatory regions (or *cis* regulatory elements) may be near, anywhere within, or at some distance from a gene, but most often are located within a few hundred nucleotides of the start of transcription.

A *hormone,* broadly defined, is a soluble substance that is secreted in a regulated manner by one cell in a multicelled organism and has defined effects on a second cell. Many but not all of these effects are to directly or indirectly modify levels or patterns of gene expression in the target cell. Thus, studies of gene expression comprise an important part of modern endocrinology.

Transcription

Messenger RNA is single stranded. Its sequence corresponds to the *coding* or *sense* strand of DNA. During transcription, it is synthesized in the 5' to 3' direction by a

Fig. 2-1 Steps in expression of a protein product of a gene. Different parts of a generic gene are diagrammed in (A). The same shadings are used in (E), but they are omitted in (B–D and F), which schematically illustrate RNA processing.

transcriptional apparatus that "reads" the complementary or *antisense* strand of DNA and synthesizes an mRNA molecule complementary to it. This process is mediated by the interactions of many proteins with defined sequences, or *elements,* of DNA.

DNA (cis) *Elements*

Promoters. Transcription is invariably controlled at least in part by sequences located in the 5' flanking region of the gene before (5' or upstream of) the start of transcription. These sequences fall into two categories. Those whose function is dependent on their location and orientation are collectively referred to as the *promoter* of the gene (although this term is also sometimes used for all transcriptional regulatory sequences in the 5' flanking region of the gene). One element of the promoter is the binding site for RNA polymerase II. In many genes this region includes a short nucleotide sequence known as a *TATA box* (TATAAA or a related sequence) approximately 30 bases upstream from the site at which transcription begins. Some genes do not contain this element but instead have one or more GC boxes (GGGCGGGG); often these are "housekeeping" genes that are transcribed at a relatively constant level in different cell types.

Enhancers and Silencers. The *cis* elements that increase transcription independently of their position and orientation are termed *enhancers,* whereas those that decrease transcription are *silencers.* Such elements can be located within a gene itself, usually in an intron, or at some distance (up to thousands of nucleotides) from a gene. When tested using reporter constructs (see below), such elements are functional even when inserted backward or 3' of the reporter gene, or even when the reporter gene is expressed from a different (heterologous) promoter.

Locus-Control Regions. In situ, locus-control regions are required to establish a tissue-specific open chromatin domain (see below) in the vicinity of a particular locus and thus permit appropriate tissue-specific expression; the first one identified is in the β-globin cluster. The open chromatin configuration is detected experimentally as tissue-specific hypersensitivity of DNA to digestion with deoxyribonuclease (DNase) I. In transgenic mice, locus-control regions direct high level tissue-specific expression that is independent of the site of chromosomal integration but dependent on copy number. Locus-control regions can exert effects over tens of kilobases and may consist of complex DNA elements themselves spaced over several kilobases. In addition to their effects on chromatin, elements within certain locus-control regions can act as transcriptional enhancers in reporter constructs, and so the distinction between these categories is not absolute.

DNA Methylation. In addition to defined DNA *cis* elements, modification of DNA by cytosine methylation at CpG dinucleotides is associated with gene inactivation. Each such dinucleotide is paired with another on the opposite DNA strand and usually both cytosines are methylated. This serves as a signal for a DNA methylase to methylate the cytosines on daughter strands whenever DNA is replicated. This minimizes expression of permanently inactivated genes when differentiated cells divide. Conversely, hypomethylation of DNA in CpG-rich regions in the 5' ends of genes is associated with active transcription. In some genes, the copies derived from each parent (i.e., the parental *alleles*) are differently and permanently methylated, or *imprinted,* leading to differences in gene expression. Several diseases such as Prader-Willi syndrome are caused by heterozygous deletion of imprinted genes because the remaining gene copy has been permanently inactivated by imprinting.

Protein Factors

Chromatin. Within chromosomes, eukaryotic DNA is organized into *nucleosomes,* each consisting of eight positively charged histone molecules (two each of histones H2A, H2B, H3, and H4) with 160–200 bp of DNA wound around it. Higher-order winding organizes nucleosomes into chromatin. This organization renders DNA relatively inaccessible to transcription factors, so that transcription is enhanced by remodeling of nucleosomes to permit assembly of transcription complexes. This remodeling or activation is mediated in part by acetylation of histones. Histone molecules interact with DNA and with each other in part via positively charged amino terminal domains, and acetylation of lysine residues in these domains reduces their positive charge. Conversely, deacetylation of histones represses transcription.

General Transcription Factors. The promoter of a gene is bound by general transcription factors (TFs) to form a transcription initiation complex that ultimately has a molecular weight of greater than 2 million (Fig. 2-2). Although preformed complexes may exist, stepwise assembly is usually postulated. TFIID binds to the TATA box. The TFIID is a complex of proteins consisting of TATA-binding protein (TBP) and at least a half dozen TBP-associated factors. This complex separates the DNA strands, allowing TFIIA and TFIIB to bind adjacent to the TATA box. This is followed by binding of TFIIF-α and RNA polymerase II. Transcription begins following binding of TFIIE, TFIIH, and TFIIJ and subsequent release of RNA polymerase II from the initiation complex.

The RNA polymerases I and III transcribe genes for ribosomal RNA and small RNAs (such as transfer RNAs), respectively. They are not regulated in the same way as RNA polymerase II, and they bind distinct sets of transcription factors.

Transcriptional Regulatory Factors. Many different factors bind to enhancer elements including nuclear hormone receptors and factors phosphorylated by kinases that are activated by hormone-dependent signaling pathways. These are described in greater detail in Chapter 3. In general, each consists of a DNA binding domain and at least one activation domain that interacts with elements of the transcriptional apparatus. Almost all DNA-binding domains include an α-helical protein segment that fits into the major groove between two turns of the DNA helix. Many of these domains (including those of nuclear hormone receptors) are stabilized by chelated zinc atoms and are termed *zinc fingers. Leucine zipper* domains have leucine residues every seventh position in the α-helix, which results in them all being on the same side of the helix. An example of such a protein is SREBP-1 (sterol regulatory element binding protein-1), which mediates transcriptional regulation by sterols.

Homeodomains are 60 amino acid motifs that are most often found in transcription factors regulating embryonic development. Examples of such factors in

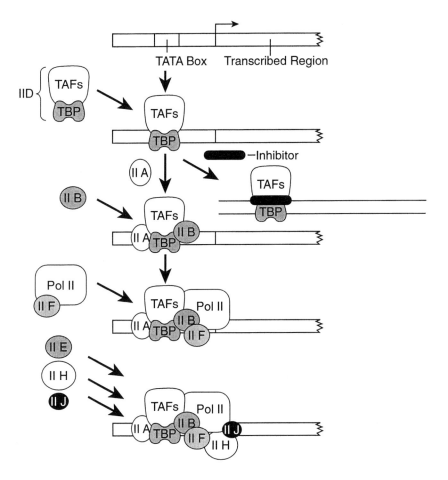

Fig. 2-2 Diagram of the sequential assembly of a transcription initiation complex. TBP, TATA-binding protein; TAFs, TBP-associated factors; II A-J, transcription factors II A-J; Pol II, RNA polymerase II. Adapted from Lodish et al., 1995.

mammals include Pit1 (defective in some cases of panhypopituitarism) and HESX1 (defective in some cases of septooptic dysplasia).

Many transcription factors bind DNA at adjacent sites as homo- or heterodimers. Factors that bind DNA elements separated by hundreds of bp may nevertheless be in physical contact because DNA is not completely rigid and can form loops. Enhancer factors may interact with general transcription factors to promote the assembly of the preinitiation complex. In addition, they interact with large complexes of proteins that act as *co-activators* or *co-repressors*. Co-activators may interact with general transcription factors to stabilize the preinitiation complex, and several also have a histone acetyltransferase activity. Others have ATPase activity and apparently remodel higher-order structures (involving many nucleosomes) in chromatin. Conversely, co-repressors destabilize the preinitiation complex, may have histone deacetylase activity, and also may remodel higher-order chromatin structures. Several co-repressors have a ubiquitin ligase activity that may target other transcriptional factors for degradation by the proteosome. The individual proteins in co-activator and co-repressor complexes have overlapping and somewhat redundant activities, so that functional specificity may result from particular combinations of factors. Clearly, co-activators and co-repressors act to integrate signals from different pathways (such as intracellular second messengers and ligands for nuclear hormone receptors) into coherent effects on expression of particular genes.

Processing of RNA

The primary RNA transcript of a gene is modified in several ways in the nucleus before being exported as mRNA to the cytoplasm where it is translated into protein (Fig. 2-1).

Cap Structure. The first posttranscriptional event during the course of RNA maturation is the addition of a cap, a methylated structure at the 5′ end of the RNA molecule. The cap structure is formed by addition of a guanosine to the 5′ end of the mRNA through an unusual 5′,5′ triphosphate bond followed by methylation of this guanosine in the N-7 position and subsequent methylation of the adjacent nucleotide(s). This structure is required for export of mRNA from the nucleus, and it also facilitates the binding of eukaryotic RNA to ribosomes and thus enhances the initiation of translation.

Poly(A) Tail. Eukaryotic transcription does not terminate at well defined sequences. However, the transcript is clipped 12–16 bases downstream from a consensus poly(A) addition site, AAUAAA or AUUAAA. Then a nucleotide sequence consisting entirely of repeated adenosines is added to the 3′ end of the RNA. It may play a role in RNA stability. Poly(A) tails generally range between 50 and 250 bases and are found in virtually all mRNAs except those coding for histones.

Splicing of Introns. A key aspect of the maturation of RNA is the removal of introns by "splicing." This process is mediated by *spliceosomes,* which are large complexes of small RNA molecules and proteins called *snRNPs* (*small nuclear ribonucleoproteins,* pronounced "snerps"). The RNA molecules in snRNPs recognize specific sequences at intron–exon boundaries, thereby signaling precisely where the RNA sequence cleavage will occur. Consensus sequences are found at both the 5′ (splice donor) and 3′ (splice acceptor) ends of introns. The last nucleotide of the exon is usually a G, and the first two nucleotides of the intron are almost invariably GT. The last two nucleotides of the intron are almost invariably AG; this is usually proceeded by several pyrimidine (C or T) nucleotides.

Intron excision consists of two transesterification reactions. In the first, a phosphate ester bond at the splice donor is transferred to the 2′ hydroxyl group of a specific adenosine located approximately 50 nucleotides 5′ of the splice acceptor, leaving the intron in a looped or "lariat" configuration and a free 3′ hydroxyl at the end of the splice donor. Then a phosphate ester bond at the splice acceptor is transferred to the splice donor.

The reason for the presence of intervening sequences in eukaryotic genes has not been established. However, in some genes they serve to separate specific structural and/or functional domains of the resultant protein. This may facilitate evolution by allowing segments coding for such domains to be transferred from one gene to another by genetic recombination. When genes encoding the same protein are compared among different species, the nucleotide sequences within introns are much less similar than coding sequences, suggesting that the exact sequence of an intron is relatively unimportant except for sequences involved in splicing.

Translation

Within the nucleotide sequence of the mature mRNA transcript lies an *open reading frame,* which is *translated* into protein by the ribosomal protein synthesis apparatus that reads the mRNA nucleotide sequence in *triplets* or *codons* (Fig. 2-3). Translation begins at an initiator methionine codon (AUG) in an adequate sequence *context* for initiation, the most important feature of which is a purine (an A or G) three nucleotides 5′ of the AUG. The ribosome reads the subsequent sequence without internal punctuation until it reaches a stop codon (UAA, UGA, or UAG), at which point the ribosome disassociates from the mRNA. Because there are four ribonucleotides, the *genetic code* consists of 64 codons. Besides the initiator and stop codons, there are 60 other codons to encode 19 other amino acids, and thus an average of three codons (range 1–6, usually 2–4) can encode each amino acid. The code is thus *degenerate.*

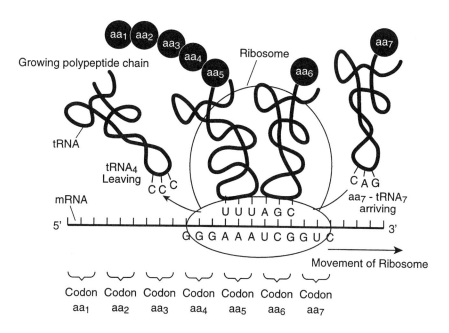

Fig. 2-3   Ribosomal protein synthesis. *A,C,G,* and *U* are nucleotides in RNA; they are illustrated in mRNA only in the region in contact with the ribosome, and only in tRNA in the region of the anticodon, which interacts with mRNA through complementary base-pairing. *aa₁₋₇* represent successive amino acids in the nascent polypeptide. Adapted from Lodish et al., 1995.

Codons are actually read by small *transfer RNA* (tRNA) molecules that are specific for each amino acid. A tRNA molecule is charged with the appropriate amino acid at its 3' end by a specific *aminoacyl tRNA synthase*. The tRNA molecule has an *anticodon* that is complementary to the codon. Degeneracy in the code lies mostly in the third nucleotide of the codon (e.g., alanine may be encoded by GCA, GCC, GCG, or GCT); the interaction between the first nucleotide of the tRNA's anticodon and the third nucleotide of the mRNA's codon is relatively weak or "wobbly," permitting a single tRNA to accommodate degeneracy in the third position of the codon.

Posttranslational Processing

Many proteins of interest to endocrinologists are either secreted from cells (such as peptide hormones) or are integral membrane proteins (such as many hormone receptors). Such proteins are synthesized on ribosomes bound to the *endoplasmic reticulum* and undergo posttranslational processing.

All such proteins contain an N-terminal segment termed a *signal peptide* that contains approximately 20 amino acids, most of which are hydrophobic. Synthesis of such proteins begins on free ribosomes, but after the first 70 or so amino acid residues have been synthesized, the N-terminus is bound by a ribonucleoprotein complex, the *signal recognition particle*. This is then bound by the signal recognition particle receptor, which is inserted in the membrane of the endoplasmic reticulum and recruits specific proteins to form a transmembrane channel to begin transporting the protein across the membrane of the endoplasmic reticulum as it is being synthesized (Fig. 2-4).

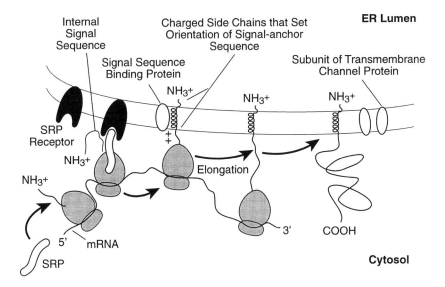

Fig. 2-4   Insertion of a nascent polypeptide into the membrane of the endoplasmic reticulum (ER). This is one of several possible modes of protein processing by the ER. The gray shapes represent ribosomes. SRP, signal recognition particle. NH_3^+ and COOH denote the amino and carboxy termini of a polypeptide. Adapted from Lodish et al., 1995.

Secreted proteins are usually synthesized as *prepeptides,* meaning that the signal peptide is cleaved by a signal peptidase shortly after it is inserted into the endoplasmic reticulum membrane. The nascent protein is then transported through the transmembrane channel. In many integral membrane proteins, the signal peptide is not cleaved; in some cases the N-terminus ends up in the lumen of the endoplasmic reticulum, whereas the orientation is reversed in others so the N-terminus remains on the cytoplasmic side of the membrane.

The nascent protein is transported across the endoplasmic reticulum membrane in an unfolded state and must then assume the correct conformation. This often requires interactions with chaperone proteins, the formation of disulfide bonds between cysteine sulfhydryl groups, and glycosylation, all of which occur within the endoplasmic reticulum. Sugars may be attached to either the amide groups of asparagines (*N-glycosylation*) or the hydroxyl groups of serine and threonine (*O-glycosylation*); glycosylation may be required for proper folding or stability of proteins and/or for proper targeting to subcellular organelles such as lysosomes.

Secretory and cell surface proteins are transported in specific vesicles to the *Golgi apparatus* where they may undergo additional processing such as modification of glycosylation. They are sorted within the Golgi apparatus into vesicles containing proteins destined for the cell surface, those for proteins that are continuously secreted (such as albumin) and those for proteins that are secreted in a regulated manner such as insulin. Sorting is an energy-requiring process involving specific guanosine triphosphate (GTP)-binding proteins.

Certain peptide hormones such as insulin are synthesized as *preprohormones;* they require additional proteolytic steps that usually take place within secretory vesicles. Some preprohormones contain multiple peptide hormones within their primary sequence, such as pro-opiomelanocortin (POMC), the precursor for ACTH α-, β-, and γ-melanotropin (MSH), γ-lipotropin (γ-LPH), and γ-endorphin (see Chapter 6).

Some proteins, particularly enzymes like cytochromes P450, are synthesized as *apoproteins* requiring addition of functional groups like heme before they are active. This typically occurs at the site (e.g., mitochondria) at which the enzyme is to function. Many additional types of posttranslational processing exist, including phosphorylation at serine, threonine or tyrosine residues, binding of lipids, and chemical modification of amino acids (e.g., hydroxylysine residues in collagen).

CLONING AND RELATED TECHNIQUES

Although many different molecular genetic techniques have been used to analyze the structure and function of hormones, they can be classified into a small number of broad categories.

Hybridization

Southern blot hybridization (Fig. 2-5) identifies DNA segments corresponding to a specific *probe* segment in a more complex mixture of DNA such as total human DNA. The DNA is treated with a *restriction endonuclease,* an enzyme that can digest DNA at a defined sequence 4–8 bp in length. The DNA is fractionated on the

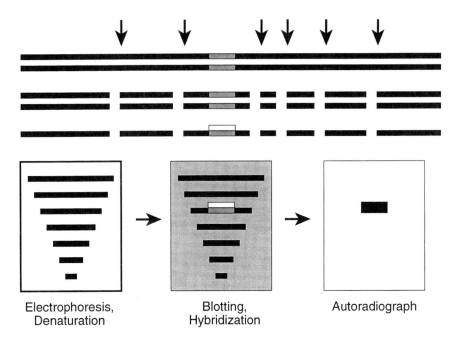

Electrophoresis, Denaturation	Blotting, Hybridization	Autoradiograph

Fig. 2-5 Schematic of Southern blot hybridization. The double line at the top of the figure represents DNA; the shaded segment denotes the DNA segment to be detected. Arrows denote digestion by a restriction endonuclease; the products of digestion are the second set of double lines. The DNA fragments are then denatured (rendered single-stranded, denoted by single lines) and hybridized with a labeled probe, represented by a short white line. The three rectangles at the bottom of the figure denote (from *left* to *right*) DNA fragments within an agarose gel, DNA fragments after transfer to a membrane and hybridization, and an autoradiogram of the hybridized membrane.

basis of size by electrophoresis in an agarose gel; the smaller the size of the fragment, the faster it migrates. The DNA is then denatured (rendered single stranded) by treating the gel with alkali and transferred to a nylon membrane by blotting; this preserves the spacial information in the gel (i.e., how far each fragment has migrated). Next, the membrane is hybridized with the probe, which is a labeled segment of cloned DNA that is rendered single stranded by boiling. During the hybridization, the two strands of the probe may reanneal, but some probe molecules will instead anneal to complementary fragments of DNA immobilized on the membrane. After washing the membrane, these bound probe molecules can be detected as distinct bands. If the probe has been radioactively labeled, the membrane is autoradiographed. As an alternative to radioactivity, it is also possible to label the probe chemically with groups such as biotin or digoxigenin. These groups are detected by binding with a specific antibody that is linked to an enzyme like alkaline phosphatase. This can mediate a chemoluminescent reaction that is detected by exposure to film.

Northern blots are conceptually similar, except that RNA is subjected to electrophoresis instead of DNA (see below).

Cloning

As applied to DNA (rather than cells or whole organisms), *cloning* refers to the isolation of a desired segment of DNA so that it can be indefinitely replicated within an easily grown *host* organism such as *Escherichia coli* bacteria and large quantities obtained thereby. This involves *ligation* of the desired insert in a *vector* that contains sequences required for DNA replication in the host, and some marker gene that permits identification and selection of cells carrying the vector (Fig. 2-6). Vectors usually have a series of recognition sites for restriction endonucleases so that DNA insert can be ligated to the vector after the vector is digested with the enzyme. In some cases digestion with a restriction endonuclease yields DNA molecules with short (2–4 nucleotides) single stranded segments at the ends; in such cases, DNA molecules can be ligated only if they have compatible, complementary ends.

Many vectors are *plasmids,* circular DNA molecules that replicate separately from the bacterial chromosome. Plasmid vectors usually carry at least one gene for antibiotic resistance, allowing bacterial cells carrying the plasmid to be selected by growth in medium containing the appropriate antibiotic. Other vectors are *bacteriophage,* viruses that infect bacteria. Bacteria infected with bacteriophage can be readily identified on culture plates as plaques of bacterial lysis or poor growth.

Whereas intact bacteriophage can infect bacteria in culture, plasmids cannot enter bacteria unless the bacteria have been chemically treated to make them *competent* to take up DNA. Bacteria that have absorbed the plasmid are selected by plating on the appropriate antibiotic.

Some vectors have additional desirable properties such as the ability to grow in mammalian cells or to direct the synthesis of a protein encoded by the insert in bacterial, yeast, insect, or mammalian cells.

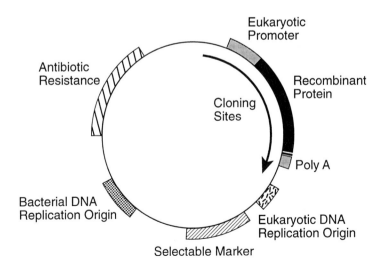

Fig. 2-6 Schematic of a plasmid vector used for expression of a cDNA encoding a recombinant protein. A plasmid is a double-stranded circular DNA molecule; this is not shown. Segments with specific functions are denoted by various shadings.

Polymerase Chain Reaction (PCR)

As long as the sequences at the ends of a DNA segment are known, it may not be necessary to clone the segment into a vector to obtain large quantities of it. Instead, the segment can be replicated in vitro (Fig. 2-7). It is rendered single-stranded (i.e., *denatured*) by heating and then a short (usually 17–21 bp) synthetic oligonucleotide "primer" is annealed near the 5' end of each original strand, creating a short double-stranded segment. The primer (and thus the double-stranded region) is extended using a DNA polymerase that incorporates deoxynucleotide triphosphate (dNTP) precursors (i.e., dATP, dCTP, dGTP, dTTP) complementary to the original strand. Thus, there will be two completely double stranded DNA molecules at the end of this process for every original molecule in the reaction. These two molecules are again denatured by heating, primers again annealed, and each molecule copied by the polymerase, yielding a total of four molecules. Because the number of molecules doubles with every cycle, any desired quantity of DNA can be obtained by running a reaction of appropriate size for a sufficient number of cycles.

In practice, PCRs are run in a *thermocycler,* which can raise and lower temperatures in a heating block to temperatures optimal for DNA denaturation, primer annealing, and strand extension. A special DNA polymerase is used that can withstand high temperatures without itself being denatured.

Analysis of DNA Sequence

Almost all sequence analysis uses the Sanger ("dideoxy" or "chain termination") method (Fig. 2-8). As with PCR, sequencing reactions involve extension of a primer annealed to a single stranded "template" DNA molecule. As originally conceived, four reactions (*A, C, G,* and *T*) are run, each containing a "dideoxy" analog of one of the four dNTPs in addition to all four dNTPs. When one of the dideoxy molecules is incorporated instead of the corresponding dNTP, the newly synthesized DNA strand can no longer be extended. The concentration of the dideoxy analog is adjusted so that a dideoxy molecule is likely to be incorporated at any of the first 100

Fig. 2-7 Polymerase chain reaction (PCR). A double-stranded DNA molecule (black double line) is denatured, and complementary primers (gray arrows) are annealed to each strand. These are extended by a DNA polymerase to yield two completely double-stranded molecules (black plus gray lines at the bottom of the figure), corresponding to each starting molecule. Each of these is then subjected to the same procedure.

Fig. 2-8 DNA sequencing. *Left,* illustration of a sequencing reaction. A short, single-stranded *primer* (actually, primers are usually 15–20 nucleotides long) is annealed to a complementary and longer single-stranded *template* molecule. The primer is then extended with a DNA polymerase until a "dideoxy" *terminator* nucleotide (the circled *G* in the figure) is randomly incorporated into the elongating DNA strand, at which point elongation stops. This produces a collection of terminated strands of various lengths that can be resolved by electrophoresis (*right*). A set of four reactions is usually run, one for each of the four dideoxy nucleotide terminators.

to 200 positions where the corresponding dNTP would normally be used. Thus, when completed, the reaction contains an assortment of newly synthesized chains of different lengths, each length corresponding to the location of the appropriate base. The chains of various length are resolved by gel electrophoresis, with the four A, C, G, and T reactions in adjacent lanes. If a radioactive dNTP was included in the reactions, the fragments could be detected by autoradiography. They appear as a ladder with a band in one of the four lanes at each "rung." By reading from the bottom of the gel (fastest migrating and smallest fragments), the sequence of the template can be deduced, starting from a point near the primer.

Most large laboratories and core facilities now carry out DNA sequencing using automated equipment. In the most widely used protocol, each template is analyzed in a single reaction that includes a mix of all four dideoxy analogs, each labeled with a fluorescent dye of a different color. Sequencing reactions are resolved by conventional gel electrophoresis, but fragments are detected by photomultipliers as they pass the bottom of the gel; the color at which each fragment fluoresces indicates which dideoxynucleotide is incorporated at the end. The sequence information is captured directly by a computer.

ANALYSIS OF GENOMES

The complement of DNA present in the nucleus of a single cell of an organism is termed the *genome;* the human genome consists of approximately 3 billion bp of *genomic* DNA in haploid cells (sperm and ova). This includes approximately 100,000 genes, structural chromosome components such as centromeres and telomeres, and intergenic segments without apparent function.

Mapping

It is often desirable to determine what chromosomal segment a particular gene is on and then determine the gene's exact position relative to other genes. There are several ways in which this is done.

Cytogenetic Mapping
Once a gene has been cloned, it is fluorescently labeled and hybridized to metaphase spreads of chromosomes. The chromosome(s) to which the labeled probe hybridizes and the approximate location on the chromosome can be determined with a suitable microscope. This technique, *fluorescent in situ hybridization* (FISH), has supplanted earlier, more laborious, and less sensitive approaches using radioactive probes.

Genetic Mapping
Genetic mapping and radiation hybrids (see the next section) are used to map the position of a gene relative to other DNA segments of known location. Such segments, or marker loci, need not be and usually are not themselves genes. Most often they are anonymous segments termed *sequence-tagged sites* of a few hundred base pairs that can be readily amplified by PCR. Usually each segment contains a region consisting of several (10–20) copies of a dinucleotide (such as CA), trinu-

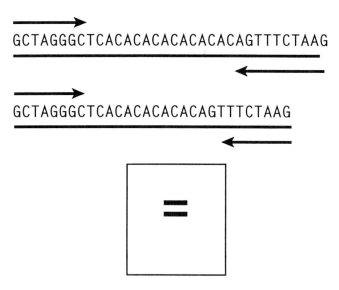

Fig. 2-9 Illustration of CA repeat polymorphisms. The CA repeat regions often vary in length between individuals. This can be detected by PCR using primers (arrows) complementary to unique regions flanking the repeat. Bands of differing sizes containing different numbers of repeats are detected by electrophoresis, illustrated schematically at the bottom of the figure.

cleotide (such as CAG) or tetranucleotide sequence (Fig. 2-9). Many of these *microsatellite* repeats vary in copy number between individuals, so that the length of the corresponding PCR-amplified segment also varies. Such length variations can be detected by electrophoresis through the same type of gel used for DNA sequence analysis. If there are a sufficient number of length variants (i.e., alleles) at a given locus, most individuals will be heterozygous for different alleles, permitting their two chromosomes to be distinguished in parents or offspring. To determine the location of a new polymorphic locus of interest, the pattern of inheritance (or segregation) of its alleles in several large kindreds is compared with the pattern of inheritance of each of the many marker loci already in the database for those kindreds. A collection of DNA samples from such kindreds is maintained by the Center for the Study of Human Polymorphism (CEPH) in France.

Somatic Cell Hybrids
When a cultured human cell is fused with a mouse cell to produce a hybrid, human chromosomes are preferentially lost. The human chromosomes retained by each line in a panel of hybrid cell lines are identified, following which the chromosomal location of any new gene or marker locus can be determined by seeing which cell lines retain the human version of the locus. In the past, this was done by Southern blot hybridization, but today it is almost always done by PCR using primers that are specific for the human version of the locus.

Although this method originally utilized cell lines with one or more intact human chromosomes, more recent panels have used *radiation hybrids* in which the human chromosomes have been extensively fragmented with high-energy radiation. Thus, each line contains many small segments from different human chromosomes. Although more lines are required for a complete panel, this permits very high resolution (within a few million bases) mapping of any human gene locus.

Cloning and Physical Mapping
Several different types of vectors are used to clone segments of genomic DNA; the amount of DNA that can be cloned in each is to some extent inversely correlated with the ease of in vitro manipulation of the DNA and freedom from artifactual DNA rearrangements or chimerism (cloning of unrelated DNA segments in the same vector molecule). Those that can be grown in *E. coli* include: *bacteriophage lambda*, which contains inserts of 15,000 to 20,000 bp (15–20 kb) of DNA; specialized plasmid vectors called *cosmids; bacteriophage P1,* with inserts of 100 kb, and *bacterial artificial chromosomes* (BACs) with inserts of a few hundred kb. *Yeast artificial chromosomes* (YACs) can carry far larger inserts of up to 2000 kilobases. By determining content of sequence tagged sites and mapping restriction enzyme recognition sites on each clone, many BAC and YAC clones of the human and mouse genomes have been conceptually assembled into long, overlapping *contigs* covering many megabases of DNA including several complete smaller chromosomes.

Thus, a particular gene segment can be mapped very precisely by demonstrating its presence on one or more clones within a contig.

The *Human Genome Project* is an ongoing effort to determine the DNA sequence of the entire human genome. The initial step in this project was the development of a detailed genetic map of the genome; this map is now complete but continues to be refined by the addition of new markers. The next step was complete coverage of the genome by contigs of clones; this phase is still in progress at this time. Finally, the DNA sequence of each clone in each contig is determined.

The sequence data are then analyzed by computer to identify putative coding exons based on the presence of intron splice donor and acceptor sequences and possible open reading frames. The predicted amino acid sequence encoded by each exon is compared with sequences already in the database to see whether it represents the human homolog of a protein previously identified in some other species, or is a member of a known gene family (such as cytochrome P450 enzymes or nuclear hormone receptors), or at least contains an amino acid motif (such as a nucleotide cofactor binding site) of known function.

At present, most data from Human Genome Project laboratories are made available on the Internet soon after they are generated, although the fragmentary nature of much of the data limits their usefulness to some extent.

ANALYSIS OF EXPRESSED GENE PRODUCTS

Complementary DNA, or *cDNA,* corresponds in sequence to mRNA. It is synthesized *in vitro* by incubating mRNA with an RNA-dependent DNA polymerase (*reverse transcriptase* derived from a retrovirus) in the presence of deoxynucleotide triphosphates. It differs from genomic DNA in two important ways. Whereas genomic DNA is essentially identical in all cells in the body (excluding immunoglobulin and T-cell receptor gene rearrangements in cells of the immune system), the cDNA that is synthesized using mRNA from a particular cell type will mirror the abundance of the different mRNA transcripts in those cells. Thus, a different *library* of cDNA must be synthesized from each organ, tissue or cell line of interest. Second, cDNA does not contain introns, because these were spliced out of mRNA before exportation from the nucleus. Hence, any efforts to express human proteins in bacterial cells must use cDNA (in a suitable expression vector) because bacteria lack the cellular machinery required to splice introns out of genes.

Screening

There are several ways to isolate a desired clone from a library of many clones of cDNA or genomic DNA. At present, cDNA libraries from many human and mouse tissues and genomic libraries from many species are commercially available.

Hybridization

Often, some sequence information is already available. This is the case if one is trying to use a cDNA clone (often containing less than the full sequence) to isolate a longer cDNA clone, a homologous cDNA in a different species, cDNAs encoding related proteins, or the corresponding genomic gene. The underlying principle is identical to that used for Southern or Northern blots. A nylon filter is dropped onto a culture plate containing bacterial colonies or bacteriophage plaques, so that a replica of the plate is transferred to the filter. The DNA in the bacteria on the filter is released and denatured by treatment with alkali and is hybridized with a labeled probe. Successful hybridization is detected as a spot on autoradiography film. By aligning the film with the plate, the corresponding colony or plaque is identified.

A special application of this technique is used when only a peptide sequence is available. Because of degeneracy in the genetic code, a mixture of synthetic DNA probes may need to be used containing all (or at least the most likely) combinations of sequences that could encode the peptide. However, if the sequence is sufficiently long, a few errors may be better tolerated and a single "guessmer" may be similar enough to the actual sequence to hybridize successfully.

In recent years, this technique has been partially supplanted by PCR screening techniques.

Polymerase Chain Reaction

There are several variations of PCR screening; the following approach is used by large laboratories and commercial services. Robotic devices are used to pick individual bacterial colonies and transfer them to microtiter plates so that each clone has a unique three-dimensional "address" consisting of a particular plate and the column and row on that plate. For large libraries, a fourth "dimension" can be used consisting of groups of plates. Pools of DNA are generated robotically to identify each component of the address (e.g., "row" pools each consist of all clones in each row of every plate in the collection and "column" pools each consist of all clones in each column of every plate). The PCRs are run using DNA from each pool and a primer pair derived from the desired sequence. Approximately 40 PCRs are required to screen a 10,000-clone library; if there is a single positive clone in the library, there will be four reactions that will yield a product, one corresponding to each dimension in the clone's address.

Immunologic Screening

Immunologic screening might be feasible if an antiserum to the desired protein product is available. A cDNA library is constructed in a vector (usually a derivative of bacteriophage lambda) in which cDNA inserts are expressed as fusion proteins with a bacterial protein such as β-galactosidase. A filter is dropped onto each culture plate as for hybridization screening, but it is processed differently and then incubated with antiserum. Replicas of plaques expressing the desired protein will bind the antibody, which is detected using a labeled second antibody.

It is necessary that the cDNA insert be in the same orientation and reading frame as the gene for the fusion protein or it will not be translated correctly by the bacterial protein synthesis apparatus. This will occur by chance in only one-sixth of the clones (one-half chance of being in the correct orientation $\times$ one-third chance of being in the correct reading frame), but some methods of cDNA library construction force all clones into the correct orientation. In any case, this drawback is overcome by simply screening more clones.

Expression Screening

In some cases the desired protein has not been purified and little structural information is available. In such cases the cDNA must be cloned based on some property that it confers on cells such as a novel enzymatic activity.

A typical strategy is to transfect plates of mammalian cells with pools of 1000 clones and assay each plate for the desired activity. If such a plate is detected, the pool of 1000 clones is divided into 10 subpools of 100 clones, which are again transfected. If a subpool conferring the activity is detected, it is successively subdivided and rescreened until a single clone is isolated.

Expressed Sequence Tags

Whereas the Human Genome Project aims to sequence the entire genome, a related project is partially sequencing thousands of cDNAs from each of many different cell types. At this time, there are over 50,000 such *expressed sequence tags (ESTs)* available. As there are an estimated 100,000 genes, this implies that a great many genes have already been identified. This approach complements the Human Genome Project, because identification of an EST within a putative gene confirms that the gene is transcribed in a particular tissue. Conversely, ESTs are generally not full-length cDNA sequences and can usually be extended using the corresponding genomic sequence.

GENETIC DISEASES

Two general approaches have been used to determine the etiology of genetic diseases. In many cases, a *candidate gene* is immediately apparent. For example, a gene encoding an enzyme is likely to carry mutations in cases of deficiency of that enzyme. In such cases, the cDNA encoding the enzyme is usually isolated first (see the sections on screening of cDNA libraries) and used to identify the corresponding chromosomal gene. The gene is then analyzed as described below to detect mutations. These mutations are then re-created in cDNA, which is expressed in cultured cells to determine the effects of each mutation on functioning of the encoded protein.

In diseases where a candidate gene is not available, the disease locus is mapped by linkage analysis (see the following section) and the affected gene identified by positional cloning approaches.

Linkage Analysis

Many diseases of interest to endocrinologists are inherited in a *Mendelian* manner (i.e., the disease segregates in the kindred as a single locus with a well defined mode of inheritance). If the gene causing a particular disease is unknown, or if mutations in a candidate gene cannot be identified, it may be possible to determine the location of the affected gene by linkage studies. Consider an autosomal recessive disease such as congenital adrenal hyperplasia due to 21-hydroxylase deficiency, which was originally mapped by linkage analysis (however, the cDNA encoding the 21-hydroxylase enzyme was identified by immunologic screening). All affected individuals in a given kindred should have identical alleles at the disease locus, and all unaffected individuals should differ from the affected individuals at that locus; thus, testing of a few hundred markers will yield the approximate location of the disease gene. If a marker locus (e.g., for 21-hydroxylase deficiency, the gene encoding the transplantation antigen HLA-B) is at a small genetic distance from the disease locus, affected individuals will likely still be identical at both the marker locus and the disease locus. However, there is a slight chance that they will not be identical at the marker locus because of a genetic recombination between the disease locus and the marker locus. Thus, if affected individuals in the same kindred are not identical at any particular locus, this might have occurred because both the marker and the disease locus are linked but were separated by a recombination, or it might mean that the marker locus was not linked at all to the disease (for example, the marker might be on a different chromosome). The log of the ratio of the probabilities of either of these explanations being true is referred to as a *LOD score*. A LOD score of 3 (meaning that it is 1000 times more likely that two loci are linked than that they are not linked) is usually considered to confirm linkage.

The use of microsatellite markers has dramatically reduced the effort required for such an analysis.

Positional Cloning

Once a disease locus has been genetically mapped, genomic clones are isolated that span the entire interval between the closest linked marker loci; this is often an interval of at least a megabase of DNA corresponding to approximately a 1% chance of recombination between the disease gene and a marker locus. If a sufficient number of affected families are available, it may be useful to isolate and map additional polymorphic marker loci from the clones in the hope that some of the markers will be separated from the disease locus by genetic recombination in one or more affected individuals. If so, this can decrease the amount of DNA that must be analyzed.

If the disease gene is known to be expressed in a particular tissue, hybridization or other techniques can sometimes be used to identify cDNAs in that tissue that correspond to genes on each clone. It may be necessary to sequence all or most of the interval to identify genes. Eventually, one or more candidate genes are identified based on their pattern of expression or likely functions based on the predicted amino acid sequences. Each such gene is then scanned for mutations in affected individuals (see the following section).

Positional cloning was initially extremely laborious (e.g., identification of the gene causing cystic fibrosis) but has become easier with progress of the Human Genome Project. The necessary clones are often already available and in many cases have been sequenced, and/or expressed sequence tags (ESTs) have been mapped. Even if this has not yet been done, DNA sequencing technology has improved to the point that determining the sequence of a megabase of DNA is within the capabilities of a properly equipped medium-sized laboratory.

Detection of Point Mutations

To prove that mutations in a gene cause a disease, it is first necessary to identify such mutations. If the gene of interest is relatively small and the number of patients to be analyzed is small, it is usually most straightforward to sequence the gene in each patient. If larger numbers of samples need to be analyzed, a method to scan for mutations may save a great deal of time and labor. Such methods usually involve amplification of DNA segments using PCR. All work best on segments of a few hundred nucleotides.

The most commonly used methods make use of the fact that changes in nucleotide sequence may change the way in which DNA fragments migrate during electrophoresis (Fig. 2-10). For example, the conditions under which complementary DNA strands separate, or "melt," may be affected. This is detected by subjecting the DNA to *denaturing gradient gel electrophoresis*—that is, electrophoresis under conditions in which the DNA becomes more likely to be denatured the farther it migrates in the gel, often by using a special apparatus that maintains the bottom of the gel at a higher temperature. As the DNA migrates down the gel, it eventually reaches a point at which the two strands begin to separate, or *denature*. Once a molecule is partially denatured, its mobility is drastically decreased. Thus, molecules with a mutation will stop at a different position in the gel from normal molecules, and this is detected by autoradiography.

In the related *single-stranded conformation polymorphism* technique, radioactively labeled double-stranded DNA is denatured by heating and then quickly cooled so that the complementary strands cannot reanneal. Each single DNA strand will snap into its most energetically favorable conformation. This will include base-pairing of nucleotides on the one strand, and thus the conformation may vary if the sequence has changed due to a mutation. The DNA strands in different conformations often migrate differently in the gel.

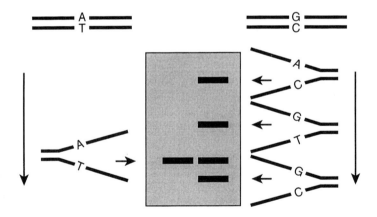

Fig. 2-10 Denaturing gradient gel electrophoresis. *Top,* two otherwise identical double-stranded DNA molecules differ at a single position (A-T or G-C). If a homogenous collection of such molecules (*left*) is subjected to electrophoresis through a denaturing gradient, they will all migrate (vertical arrows) to the same position in a gel (*center*). If a mixture of the two sequences is denatured to separate the strands and allowed to reanneal (*right*), four bands will be seen in the gel. The top two are *heteroduplexes* consisting of molecules with mismatched bases. These are relatively unstable and denature easily, so that they migrate slowly. The two molecules with fully complementary bases denature under slightly different conditions and thus migrate to slightly different positions in the gel.

Detecting a Known Mutation

In many cases previous work has identified mutations causing a particular disease, and an investigator wishes to determine the frequencies of these mutations in a different or larger population. This is often less difficult than identifying the mutations in the first place. Usually, segments of the gene of interest are amplified by PCR.

It may be possible to use single-stranded conformation polymorphisms or DNA sequencing on a routine basis. These may be the methods of choice for rare disease in which each family carries a different mutation. Other approaches are specifically useful for detecting limited numbers of known mutations; three are described below.

Restriction Fragment Length Polymorphisms

Southern blots are a way to detect deletions or duplications of DNA, which will change the number or size of hybridizing fragments. They usually cannot detect smaller changes of DNA sequence. The exception to this is if a change in DNA sequence forms or destroys a recognition site for a restriction endonuclease, because this will change the size of a DNA fragment produced by digestion with that enzyme. This is referred to as a *restriction fragment length polymorphism* (RFLP) (Fig. 2-11). Because there are dozens of different restriction enzymes and recognition sequences, it is not unusual to find a suitable enzyme to detect a particular sequence change, but it is laborious to screen all known enzymes blindly. It is often more useful to identify mutations using other techniques and to use a RFLP (if one exists) for routine identification.

Ever since the advent of PCR, it has become common to detect RFLPs by amplifying the appropriate segment of DNA, digesting it with a restriction enzyme,

Fig. 2-11 Restriction fragment-length polymorphism (RFLP). *Top,* two otherwise identical double-stranded DNA molecules differ at a single position (G-C or A-T). The former (*left*) is part of a GGCC sequence that is digested by a restriction endonuclease, whereas the latter (*right*) is part of a GGAC sequence that is not digested. Thus, fragments of different sizes are produced (*center*); these are detected by electrophoresis (*bottom*).

and subjecting the fragments to electrophoresis. Because PCR produces relatively large quantities of DNA, the polymorphism can be detected by examination of gels stained with a DNA dye such as ethidium bromide; radioactive labeling or hybridization is unnecessary.

Allele-Specific Oligonucleotide Hybridization

The PCR-amplified DNA samples are denatured and blotted to a nylon membrane. The membrane is then hybridized with short (~20 nucleotides) single-stranded probes that are radioactively or chemically labeled. For each mutation, two probes are made, one corresponding to the normal sequence, and the other to the mutant sequence. The probes are hybridized separately to duplicate samples under conditions in which only a perfectly matched probe will hybridize. Thus, homozygous normal, heterozygous mutant, and homozygous mutant samples will hybridize with only the normal probe, with both probes, or with only the mutant probe, respectively (Fig. 2-12).

This hybridization process can be reversed, with a fluorescently labeled PCR product hybridized to oligonucleotides immobilized on a solid substrate, or "gene chip." This permits simultaneous detection of many different mutations. This technology is now being used on a large scale to scan hundreds of genes from dozens of individuals for *single nucleotide polymorphisms,* or *SNPs*, with the idea that such polymorphisms can be used for association studies of common diseases (see below).

Allele-Specific PCR

Two PCRs are run. They have one primer in common, but the "allele-specific" primers at the other end differ in the two reactions; one recognizes the normal sequence, and the other the mutant sequence. Under appropriate PCR conditions, only a perfectly matched primer will work in the PCR. Thus, one or the other allele-

Fig. 2-12   Allele-specific oligonucleotide hybridization. *Top,* two otherwise identical double-stranded DNA molecules differ at a single position (A-T or G-C). These are denatured and hybridized with a labeled single-stranded probe that is complementary to and will hybridize with one of these sequences; this is detected by autoradiography (*bottom*).

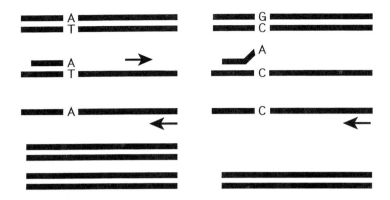

Fig. 2-13 Allele-specific PCR. *Top,* two otherwise identical double-stranded DNA molecules differ at a single position (A-T or G-C). They are subjected to PCR using one primer that is complementary to both molecules (arrow at the right of each molecule), and a second primer (short strand ending in *A*), which is complementary only to one. Thus, only the molecule on the left can be amplified by PCR under these conditions.

specific reaction (or both, if the sample is from a heterozygote) will yield a detectable product depending on the genotype of the sample (Fig. 2-13).

Categories of Disease-Causing Mutations

Mutations are usually classified by their effects on gene function. We give some examples of frequently occurring types of mutations as they occur in the *CYP21* gene encoding steroid 21-hydroxylase (Fig. 2-14). Such mutations cause congenital adrenal hyperplasia, a defect of cortisol biosynthesis (see Chapter 8).

Deletions and Other Rearrangements

Obviously, deletion of all or part of a gene prevents synthesis of a functional protein. Typically, such mutations are generated by recombinations between duplicated gene segments. For example, CYP21 lies on a duplicated segment of 30 kb; the duplicate copy of CYP21 is a nonfunctional *pseudogene* containing several inactivating mutations. Approximately 20% of mutations involving CYP21 are deletions of all or most of the normally active copy of the gene. Other mutations are *gene conversions,* which are transfers of segments containing deleterious mutations from the pseudogene to the normally active gene.

Mutations in Coding Sequences

A *missense* mutation changes an amino acid incorporated into the protein. For example, the mutation of ATC to AAC in codon 172 of CYP21 changes the corresponding amino acid from isoleucine to asparagine; this reduces enzymatic activity to 1% of normal and causes congenital adrenal hyperplasia.

A *nonsense* mutation generates a premature stop codon and prevents synthesis of a functional protein. The mutation of CAG to TAG in codon 318 of CYP21 results in synthesis of a truncated unstable enzyme leading to a severe form of adrenal hyperplasia.

Fig. 2-14 Examples of different mutations causing 21-hydroxylase deficiency. Nucleotide sequences with corresponding amino acid sequences are shown surrounding each mutation; coding sequences are grouped into triplet codons. Each normal sequence is on the left with the mutant sequence on the right. Changed amino acids are in bold. The insertion causing a *frameshift mutation* is a *T* marked by an arrowhead. The actual *splicing mutation* is shaded; this activates a cryptic splice acceptor site (boxed *AG* in the bottom sequence), causing retention of an extra 19 nucleotides of intron sequence in mRNA.

A *frameshift* mutation inserts or deletes a number of nucleotides not divisible by 3. Because mRNA is translated in codons of three nucleotides without internal punctuation, this causes the ribosome to shift to an incorrect grouping of nucleotides (i.e., a shift in the reading frame), and thus the resulting protein sequence becomes completely abnormal at the point of the mutation. An insertion of a single extra T nucleotide in a run of seven T nucleotides beginning at codon 246 of CYP21 is an example of such a mutation.

Mutations Affecting Splicing
Mutations that affect the GT or AG sequences at the beginning or end of an intron prevent removal of the intron and result in its retention within mRNA. Attempts by the ribosome to translate the inserted sequence usually lead to a nonfunctional protein. Other mutations within the intron can activate a normally nonfunctional or *cryptic* splice site with the same result. For example, mutation of an A to a G 13 nucleotides before the end of the second intron of CYP21 leads to abnormal splicing and the retention of 19 extra nucleotides within CYP21 mRNA. This shifts the reading frame of translation and renders the resulting protein nonfunctional.

Genetics of Common Diseases

Many common diseases such as hypertension or obesity are presumed to have multiple genetic susceptibility traits as well as environmental or lifestyle etiologies. Genetic analysis of such disorders is consequently more difficult than for Mendelian traits. Two complementary strategies are used: *linkage analysis* and *association stud-*

ies. These methods have a number of difficulties in common as well as some that are unique to each approach. First, traits such as blood pressure may result from the interplay of so many factors that it is difficult to identify any but those genetic loci with the strongest influence. This problem can be addressed by examining *intermediate phenotypes* that are presumed to influence the trait under study but are probably controlled by fewer genetic factors. For blood pressure, examples are levels of regulatory hormones such as renin and aldosterone. Second, some loci may influence the trait only at certain ages or in one sex or in a particular race. This can be addressed by stratifying the study population so that particular subsets of the population are analyzed individually. Third, some loci may have an effect only in combination with particular alleles at another locus, a phenomenon termed *epistasis.* This may require very large study populations to detect.

Affected Pedigree Member Analysis

It is difficult to study common multifactorial diseases by conventional linkage analysis of affected kindreds because these diseases do not segregate in simple ways. *Affected pedigree member* (affected sib pair) analysis is a powerful technique for addressing these problems. Two siblings will, on average, share 50% (one-half) of alleles at any given locus. If both sibs are affected by a disease, and a gene near a particular locus contributes to the development of that disease, then the sibs will, on average, share >50% of alleles. Similar analyses apply to pedigree members who are not full siblings.

The power of this approach is limited in several ways. Most obviously, traits such as blood pressure are normally distributed, and thus division of a population into unaffected and affected individuals requires an arbitrary cutoff value. This problem can be obviated by use of *quantitative trait locus analysis,* which makes use of kindreds in which sibs differ widely for a trait, and genetic differences between the sibs are sought. Second, linkage techniques have the greatest power when known candidate genes (e.g., components of the renin–angiotensin system for blood pressure) are analyzed. Although a "genome scan" may be carried out, analysis of (for example) 100 markers means that it is not unlikely that uncorrected p values of 0.001 (corresponding to a LOD score of 3) will occur by chance. Studies of quite large populations (or several independent populations) may be required to obtain significant p values after correction for multiple comparisons.

Association Studies

Simple (often single nucleotide) polymorphisms are sometimes detected that might affect the function of a gene, perhaps because they change coding sequences or are reasonably supposed from their location in the promoter to influence gene expression. If a polymorphism is in a plausible candidate gene for a particular disease, one can determine whether the frequency of the polymorphism differs between unaffected controls and affected individuals. In the case of a continuously variable trait such as blood pressure, one can see whether levels of the trait differ in individuals who do or do not carry the polymorphism; if the polymorphism is frequent, those homozygous for the polymorphism can be compared to those who are heterozygous as well as to those who are not carriers.

A common problem with association studies is that the control and affected populations may not be strictly comparable. For example, whites tend to have lower blood pressure than do blacks and may also differ from blacks in frequencies of many polymorphisms in various genes. Studies of blood pressure in American blacks may thus be easily confounded by the degree of white admixture in the black population. This problem can be obviated to some extent by population-based studies (e.g., examining blood pressure in all members of a single study population rather than comparing affected and control groups) or by studying relatively homogenous populations (e.g., Africans from one tribe in a single locale). Other study designs might be useful; in *transmission disequilibrium* studies, for example, one examines the parents of an affected individual and compares alleles on the chromosomes inherited by the affected child with the parental chromosomes that were not inherited.

A second problem is the phenomenon of *linkage disequilibrium;* that is, particular alleles at polymorphic sites within a gene, or even within adjacent genes, may be nonrandomly associated with each other. Thus, one cannot infer causation from a positive association between a polymorphism and a trait without careful studies of the functional effects of that polymorphism, because an unsuspected associated polymorphism may actually be responsible for the observed physiologic effects.

ASSAYING GENE EXPRESSION

Because most hormones directly or indirectly influence patterns of gene expression, it is often useful to determine levels of expression of various genes under different circumstances in a particular tissue or cell type.

Northern Blots

In one of the oldest and most widely used methods for analyzing gene expression, mRNA is size-fractioned by electrophoresis through agarose and blotted to a nitrocellulose or nylon membrane. It is then hybridized with a radioactively labeled DNA or RNA probe corresponding to the gene of interest, washed, and exposed either to X-ray film or to a reusable and charge-coupled imaging cassette that can be electronically scanned. The intensity of each hybridizing band is a measure of the level of gene expression, and the electrophoretic mobility of each band is proportional to its size.

Ribonuclease Protection Assays

Alternatively, a highly radioactive RNA probe complementary to the mRNA of interest can be hybridized in solution with a cell or tissue RNA sample and then digested with ribonucleases that destroy single-stranded but not double-stranded RNA. Thus, probe molecules will remain intact only when they are bound to complementary mRNA molecules; they are detected by electrophoresis and autoradiography. This method is more sensitive but somewhat more technically demanding than Northern blots.

Reverse Transcriptase–Polymerase Chain Reaction (RT-PCR)

The PCR is able to amplify DNA with single-molecule sensitivity. Although it cannot directly use mRNA as a starting material, mRNA can be reverse-transcribed into cDNA and the cDNA molecules of interest amplified using specific primers. There are two ways in which RT-PCR can be used to quantitate mRNA.

Keep Amplification in the Exponential Phase of the PCR
The intensity of an amplified fragment is directly proportional to the amount of starting DNA as long as the PCR has been run for few enough cycles that starting materials such as primers are not limiting and each cycle of PCR amplifies DNA with equal efficiency. The number of cycles for which this is the case varies with the abundance of the cDNA of interest, so it is often necessary to remove aliquots of the PCR every few cycles. After electrophoresis through agarose, the abundance of the amplified fragment is assayed by staining the DNA. To provide a basis for comparison, an unrelated cDNA of known constant abundance (a "housekeeping" gene) is usually amplified in the same PCR using a second set of primers. This approach is simple but only semi-quantitative.

Competitive PCR
To obtain more accurate quantitation, a competitive template is constructed that is identical in sequence to the cDNA of interest at both ends but different in length so that it can be resolved from the cDNA by electrophoresis. Different amounts of the competitor are added to duplicate RT–PCRs. When the competitor is present in amounts greatly in excess of the actual cDNA of interest, the competitor will be preferentially amplified whereas the opposite will occur when the competitor is present in very small amounts compared to the actual cDNA. Equal amounts should be amplified when the molar amounts of the competitor and actual cDNA are equal.

Arrays of DNA

It is now possible to covalently bind many thousands of different cDNAs to a glass "chip." An RT–PCR is run with fluorescent deoxynucleotide triphosphates and the fluorescent cDNA hybridized with the immobilized material on the chip. The intensity of fluorescence at each position is read by specialized equipment. Thus, the abundance of thousands of different mRNAs in a sample can be determined simultaneously. As cDNAs corresponding to many (perhaps most) genes have now been identified as expressed sequence tags, this means that most changes in gene expression occurring with (for example) treatment of a cell line with a particular hormone can be identified in a single experiment. This technology is currently under intensive development, and it is likely to revolutionize studies of gene expression.

Analysis of Transcriptional Regulation

Whereas the preceding methods ascertain mRNA abundance, other approaches are required to identify sequences within a gene that regulate its expression. This process, colloquially known as "promoter bashing," makes use of several complementary techniques.

Reporter Constructs

A *reporter gene* encodes a product the level of which can be easily and accurately measured. One of the most widely used is luciferase, an enzyme from fireflies. Luciferase levels are determined by lysing cells, adding luciferin and ATP (the substrates for luciferase), and measuring light output with a luminometer. This gene has been cloned into vectors that have restriction enzyme sites immediately 5′ of the gene into which fragments may be directionally cloned. To identify cis elements in the 5′ flanking region of the gene, a series of constructs are made containing various portions of the promoter region of interest (typically 100–2000 bp) in a reporter vector. Most often a *serial deletion* approach is used in which the constructs have inserts with a common 3′ end (the normal transcriptional start site) but different 5′ ends. As successively shorter segments of 5′ flanking sequences are included, levels of transcription (measured by luciferase activity) are likely to change in a stepwise manner. A decrease in activity suggests that a positive regulatory (enhancer) element has been deleted, whereas an increase in activity implies deletion of a negative regulatory (silencer) element. These elements can be further characterized by *footprinting* and *gel mobility shift assays*.

Identification of Trans-Acting Factors

The DNAse I Footprinting. Once genetic regions that influence transcription have been identified by serial deletion or mutation of reporter constructs, proteins that interact with them are identified. One approach makes use of the fact that proteins bound to DNA can protect DNA from digestion by deoxyribonuclease I (DNAse). A DNA segment of a few hundred base pairs is radioactively labeled at one end, incubated with an extract of nuclear proteins, and digested with DNAse I under conditions where each DNA molecule is cut an average of once. If no protein binds the DNA, a rather even distribution of fragment sizes is observed by autoradiography after the mixture is size-fractionated by electrophoresis through a polyacrylamide gel. However, if a segment is protected from digestion because a protein is bound, there will be a corresponding region of reduced intensity on the gel, termed a "footprint," because molecules of that size will be underrepresented in the DNAse I digestion reaction.

Electrophoretic Mobility Shift Assays. Double-stranded probes for each region of interest are synthesized and radioactively labeled. These probes can be complementary oligonucleotides, each approximately 20 nucleotides long or somewhat longer (perhaps 100 bp) restriction fragments or PCR products. Probes are incubated with nuclear extracts. Protein–DNA interactions decreased mobility of the radioactive DNA upon electrophoresis under nondenaturing conditions, detected as slower migrating bands on autoradiography. In some cases, multiple bands may be observed even with quite short probes, reflecting interactions of multiple factors with each other as well as with a particular DNA element.

Whereas footprinting analysis identifies regions of protein–DNA interaction with single-nucleotide resolution, it cannot detect complex interactions as is possible with gel retardation assays. Thus, it is useful to carry out both types of analysis.

IN VITRO EXPRESSION OF PROTEINS

Methods exist for expressing recombinant polypeptides in bacteria, yeast, or cultured insect or mammalian cells (the latter three categories are examples of *eukaryotic* cells, meaning they have a nucleus). These systems vary in their complexity and in the expected yield of protein. The system chosen to express a functional protein depends on the purpose of the experiment. A report of cloning of cDNA encoding a particular enzyme often includes a formal demonstration that the encoded enzyme indeed has the expected activity. If a detailed kinetic analysis is not desired, this requires only a relatively small amount of enzyme, and purification is not necessary. A technically simple system such as transfection of a plasmid into mammalian cells is often used. Large amounts of protein may be required for biochemical research (e.g., X-ray crystallography) or for the manufacturing of pharmaceuticals. If posttranslational modifications such as glycosylation are not required for activity, bacterial systems can be scaled up to yield kilogram quantities of proteins. Certain eukaryotic expression systems, such as baculovirus infecting insect cells, have also been employed for large-scale production.

Bacterial Expression Systems

The general advantages of such systems include a very high yield of protein, inexpensive culture media, and ease of purification. Lack of posttranslational modifications (e.g., glycosylation) can be either an advantage (if, for example, it is desired to crystallize the protein) or a disadvantage if such modifications are required for function. Some proteins are difficult to express in bacteria or else they cannot be synthesized in the proper conformation. Bacterial systems cannot be used to express genomic DNA fragments containing introns because they lack the RNA processing apparatus necessary to splice introns.

Bacteriophage lambda derivatives are used for construction of cDNA libraries that are to be screened by testing for expression of recombinant proteins (see above). Plasmids are used for most other purposes. If a particular recombinant protein is not deleterious to growth of *E. coli,* a host–vector combination may be used in which the vector's promoter is always active, recombinant mRNA is always being transcribed, and recombinant protein always synthesized. However, in many cases bacteria do not tolerate the presence of large amounts of recombinant protein, and thus it is impossible to grow bacteria while the protein is produced. Therefore, it is often desirable to *repress* transcription from the plasmid's promoter until large numbers of bacteria have been grown, following which the promoter is *induced* to allow high levels of transcription for a few hours. Different promoters are induced by changes in temperature, the absence of a nutrient (such as an amino acid), or the presence of a moderately toxic chemical.

Because foreign proteins are sometimes poorly tolerated by bacteria, many vectors contain all or part of a gene for a bacterial protein, followed by restriction enzyme sites into which DNA encoding the desired polypeptide may be inserted. If the translational reading frame of the DNA insert is the same as that of the bacterial gene, a *fusion protein* is synthesized consisting of the bacterial polypeptide at the N-

terminus followed by the foreign polypeptide. Such fusion proteins may be synthesized at higher levels and may be resistant to degradation by bacterial proteases.

Some vectors encode recognition sites for specific proteases such as the clotting factors Xa or thrombin, so that the bacterial portion of the fusion protein can
be cleaved off from the recombinant portion, yielding the desired native protein. It
is obviously necessary that the recombinant protein not itself contain sequences
cleaved by the proteases.

Mammalian Cell Expression Systems

Expression of a mammalian protein in mammalian cells is the approach most likely
to yield a functional protein with all necessary posttranslational modifications including appropriate protein folding. Genomic DNA containing introns may be expressed in mammalian cells. However, mammalian cells require much more
expensive culture media than do bacteria; they grow much more slowly, require manipulation under strictly sterile conditions, and may carry human pathogens, particularly viruses. It is difficult to get the high levels of expression obtainable with
optimized bacterial systems.

Transfection with Plasmids

This is technically the simplest method for introducing extraneous DNA into a cell.
Plasmid vectors that can be used for eukaryotic expression are conceptually similar
to those used for bacterial expression; indeed, they have the *E. coli* DNA replication origin and antibiotic resistance gene(s) necessary for growth in bacteria. In addition, they have a DNA replication origin for growth in mammalian cells and,
instead of a bacterial promoter, a promoter that is effective in mammalian cells. The
promoter and replication origin are usually of viral origin. All genetic manipulations
(e.g., insertion of recombinant DNA, mutagenesis) of such vectors are carried out
in bacteria, following which plasmid DNA is introduced into cells by one of several methods: DNA can be complexed with materials such as calcium phosphate
precipitates or cationic liposomes, which are actively taken up by mammalian cells,
or cells can be rendered permeable to DNA by exposure to electric current, a procedure termed *electroporation.*

Transient transfections are usually adequate for examining the activity of the
protein encoded by a recombinant DNA. Plasmid DNA in the nucleus is transcribed,
and mRNA is translated in the cytoplasm by the cell's ribosomes. Levels of protein
or of the corresponding activity usually reach a maximum at about 48–72 hours,
following which the plasmid is lost from the majority of cells as they divide. If it
is desired that the cell express transfected DNA for more than a few days, clones
of permanently transfected cells can be selected in which the transfected DNA is
integrated into chromosomal DNA. Unless the expressed DNA produces a change
in phenotype that can be selected for, it is necessary to simultaneously transfect
DNA that encodes a selectable characteristic, such as resistance to neomycin and
related antibiotics that are toxic to mammalian cells.

Infection with Viruses

Viral vectors often permit higher rates of expression than do plasmids because they
infect almost all cells in a culture, whereas transfection protocols usually affect a

minority of cells. However, many viruses require complex construction steps and/or packaging of DNA into intact virions prior to use, and many are actual or potential human pathogens that need to be handled with caution. Some useful viruses such as *vaccinia* and *adenovirus* have DNA genomes. *Retroviruses* have RNA genomes and copy their genome into DNA using a virally encoded reverse transcriptase. Because intact retroviruses infect a very high proportion of cells, and retroviral genomes are efficiently integrated into mammalian chromosomes, this is a preferred method for trials of *in vivo* gene therapy.

Invertebrate Cell Expression Systems

Yeast

Saccharomyces cerevisiae may be transformed with plasmids that have a yeast origin of DNA replication, a promoter that permits transcription in yeast, and a selectable marker gene. Because they are eukaryotic cells (and are thus structurally and metabolically closer to mammalian cells than to bacteria) but grow rapidly and in simple culture media, yeast combine many of the advantages of both bacterial and mammalian cell expression systems. However, not all mammalian proteins function the same way in yeast as in mammalian cells, and so functional studies in yeast must be interpreted cautiously.

Baculovirus

This is a virus that infects *Spodoptera frugiperda* insect cells. Foreign DNA is inserted into the vector by homologous recombination using a shuttle plasmid, a relatively cumbersome method. Very high levels of expression can be achieved, and most required posttranslational modifications are made to expressed proteins. Baculovirus has the advantage of not being a pathogen for humans, and its host cells are more robust than most mammalian cells.

TRANSGENIC MICE AND KNOCKOUTS

Although studies of human genetic diseases have yielded great insights into the functions of many genes, the number of genes of interest far exceeds the number of known genetic diseases. Thus, techniques have been developed to introduce any desired genetic modification into mice. These fall into two categories. To make a *transgenic mouse,* DNA is injected into the male pronucleus of fertilized eggs; in some cases, DNA will be randomly integrated into mouse chromosomes. The eggs are then implanted in "pseudopregnant" female mice that have been hormonally treated to be receptive to implantation. If the procedure is successful, most cells in each resulting mouse, including at least some germ cells, will contain the transgenic DNA so that breeding of a founder mouse will establish a line in which all mice carry the transgene. This technique can be used to express particular proteins at higher levels or under different regulation than normal or to express proteins that are not normally carried by mice. For example, mice lacking a particular cell lineage (e.g., growth hormone secreting cells in the pituitary) can be created by expressing a toxin under the control of a promoter specific for those cells (e.g., diphtheria toxin controlled by the growth hormone promoter).

Knockout mice, in which a particular gene is inactivated, are produced by a related but more complicated technique. Mouse embryonic stem cells are grown in culture and transfected with a targeting construct that contains several kilobases of a murine gene of interest with a portion replaced by a selectable marker (such as a gene coding for resistance to the toxic drug neomycin). Most of the time, this construct will integrate into random locations in the genome, but occasionally it will integrate into the corresponding gene by homologous recombination. Successfully transfected cells are selected by growth in the appropriate toxic drug, and cells in which one copy of the endogenous gene has been replaced by the targeting construct are identified using other selection techniques or genetic analysis by PCR. Such a cell line is grown and cells are then injected into early mouse embryos at the blastocyst stage. The embryonic stem cells will grow and differentiate along with the other cells in the embryo so that the resulting mouse will be a chimera for the targeted cells. Again, breeding the founder should yield some mice carrying a single copy of the targeted gene in all cells including the germline. Breeding of two such heterozygous mice will produce mice (one-fourth of the total offspring) that are homozygous for the targeted, inactivated gene, and thus effects of loss of function of the gene can be assessed (of course, loss of some genes will be lethal and no homozygous offspring will be obtained).

SUGGESTED READING

Ausubel FM, Brent R, Kingston RE, Moore DD, Seidman JG, Smith JA, and Struhl K: *Current Protocols in Molecular Biology,* Wiley, New York, 1994.

Dracopoli NC, Haines JL, Korf BR, Moir DT, Morton CC, Seidman CE, Seidman JG, and Smith DR: *Current Protocols in Human Genetics,* Wiley, New York, 1994.

Lodish HF, Baltimore D, Berk A, Zipursky SL, Matsudaira P, and Darnell J: *Molecular Cell Biology*, New York, Scientific American Books, 1995.

Sambrook J, Fritsch EF, and Maniatis T: *Molecular Cloning: A Laboratory Manual,* Cold Spring Laboratory Press, Cold Spring Harbor, NY, 1989.

3

Mechanisms of Hormone Action

CAROLE R. MENDELSON

The capacity of a cell to respond to a particular hormone depends upon the presence of cellular receptors specific for that hormone. After binding the hormone, the receptor is biochemically and structurally altered, resulting in its activation; the activated receptor then mediates all of the actions of the hormone on the cell. The steroid and thyroid hormones as well as retinoids and 1,25-dihydroxyvitamin D_3 diffuse freely through the lipophilic plasma membrane of the cell and interact with receptors that are primarily within the nucleus. Upon activation, the receptors alter the transcription of specific genes, resulting in changes in the levels of specific mRNAs, which are, in turn, translated into proteins. Hormones that are water soluble, such as the peptide and polypeptide hormones, catecholamines, and other neurotransmitters, as well as the relatively hydrophobic prostaglandins, interact with receptors in the plasma membrane. After hormone binding, the activated membrane receptors initiate signal transduction cascades that result in changes in enzyme activities and alterations in gene expression.

In this chapter, the properties of various classes of receptors that are localized within the plasma membranes of target cells and the signal transduction mechanisms that mediate interactions with their ligands will first be addressed. This will be followed by consideration of the structural properties of the nuclear hormone receptors, the events that result in their activation, and the mechanisms whereby the activated nuclear receptors alter the expression of specific genes. Finally, a number of endocrine disorders that are caused by alterations in the number and/or function of plasma membrane and nuclear receptors will be reviewed.

RECEPTOR PROPERTIES

The function of a receptor is to recognize a particular hormone among all the molecules in the environment of the cell at a given time, and, after binding the hormone, to transmit a signal that ultimately results in a biological response. Hormones are normally present in the circulation in extremely low concentrations, from 10^{-11} to 10^{-9} M. The receptor must therefore have an affinity for the hormone that is of a magnitude appropriate to the circulating levels. The receptor must also bind the hormone with high specificity, so that it has a greater affinity for a particular biologically active molecule rather than a related but less biologically active species.

The affinity of the receptor for a particular ligand in relation to its affinity for other related molecules determines the specificity of the hormone–receptor interaction.

The affinity of a hormone for its receptor results from noncovalent binding, primarily in the form of hydrophobic interactions that provide the driving force for the binding reaction, and from electrostatic interactions. The latter, which occur between oppositely charged groups on peptide hormones and their receptors, are important for hormone–receptor specificity. The affinity of a hormone–receptor interaction is defined in terms of the *equilibrium dissociation constant* (K_d). In a system in which there is a single class of binding sites with no interactions among receptors, the K_d is defined as the concentration of hormone, at equilibrium, that is required for binding to 50% of the receptor sites. The affinity can also be expressed as the *equilibrium association constant* (K_a), which is the reciprocal of the K_d.

The binding of hormone to receptor is a saturable process; there are a finite number of receptors for a given hormone on a target cell. In addition, the binding of hormone to receptor must either precede or accompany the biological response, and the magnitude of the biological response must be associated, in some manner, with receptor occupancy. Hormones or analogues that bind to receptors and elicit the same biological response as the naturally occurring hormone are termed *agonists*. Molecules that bind to receptors but fail to elicit the normal biological response are termed *competitive antagonists,* as they occupy the receptors and prevent the binding of the biologically active molecules. Molecules that bind to receptors but are less biologically active than the native hormone are termed *partial agonists*. The term *partial antagonist* also applies because partial agonists bind to receptors and prevent the binding of the fully biologically active native hormone.

RELATIONSHIP OF BINDING TO BIOLOGICAL RESPONSE

The biological response of a target cell to a hormone is determined by a number of factors, including the concentration of hormone, the concentration of receptors, and the affinity of the hormone–receptor interaction. Normally, the concentration of a particular hormone in the circulation is much lower than the K_d of the hormone–receptor interaction. Therefore, the receptors on a target cell are almost never saturated, and an increase in the concentration of circulating hormone results in an increase in the number of occupied receptors.

In a number of examples of peptide hormone binding to cell surface receptors, the response of the target cell to the hormone is directly proportional to the number of receptor sites that are occupied—that is, the binding and biological response curves are superimposable over the entire range of hormone concentrations, and a maximum biological response is achieved when 100% of the receptor sites are occupied (Fig. 3-1). If the number of cellular receptors is reduced without a change in the K_d, both the binding and biological response curves are reduced and remain superimposable.

In the majority of examples, however, the maximum biological response of a target cell is achieved at concentrations of hormone lower than those required to fully occupy all of the receptors on that cell. For example, in isolated adipocytes, maximum stimulation of glucose oxidation is achieved at concentrations of insulin

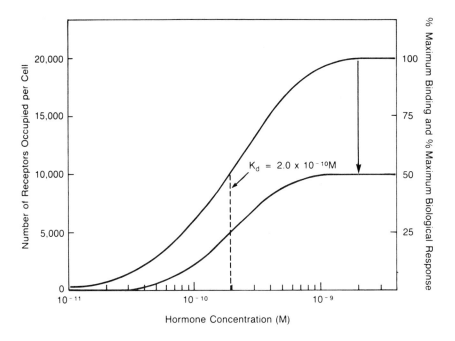

Fig. 3-1 Hormone binding and biological response curves when no spare receptors are present. In this example, the hormone binding and biological response curves are superimposed over the entire range of hormone concentrations. A 50% decrease in receptor number with no change in the K_d of the hormone–receptor interaction will result in an equivalent reduction in the maximum biological response.

that occupy only 2%–3% of the cellular receptors. In Leydig cells, maximum stimulation of testosterone synthesis occurs at concentrations of gonadotropin that occupy only 1% of the cellular receptors. In these systems, >97% of the receptors are referred to as *spare receptors*. The term "spare receptors" does not imply that these receptors are not being utilized, but rather that a maximum biological response is achieved when all of the receptors on a target cell are occupied on average <3% of the time. The degree of spareness of receptors for a particular hormone on a target cell can vary from one cellular response to another, resulting in a different dose-response curve for each biological response of a cell to a given hormone.

Let us consider the hormone-binding (Fig. 3-2A) and biological response (Fig. 3-2B) curves for a hypothetical target cell that contains spare receptors for a particular biological response. The cell normally contains 20,000 receptors for the hormone. In this example, 75% of these receptors are considered to be spare receptors, as a maximum biological response is achieved at concentrations of hormone required to occupy only 5000 receptor sites per cell. When the number of cellular receptors is reduced by 50% and 75% without a change in receptor affinity, the maximum biological response remains unchanged; however, maximum response is achieved at progressively increased concentrations of hormone. When the number of cellular receptors is reduced further, by 88%, the maximum biological response is reduced proportionately. From this example, one can see that the greater the pro-

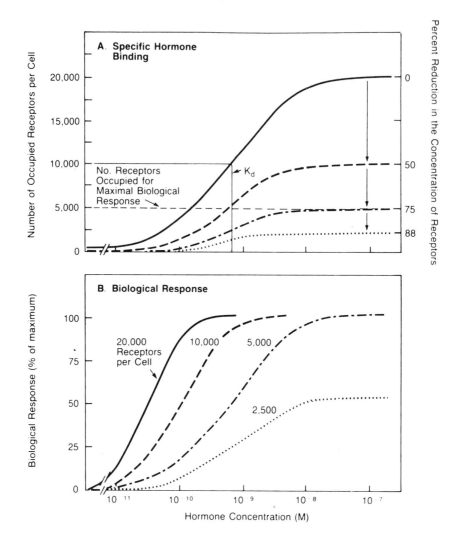

Fig. 3-2 Hormone binding (A) and biological response (B) curves when spare receptors are present. In this example, when the target cell contains its full complement of 20,000 receptors, a maximum biological response is achieved at concentrations of hormone required to occupy only 25% of the cellular receptors. When the number of cellular receptors is reduced to 10,000 or 5,000 without a change in the K_d, a maximum biological response can still be achieved, albeit at progressively increased concentrations of hormone. When the number of cellular receptors is decreased by 88%, the maximum biological response is reduced by 50%.

portion of spare receptors for a particular biological response, the more sensitive is the target cell to the hormone—that is, the lower the concentration of hormone required to achieve half-maximum biological response. In addition to increasing the sensitivity of the target cell to the hormone, spare receptors also serve to prolong the biological response of a cell to short bursts of circulating hormone. The hormone–receptor complexes in excess of those required for the maximum biological response will maintain the response for longer periods as the concentration of hormone in the circulation declines.

PEPTIDE AND POLYPEPTIDE HORMONES, NEUROTRANSMITTERS, AND PROSTAGLANDINS

Receptor Structure and Function

Receptors for peptide and polypeptide hormones, catecholamines, and other neurotransmitters and prostaglandins are integral membrane proteins that are interspersed within the phospholipid bilayer of the plasma membranes of target cells. Because these receptors are soluble in aqueous media only in the presence of detergents, they have proved difficult to purify and, until ~15 years ago, little was known of their structure. Most of the cellular components that are involved in the initial response of the target cell to such hormones are also present either within or associated with the inner leaflet of the plasma membrane.

Cell surface receptors for some nonhormonal ligands, such as low-density lipoprotein (LDL), transferrin, the asialoglycoproteins, IgA/IgM, toxins, and viruses also are integral membrane proteins. The function of these receptors is to translocate the respective ligands to intracellular sites where the ligands themselves act to alter cellular function. For these systems, the information is contained within the ligand itself, and the receptor serves merely to facilitate the delivery of the ligand to its site of action within the cell. An example of a nonhormonal ligand that operates through such a system is cholera toxin, which binds to ganglioside G_{M1} receptors on the plasma membrane. The receptor serves to concentrate the toxin molecule and to facilitate its translocation to sites within the plasma membrane where the toxin causes the activation of adenylyl cyclase (see below).

By contrast, in the case of receptors for peptide and polypeptide hormones, prostaglandins, and neurotransmitters, the hormonal ligand merely activates the receptor, which in turn transmits various signals that result in altered cellular function. In fact, antibodies against the insulin and thyrotropin (thyroid-stimulating hormone, TSH) receptors can activate the respective receptors and mimic the actions of the hormones themselves. It is probable, therefore, that the hormone causes some conformational change in the receptor, which in turn transmits a signal that results in the generation of a biological response.

The primary structures of a large number of cell surface receptors for hormones and other bioactive molecules have been determined by the use of recombinant DNA techniques. Figure 3-3 diagrammatically shows the structures of representative members of different families of receptors that differ in structure and function. Shown are the β-adrenergic receptor, as a member of the large superfamily of G-protein-linked receptors, receptors for epidermal growth factor (EGF), insulin and platelet-derived growth factor (PDGF), which are members of the tyrosine kinase receptor superfamily, the growth hormone (GH) receptor, which associates with a soluble tyrosine kinase and is a member of the cytokine receptor superfamily, and the atrial natriuretic peptide (ANP) receptor, a member of the family of receptor guanylyl cy-

Fig. 3-3 Schematic representation of the proposed structures and plasma membrane orientations of the β-adrenergic, EGF, insulin, PDGF, GH, and ANP receptors. All six receptors are transmembrane proteins oriented so that their carboxy termini are in the cytoplasm. The β-adrenergic receptor shown with its associated G protein complex crosses the plasma membrane seven times, whereas the other receptors cross the plasma membrane only once. The receptors for insulin and PDGF all contain intrinsic cytoplasmic tyrosine kinases, shown by the open areas. The hatched areas represent regions of the EGF and insulin receptors enriched in cysteine residues. The open areas represent domains with a high degree of sequence similarity to tyrosine kinases of the *src* gene family. The filled-in region of the ANP receptor has homology to soluble guanylyl cyclase. Solid circles represent individual cysteine residues. The cytoplasmic domain of the GH receptor is shown in association with the Janus kinase JAK2, a cytoplasmic tyrosine kinase that associates with the ligand-bound receptor and mediates signal transduction.

clases. All of these receptors are glycoproteins that cross the plasma membrane either once (receptors for EGF, insulin, PDGF, ANP, and GH) or several times (β-adrenergic receptor).

Guanine Nucleotide-Binding Protein (G Protein)-Linked Receptors

The β-adrenergic receptor, a protein that mediates some of the actions of the catecholamines, epinephrine and norepinephrine, is a member of a large family of related receptor molecules all containing seven hydrophobic regions, each of which forms an α-helix of sufficient length to span the plasma membrane. These receptor molecules are therefore likely to cross the plasma membrane seven times (Fig. 3-3). This G-protein-linked receptor family includes the β- and α-adrenergic receptors, the muscarinic cholinergic receptors, receptors for vasopressin, angiotensin II, serotonin, substance P, dopamine, luteinizing hormone (LH), follicle-stimulating hormone (FSH), thyroid-stimulating hormone (TSH), platelet-activating factor, prostaglandins, as well as the retinal rod outer segment protein rhodopsin, which serves as a "receptor" for light and mediates a complex signal transduction mechanism that culminates in the visual response. Each member of this receptor family interacts within the plasma membrane with a specific member of another family of proteins, the guanine nucleotide-binding proteins (G proteins). The G protein family includes G_s, which mediates adenylyl cyclase stimulation; G_i, which mediates adenylyl cyclase inhibition; G_q, which mediates phospholipase C activation; and G_t (transducin), a protein of the rod outer segment that mediates activation of cyclic GMP phosphodiesterase, resulting in the closure of Na^+ channels in the rod cell membranes to produce the visual response. All of the G proteins are heterotrimers composed of α-, β-, and γ-subunits. The α-subunit is unique to each G protein, whereas the β- and γ-subunits are similar. Some 20 different α-subunit proteins have now been characterized, as well as several related β- and γ-subunit proteins. The binding of the catecholamines epinephrine and norepinephrine to β-adrenergic receptors promotes interaction of the receptors with the stimulatory guanine nucleotide-binding protein of adenylyl cyclase (G_s). Interaction of the β-adrenergic receptor with G_s promotes the activation of adenylyl cyclase (see below).

Nicotinic Acetylcholine Receptors

In higher vertebrates, there are two basic subtypes of acetylcholine receptors, *muscarinic* and *nicotinic*. Muscarinic receptors are members of the seven-transmembrane domain receptor family, are localized in cells throughout the body, and interact with G proteins. In contrast, nicotinic receptors are members of a family of ligand-regulated ion channels that serve essential roles in transmission of nerve impulses. This family also includes receptors for γ-amino-butyric acid (GABA), glutamate, and glycine. Nicotinic receptors are present in the neuromuscular junctions. Acetylcholine, which is released from the presynaptic nerve endings upon depolarization of the neuron, binds to such receptors clustered in the motor endplates of skeletal muscle. The acetylcholine receptors of electric eels and electric fish are structurally and functionally homologous to nicotinic acetylcholine receptors and are probably the best characterized of the cell surface receptors because they are present in very high concentrations in the plasma membranes of electrocytes, which are specialized cells that develop from embryonic muscle cells and generate the electric potential that such species use to stun or kill their prey. The acetylcholine receptor is composed of five similar subunits each of 50,000–65,000 molecular weight, which are the products of four different but homologous genes: the five subunits surround an ion-conducting channel. The binding of acetylcholine to the receptor results in the opening of the ion-conducting channel created by a conformational change in the subunits of the receptor, which form the walls of the ion channel. The channel predominantly transports sodium ions, resulting in a depolarization of the plasma membrane of the postsynaptic cell.

Receptors with Intrinsic Protein Tyrosine Kinase Activity

Receptors for epidermal growth factor (EGF), platelet-derived growth factors (PDGFs), fibroblast growth factors (FGFs), insulin and insulin-like growth factor-I (IGF-I) contain intrinsic protein kinases that specifically stimulate phosphorylation of tyrosine residues on target proteins (Fig. 3-3). Binding of the hormone to its receptor causes conformational changes involving receptor dimerization that lead to tyrosine kinase activation and subsequent stimulation of downstream signaling pathways mediating increased cell proliferation.

The EGF Receptor. The EGF receptor is a glycoprotein containing an intrinsic tyrosine kinase that is stimulated upon the binding of EGF and is presumed to mediate some of its actions. The receptor is composed of a single polypeptide chain of 1186 amino acids. The protein can be divided into three domains: an N-terminal extracellular domain that contains the EGF binding site, a short α-helical membrane-spanning domain of hydrophobic amino acids; and a C-terminal cytoplasmic domain that shares sequence homology with other tyrosine-specific protein kinases. The N-terminal region contains many cysteine residues, which are clustered into two regions that form an EGF-binding cleft. The EGF receptor is overproduced in a number of tumor cell lines, suggesting that overexpression of the EGF receptor gene may contribute to the phenotype of cellular transformation. It also is of interest that both the transmembrane and the cytoplasmic portion of the EGF receptor, which encodes the tyrosine kinase, have a very high degree of sequence homology with one of the transforming proteins of the avian erythroblastosis virus, the *v-erb-B* oncogene product. Viral oncogenes are derived from host cellular genes that are acquired during the course of infection. Apparently, the progenitor of the avian erythroblastosis virus acquired from host cells is the portion of the EGF receptor gene that encodes the transmembrane and cytoplasmic domain, but not the part that encodes the extracellular EGF-binding region. It has been suggested that the *v-erb-B* gene product induces cellular transformation because of the constitutive expression of the tyrosine kinase domain in the absence of expression of the regulatory EGF-binding domain.

Insulin Receptor. Insulin, a polypeptide hormone, exerts a variety of metabolic and growth-promoting effects on its target cells that are initiated by its interaction with specific plasma membrane receptors. The insulin receptor is a high-molecular-weight glycoprotein that exhibits insulin-dependent, tyrosine-specific protein kinase activity. The receptor probably exists in the plasma membrane as a tetramer consisting of two disulfide-linked heterodimers $(\alpha\beta)_2$ (Fig. 3-3). The α- and β-subunits of the insulin receptor are synthesized as part of a single precursor polypeptide chain, which is subsequently glycosylated, proteolytically cleaved, and inserted into the plasma membrane. The α-subunit contains the hormone-binding site of the receptor. The β-subunits contain the insulin-dependent tyrosine kinase activity. Tyrosine protein kinase activity also is associated with the EGF receptor and with several other growth-factor receptors, including those for IGF-I (closely related structurally to the insulin receptor), PDGFs, the colony-stimulating factor CSF-1, fibroblast growth factors (FGFs), HER-2/neu (closely related structurally to the EGF receptor), as well as a number of transforming retroviral oncogene products. Such findings are indicative of the role of tyrosine protein kinases in growth control (see Chapter 12). The α-subunit of the insulin receptor does not contain a hydrophobic membrane-spanning sequence and probably is localized exclusively on the outer face of the plasma membrane. Like the N-terminal extracellular domain of the EGF receptor, the α-chain is rich in cysteine residues.

Guanylyl Cyclase Receptors
Receptors for natriuretic peptides are transmembrane guanylyl cyclases that consist of an extracellular ligand-binding domain, a single α-helical transmembrane domain, and a cytosolic catalytic domain consisting of one region with homology to

protein kinases and another with homology to soluble guanylyl cyclases (Fig. 3-3). Atrial natriuretic peptide, released from the atrium of the heart, binds to receptors on target cells, activates guanylyl cyclase, and promotes increased production of cyclic GMP. Members of this receptor family also include receptors for heat-stable enterotoxins from *Escherichia coli* (guanylins) and sea urchin sperm receptors for a number of chemoattractant peptides produced by sea urchin eggs.

Receptors for Growth Hormone, Prolactin, and Other Members of the Cytokine Receptor Superfamily

Receptors for growth hormone and prolactin belong to a large superfamily that includes receptors for the hematopoietic growth factors, which control the proliferation, differentiation, and activity of eight lineages of blood cells that are generated from an ancestral pool of stem cells. Hematopoietic growth factors include the interleukins (IL)-2–7, IL-9–11, colony-stimulating factors G-CSF and GM-CSF, leukemia-inhibitory factor (LIF), oncostatin M-(OSM), erythropoietin, as well as ciliary neurotrophic factor (CNTF). The hematopoietic growth factors exert pleiotropic effects; that is, most of the factors are active on cells of more than one lineage, and more than one factor controls growth and differentiation of cells in any one lineage.

Conversely, growth hormone has a variety of metabolic effects and stimulates skeletal growth through induction of IGF-I. Prolactin has numerous biological effects; in mammals, its best-known action is to stimulate growth and differentiation of the mammary gland, in addition to lactogenesis. Interestingly, receptors for prolactin and growth hormone also are present on cells of the immune system. In contrast, the CNTF receptor (CNTFR) α-chain is restricted to the nervous system; CNTF supports the survival of chick embryonic ciliary ganglion cells and of sympathetic sensory and motor neurons.

The high-affinity binding forms of receptors in the cytokine superfamily are comprised of either a homodimeric complex of specific α-chains, or a heterodimeric complex of the specific α-chains with one or more β-subunits that also are members of this superfamily. The extracellular domains of these receptors share a number of common structural features, including two pairs of disulfide-linked cysteine residues in conserved positions (usually near the aminoterminal end, i.e., distal to the plasma membrane), and a WSXWS sequence (tryptophan, serine, any amino acid, followed by another tryptophan, serine) proximal to the plasma membrane. Receptors for the interferons (IFN)α/β, IFN-γ, and IL-10 are structurally related to the cytokine receptors described above, but lack this WSXWS sequence in their extracellular domains.

Unlike the cytoplasmic domains of receptors for EGF, insulin, IGF-I, PDGF, and FGF, which have intrinsic protein tyrosine kinase activity, the cytoplasmic domains of members of the cytokine receptor superfamily lack homology to known protein kinases, and have no intrinsic kinase activity. Despite this absence of a kinase domain, binding of cytokines, growth hormone, and prolactin to their receptors is followed by a rapid increase in tyrosine phosphorylation of cellular proteins and of the receptor itself. Within the plasma membrane-proximal region of the cytoplasmic domain are two regions (box 1 and box 2) that are required for mediation of the growth-promoting effects of the cytokines. As will be discussed later in this chapter, signal transduction is mediated by the activation of soluble, cytoplasmic tyrosine kinases (JAKs) that bind to the membrane-proximal cytoplasmic region. A schematic of the growth hormone receptor and its associated kinase, JAK2, is shown in Figure 3-3.

As mentioned above, in the case of all members of the cytokine receptor superfamily, high-affinity binding requires either homodimerization of the receptor α-chains (prolactin, growth hormone, G-CSF, and erythropoietin receptors), or heterodimerization with one or more β-subunits that also are members of this superfamily. The fact that some of these β-subunits are shared in common with different family members helps to explain the observed pleiotropic effects. As an example, the high-affinity binding forms of receptors for IL-3, IL-5, and GM-CSF are comprised of a heterodimeric complex of the specific α-chains with a common β-subunit. The α-chain receptors for IL-6, LIF/OSM, and CNTFR also share a common β-subunit (gp130).

Signal Transduction Mechanisms

It generally is accepted that polypeptide hormones and catecholamines exert their effects on cellular metabolism by binding to receptors on the surface of target cells and activating a membrane-associated enzyme that in turn elaborates an intracellular second messenger. This second messenger subsequently mediates the various biological effects of the hormone. This so-called second messenger hypothesis of hormone action was proposed in the early 1960s when it was discovered that the activation of glycogen phosphorylase by epinephrine and glucagon in liver slices was mediated by the formation of a heat-stable compound, which was identified as adenosine $3',5'$-monophosphate (cyclic AMP). Cyclic AMP is formed from Mg·ATP by a membrane-associated enzyme, adenylyl cyclase. According to this concept, the hormone, or first messenger, carries information from its site of production to the target cell, where it binds to specific receptors on the cell surface. This results in the activation of a membrane-bound enzyme or effector (e.g., adenylyl cyclase), which generates a soluble intracellular second messenger (e.g., cyclic AMP), which then transmits the information to the cellular machinery, resulting in a biological response. In recent years, a number of other effector/second messenger systems have been discovered that mediate the actions of a variety of hormones on cellular metabolism and function.

G Protein-Coupled Signal Transduction

As discussed previously, receptors for polypeptide hormones, prostaglandins, and neurotransmitters that cross the plasma membrane seven times are coupled to G proteins that are heterotrimers comprised of unique α-subunits and common $\beta\gamma$-subunits. The α-subunit, α_s, mediates activation of adenylyl cyclase; the α-subunit, α_i, mediates inhibition of adenylyl cyclase, and the α-subunit, α_q, mediates activation of phospholipase C-β, which ultimately results in an increase in cytosolic calcium and an activation of protein kinase C. In the cases of all G protein-linked receptors, the binding of hormone to receptor causes the receptor to interact with a specific G protein heterotrimer. This interaction causes the release of bound guanosine diphosphate (GDP) from the α-subunit and the binding of guanosine triphosphate (GTP). The GTP-bound α-subunit, which now dissociates from $\beta\gamma$, is activated and binds to various effector molecules in the cell (e.g., adenylyl cyclase, phospholipase Cβ [PLCβ]), resulting in changes in effector activity.

Hormone-Sensitive Adenylyl Cyclase. The hormone-sensitive adenylyl cyclase system has at least three components: the receptor (R_s or R_i); a form of guanine nucleotide-binding regulatory protein (G_s or G_i); and the catalytic component (C), which enzymatically converts Mg·ATP to cyclic AMP (Fig. 3-4). The guanine nucleotide-binding regulatory protein, G_s, mediates the action of hormones that stimulate adenylyl cyclase activity, whereas G_i mediates the actions of those hormones that inhibit adenylyl cyclase. All of these components can be independently isolated and recombined *in vitro* to reconstitute a functional hormone-sensitive adenylyl cyclase system. It is apparent that a number of different types of hormone receptors on a single cell can interact with the same pool of regulatory and catalytic components and that these combined interactions result either in a net stimulation or inhibition of adenylyl cyclase activity. As discussed above, G_s and G_i are heterotrimers comprised of a unique α-subunit (α_s or α_i) and a heterodimer of β- and γ-subunits. The $\beta\gamma$-subunits shared by G_s and G_i are essential for the integrated actions of stimulatory and inhibitory hormones on adenylyl cyclase activity. It has been proposed that the binding of hormone to receptor results in a conformational change that promotes the interaction or coupling of the hormone-receptor complex with the other components of hormone-sensitive adenylyl cyclase.

Receptor-Mediated Stimulation of Adenylyl Cyclase. The proposed mechanism for the hormonal activation of adenylyl cyclase, which is based on the studies from a number of laboratories, is presented in Figure 3-5. In the inactive state, the guanine

Fig. 3-4 Plasma membrane components of hormone-sensitive adenylyl cyclase. Hormone-sensitive adenylyl cyclase is composed of the following integral proteins of the plasma membrane: receptors for either stimulatory (R_s) or inhibitory (R_i) hormones, the guanine nucleotide-binding regulatory proteins G_s or G_i, and the catalytic component (C). G_s is composed of a unique α-subunit, $M_r \approx 45,000$, and β- and γ-subunits, $M_r \approx 35,000$ and 10,000, respectively. G_i has a unique α-subunit, $Mr \approx 41,000$, and β- and γ-subunits that are similar to those of G_s.

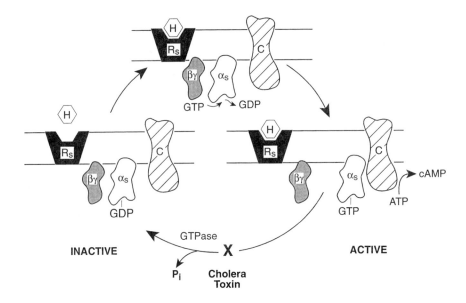

Fig. 3-5 Proposed mechanism for the hormonal activation of adenylyl cyclase, G_s, is composed of three subunits, α_s, β, and γ. In the absence of the binding of a stimulatory hormone to its receptor, the guanine nucleotide GDP is bound to α_s and adenylyl cyclase is in the inactive state. The binding of hormone to receptor facilitates the dissociation of GDP and the association of GTP with the α_s. This, in turn, results in the dissociation of α_s from the $\beta\gamma$-subunits and its association with the catalytic component (C), resulting in adenylyl cyclase activation. The activated α_s contains a GTPase, which hydrolyzes the bound GTP to GDP, resulting in a return of adenylyl cyclase to an inactive state. Cholera toxin, which inhibits the GTPase activity, causes a persistent activation of adenylyl cyclase.

nucleotide that is bound to the α_s-subunit of G_s is GDP. The binding of hormone (H) to receptor (R) is believed to promote the formation of the ternary complex, $H \cdot R \cdot G_s$, which facilitates the dissociation of GDP and the binding of GTP to the α_s-subunit. The binding of GTP to α_s results in its dissociation from the $\beta\gamma$-subunits. The $\alpha_s \cdot GTP$ then associates with the catalytic subunit (C) of the adenylyl cyclase to form the active holoenzyme ($\alpha_s \cdot GTP \cdot C$). The activated catalytic subunit then converts ATP (adenosine triphosphate) to cyclic AMP. The activated α_s contains a GTPase activity, which catalyzes the hydrolysis of GTP to GDP and terminates the cycle of adenylyl cyclase activation. Cholera toxin, which is produced by the bacterial organism *Vibrio cholera*, binds to G_{M1} gangliosides (complex glycolipids) on the cell surface and penetrates the cell membrane. Once within the cell membrane, the toxin catalyzes the adenosine diphosphate (ADP)-ribosylation of an arginine residue (Arg201) in α_s, causing inhibition of the GTPase activity (Fig. 3-5). This change results in a persistent activation of adenylyl cyclase. In intestinal mucosal cells, the binding of cholera toxin and subsequent activation of adenylyl cyclase results in the stimulation of ion (primarily Cl^-) and water secretion across the intestinal brush border, causing massive diarrhea.

Receptor-Mediated Inhibition of Adenylyl Cyclase. A number of hormones inhibit adenylyl cyclase activity. They include catecholamines that bind to α_2-adrenergic receptors, muscarinic–cholinergic agonists, and opioids. These hormones bind to cell surface receptors that interact with the inhibitory guanine nucleotide-binding regulatory protein, G_i, which is similar in structure to G_s, having three subunits, α_i, β, and γ. The $\beta\gamma$-subunits of G_i are similar to those of G_s, whereas the α-subunit is distinct. $G\alpha_i$ contains a guanine nucleotide-binding site. The binding of these hormones to their receptors promotes the exchange of GTP for GDP on α_i. This results in the dissociation of α_i from $\beta\gamma$. The inhibition of adenylyl cyclase activity appears to be mediated primarily by the interaction of the free $\alpha_i \cdot$GTP with adenylyl cyclase. Inhibition of adenylyl cyclase also is mediated, in part by the increased levels of free $\beta\gamma$, which by mass action reduce the concentration of free α_s. Islet-activating protein, one of the toxins of *Bordetella pertussis,* prevents the dissociation of $G_{i\alpha}$ from $\beta\gamma$, which results in adenylyl cyclase activation because less free α_i is available to inhibit adenylyl cyclase and less $\beta\gamma$ is free to interact with α_s. Thus, cholera toxin activates adenylyl cyclase by promoting the dissociation of G_s, whereas islet-activating protein activates adenylyl cyclase by inhibiting the dissociation of G_i.

It should be noted that the free $\beta\gamma$-subunits can themselves regulate certain cellular effectors. For example, free $\beta\gamma$ directly binds and activates a K^+-selective ion channel in heart atrial cells, and binds to and activates PLCβ, resulting in its activation. The latter is an example of an enzyme that is activated both by an activated α-subunit (in this case $\alpha_q \cdot$GTP) and by free $\beta\gamma$.

Cyclic AMP Regulation of Cellular Function

The major mechanism by which cyclic AMP regulates cellular function is through its binding to cyclic AMP-dependent protein kinases (PKA). The cyclic AMP-dependent protein kinase holoenzyme is comprised of a regulatory subunit (R) dimer and two catalytic subunits (C). The R subunit is a cyclic AMP-binding protein, whereas the C-subunit, when free of R, expresses protein kinase activity. Each molecule of R dimer binds four molecules of cyclic AMP. The binding of cyclic AMP to R causes dissociation of the inactive holoenzyme to yield two active catalytic subunits. The reaction is generally represented as

$$R_2C_2 + 4 \text{ cAMP} \rightarrow R_2 \cdot 4 \text{ cAMP} + 2 \text{ C}$$

(inactive)   (active)

The active free catalytic subunits can now catalyze the phosphorylation of a number of cellular proteins; PKA catalyzes the transfer of a high-energy phosphate from ATP to the hydroxyl groups of serine and, to a much lesser extent, threonine residues on cellular proteins. The phosphorylation of enzymes may result in changes in enzyme activity. For example, phosphorylation of hormone-sensitive lipase, cholesteryl esterase, or glycogen phosphorylase results in enzyme activation. In contrast, phosphorylation of glycogen synthase decreases enzyme activity. The specific responses of various cell types to an increase in cyclic AMP and the activation of cyclic AMP-dependent protein kinase is determined by the cellular phenotype and, therefore, by the enzymes and substrates available for regulation. Thus, a major response of a liver cell to an increase in cyclic AMP is glycogenolysis, because the liver cell expresses the enzymes to synthesize and to metabolize glycogen. Conversely, in a fat cell the primary response to an increase in cyclic AMP is lipolysis, because the fat cell expresses the enzymes for uptake of triacylglycerol precursors from the circulation, and for the synthesis and metabolism of triacylglycerols.

In addition to its PKA-mediated actions to alter the activities of various metabolic enzymes, cyclic AMP through PKA-mediated phosphorylation also regulates the transcription of specific genes in eukaryotic cells. An effect of cyclic AMP at the level of gene transcription has been found for a number of eukaryotic genes, including phosphoenolpyruvate carboxykinase (PEPCK), tyrosine aminotransferase (TAT), the human glycoprotein hormone α-subunit gene, preprosomatostatin, vasoactive intestinal polypeptide (VIP), the surfactant protein SP-A, and several forms of cytochrome P-450 involved in steroid hydroxylation.

Our understanding of the molecular mechanisms whereby cyclic AMP activates gene transcription in mammalian cells was greatly advanced by the discovery of a DNA-binding protein or transcription factor, termed *cyclic AMP response element binding protein* (CREB), which is activated by PKA-mediated phosphorylation to regulate the transcriptional activity of a number of specific genes. The CREB is a member of a family of related DNA-binding proteins, the activating transcription factors (ATF proteins), that bind to a common sequence of DNA, TGACGTCA (the cyclic AMP response element, CRE), which is palindromic; that is, it possesses a twofold rotational axis of symmetry. Increased cellular levels of cyclic AMP result in an activation of CREB through its phosphorylation on serine residues by PKA. The phosphorylated CREB homodimer bound to the CRE then recruits a family of co-activator proteins that stabilize binding of the basal transcription complex to the downstream promoter and facilitate the binding of RNA polymerase II, resulting in increased transcription of cyclic AMP-responsive genes. It should be noted, however, that the CRE does not appear to be present in the regulatory regions of all genes that are regulated by cyclic AMP. Therefore, additional cyclic AMP-responsive transcription factors and mechanisms mediate AMP regulation of eukaryotic gene transcription.

Cyclic AMP is rapidly metabolized in cells by the cyclic nucleotide phosphodiesterases, which hydrolyze cyclic AMP to form the inactive $5'$-AMP.

$$\text{cyclic AMP} \rightarrow 5'\text{-AMP}$$

The actions of a number of hormones, including insulin and catecholamines binding to α_1-adrenergic receptors, are mediated in part by an activation of phosphodiesterase and a subsequent decrease in cellular cyclic AMP levels.

Signal Transduction Mechanisms Independent of Cyclic AMP

A significant number of polypeptide hormones that bind to G protein-linked receptors exert their actions on cellular metabolism and function by mechanisms that do not involve adenylyl cyclase activation and cyclic AMP. Table 3-1 lists hormones that act by increasing cyclic AMP, by inhibiting adenylyl cyclase, by increasing phosphoinositide turnover, and by activation of intrinsic or associated tyrosine kinases. Hormones that act through cyclic AMP-mediated mechanisms include epi-

Table 3-1 Signal Transduction Mechanisms in Hormone Action

Receptors that mediate activation of adenylyl cyclase	Receptors that mediate inhibition of adenylyl cyclase	Receptors that mediate increased phospho-inositide turnover	Receptors that mediate tyrosine kinase activation
β-Adrenergic	α_2-Adrenergic	α_1-Adrenergic	Insulin
LH, FSH, TSH, hCG	Opioid	Angiotensin II	Growth factors (PDGF, EGF, FGF, IGF-I)
Glucagon	Muscarinic cholinergic—M2	Muscarinic cholinergic—M3	Growth hormone
Vasopressin—V_2		Vasopressin—V_1	Prolactin
ACTH			

nephrine and norepinephrine binding to β-adrenergic receptors, vasopressin, acting through V_2 receptors, adrenocorticotropic hormone (ACTH), glucagon, and the pituitary glycoprotein hormones, luteinizing hormone (LH), follicle-stimulating hormone (FSH), and thyroid-stimulating hormone (TSH). The glycoprotein hormone of human placental origin, namely human chorionic gonadotropin (hCG), which is highly homologous to LH and binds to LH receptors, also increases cyclic AMP formation.

In contrast, epinephrine and norepinephrine binding to α_2-adrenergic receptors, opioids, and acetylcholine binding to M2 muscarinic receptors cause adenylyl cyclase inhibition. Furthermore, epinephrine and norepinephrine binding to α_1-adrenergic receptors, vasopressin binding to V_1 receptors, and acetylcholine binding to the M3 subtype of muscarinic cholinergic receptors act by signal transduction pathways initiated by increased phosphoinositide turnover. Other hormones, such as insulin, various growth factors, growth hormone, prolactin, and other members of the cytokine receptor family act through signal transduction pathways initiated by activation of intrinsic or receptor-associated tyrosine kinases.

It is apparent that a number of G protein-linked receptors exist in different subtypes and interact with different heterotrimeric G proteins. Therefore, the same hormone may act through a cyclic AMP-mediated mechanism in one tissue and by a cyclic AMP-independent mechanism in another. As noted above, vasopressin binds to a specific subset of receptors (V_2) on cells of the kidney collecting tubules and loop of Henle to promote sodium and water reabsorption. These actions of vasopressin are mediated by increased cyclic AMP formation and cyclic AMP-dependent protein kinase activation.

Conversely, in the liver, vasopressin acts through another subset of receptors (V_1) to enhance glycogenolysis, and this effect is mediated by increased phosphoinositide turnover. The catecholamines—epinephrine and norepinephrine—bind to several subsets of receptors that are present in different relative amounts in various tissues. In liver cells, norepinephrine binds both to β- and to α_1-adrenergic receptors to increase glycogenolysis. Binding to β-receptors results in adenylyl cyclase activation, an increase in cyclic AMP, and activation of cyclic AMP-dependent protein kinase, which in turn catalyzes the phosphorylation and activation of phosphorylase kinase. The activated phosphorylase kinase catalyzes the phosphorylation and activation of phosphorylase, resulting in enhanced glycogenolysis. Phosphorylase kinase also catalyzes the phosphorylation of glycogen synthase, resulting in its inactivation. Norepinephrine, acting through α_1-receptors, promotes an increase in the levels of free cytosolic calcium ion, which causes, by mechanisms discussed below, the activation of phosphorylase kinase, and the subsequent increase in glycogen breakdown. There are five different subtypes of muscarinic acetylcholine receptors (M1–M5) that mediate different signal transduction pathways. For example, the M3 subtype is linked to G_q and mediates increased phosphoinositide turnover, whereas the M2 subtype is linked to M2, which is linked to G_i and mediates adenylyl cyclase inhibition.

Phosphoinositide Turnover. A number of hormone–receptor interactions increase free cytosolic calcium ion and activate protein kinase C, which serve important roles in the regulation of cellular function. Hormone–receptor interactions that result in the formation of these second messengers include the binding of acetylcholine to the M3 subtype of muscarinic cholinergic receptors, epinephrine and norepinephrine, to α_1-adrenergic receptors, vasopressin to V_1 receptors, and angiotensin II to receptors on liver cells. The proposed mechanism of action of such hormones is presented in Figure 3-6. The binding of hormone to receptor results in its association with a heterotrimeric G protein that contains $\alpha_q\beta\gamma$. This, in turn, promotes dissociation of GDP from α_q and the subsequent binding of GTP. The $\alpha_q\cdot$GTP causes the activation of a plasma membrane–associated phospholipase C (PLCβ), which catalyzes the hydrolysis of a specific inositol phospholipid within the plasma membrane, phosphatidylinositol 4,5-bisphosphate (PIP$_2$), to form the second messengers diacylglycerol (DAG) and inositol 1,4,5-trisphosphate (IP$_3$).

The hydrolysis of PIP$_2$ and the formation of IP$_3$ are specifically associated with an increase in the levels of free cytosolic calcium ion and the subsequent physiological response. Incubation of permeabilized cells with IP$_3$ results in a profound increase in the release of calcium ion from intracellular stores, primarily the endoplasmic reticulum. An endoplasmic-reticulum–associated receptor for IP$_3$ has been cloned and characterized. The IP$_3$ receptor has an apparent molecular weight of 260,000 and contains at least four membrane-spanning domains. It is postulated that these membrane-spanning domains form the calcium channel. In addition to mediating IP$_3$-stimulated calcium release from the endoplasmic reticulum, this receptor may act in conjunction with the dihydropyridine (DHP)-gated calcium channels to facilitate the influx of extracellular calcium into the cell. Once formed, IP$_3$ is rapidly hydrolyzed to IP$_2$, IP, and inositol by the actions of specific phosphomonoesterases. The action of the esterase that hydrolyzes IP to inositol is inhibited by lithium ion.

CALCIUM. The levels of free calcium ion in the cytoplasm are normally quite low (10^{-7} M) as compared to the levels of calcium ion in the extracellular fluid (10^{-3} M). The influx of calcium into most cells at rest is minimal, despite a large electrochemical gradient, since the plasma membranes of most cells at rest are relatively impermeable to calcium ion. Within the cell, calcium is stored in relatively high concentrations in the mitochondrial membrane, the endoplasmic reticulum (sarcoplasmic reticulum of muscle cells), and the plasma membrane. An increase in the levels of free cytosolic calcium ion can have a variety of effects on the cell, in-

Fig. 3-6 Proposed mechanism for the hormone-induced increase in free cytosolic calcium and activation of protein kinase C. The polyphosphoinositides phosphatidylinositol 4-phosphate (PIP) and phosphatidylinositol 4,5-bisphosphate (PIP_2) are formed within the plasma membrane from phosphatidylinositol (PI) and ATP in reactions catalyzed by kinases. The binding of hormone to receptor results in its association with a G protein heterotrimer containing $\alpha_q\beta\gamma$. This causes the dissociation of GDP from α_q and the association of GTP. The α_q·GTP then dissociates from $\beta\gamma$ and activates a specific phospholipase C (PLC) within the plasma membrane, which catalyzes the hydrolysis of PIP_2 to form the putative second messengers, inositol trisphosphate (IP_3) and diacylglycerol (DAG). The water-soluble IP_3 diffuses into the cytoplasm and stimulates the release of calcium from storage sites, primarily within the endoplasmic reticulum. The increased free cytosolic calcium exerts most of its effects on cellular metabolism by binding to calmodulin (Cam). The calcium–calmodulin complex binds to various enzyme or effector proteins, causing changes in their activities. One such protein is phosphorylase kinase, which is activated by an increase in cytoplasmic calcium ion. The IP_3 is subsequently hydrolyzed by specific phosphatases to form the inactive IP_2, IP, and inositol. The DAG remains within the plasma membrane, where it facilitates the activation of protein kinase C (C-Kinase) by calcium ion and phospholipid. The DAG and inositol are utilized for the resynthesis of PI.

cluding changes in cell motility, contraction of muscle cells, increased release of secretory proteins, and activation of a number of regulatory enzymes. Calcium ion exerts most of these effects in cells by binding to specific calcium-binding proteins, such as calmodulin, in nonmuscle cells, and troponin C in striated muscle cells. The binding of calcium results in the activation of these calcium-binding proteins. Calmodulin has no intrinsic activity of its own; after binding calcium ion (each molecule of calmodulin has four calcium-binding sites), it is activated and binds to various enzymes or effector molecules, causing a change in their activities.

Two enzymes that are activated by the calcium–calmodulin complex are *phos-*

phorylase kinase and *cyclic AMP phosphodiesterase*. The activation of phosphorylase kinase by cyclic AMP-dependent protein kinase is dependent upon calcium. Phos-
phorylase kinase has four subunits, α, β, γ, and δ. The δ-subunit is calmodulin, and
the γ-subunit is the catalytic component of the enzyme. The α- and β-subunits are
phosphorylated by cyclic AMP-dependent protein kinase. The phosphorylation of the
α- and β-subunits in the presence of calcium ion activates the γ-subunit and increases
the affinity of the δ-subunit (calmodulin) for calcium. In the presence of calcium ion,
the enzyme binds a second molecule of calmodulin (δ'). This in turn activates the
dephosphorylated form of the enzyme but has little effect in promoting the further
activation of the phosphorylated enzyme.

Phosphorylase kinase is an example of an enzyme that is activated by an increase either in intracellular calcium ion or cyclic AMP, or both. This provides an
example of a system in which the actions of cyclic AMP and calcium occur in the
same direction. There are other examples in which the actions of calcium antagonize those of cyclic AMP; cyclic AMP phosphodiesterase, the enzyme that catalyzes
the metabolism of cyclic AMP to the inactive 5'-AMP, is activated by the calcium–
calmodulin complex. An increase in free cytosolic calcium ion, therefore, can cause
a decrease in the levels of cyclic AMP and of cyclic AMP-dependent protein kinase
activity and a change in the activities of the enzymes that are substrates for this
kinase.

PROTEIN KINASE C (PKC). The other product of the hydrolysis of inositol phospholipids, diacylglycerol (DAG), is also believed to serve as a second messenger by
acting within the cell membrane to activate PKC. Protein kinase C is a phospho-
lipid- and calcium-dependent enzyme that catalyzes the phosphorylation of serine
and threonine residues on a number of cellular proteins. Diacylglycerol dramatically
increases the affinity of the enzyme for calcium ion and for phospholipid and therefore promotes an increase in enzyme activity at resting levels of intracellular calcium. The DAG-mediated hormonal activation of PKC can be mimicked by
incubating cells with tumor-promoting phorbol esters, which interact with the enzyme at the same site as DAG. Because phorbol esters are not rapidly degraded,
these agents cause long-term activation of PKC.

In addition to phosphorylating serine and threonine residues on a number of
enzyme proteins, PKC can alter the expression of a number of specific genes. This
action of PKC is mediated by the activation of a DNA-binding protein complex or
transcription factor known as *AP-1*, which is a heterodimer of two related proteins,
c-Fos and *c-Jun*, which are recognized as protooncogenes. The AP-1 binds to a specific DNA sequence $TGA^C/_GTCA$, which is quite similar to that recognized by the
cyclic AMP-activated transcription factor CREB. In contrast to CREB, which is activated by increased phosphorylation, AP-1 binding and transcriptional activity appear to be increased by dephosphorylation of constitutively phosphorylated amino
acid residues near the carboxyterminus and phosphorylation of other residues near
the aminoterminus of *c-Jun*. Thus, it is likely that activated protein kinase C alters
AP-1 transcriptional activity by activating both a specific phosphatase and a specific kinase.

It is thus apparent that the hormonal activation of phosphatidyinositol turnover
results in the elaboration of two important mediators, IP$_3$ and DAG, which in turn

promote an increase in intracellular calcium and activation of protein kinase C, respectively. The result is a variety of cellular responses that are dependent upon cellular phenotype and include alterations in enzyme activity and in transcription factor activation.

Phosphatidylcholine Turnover. Although numerous hormones and neurotransmitters exert their effects through PIP_2 hydrolysis, a significant number have been found to stimulate the hydrolysis of phosphatidylcholine (PC). Phospholipase C-mediated hydrolysis of PC yields DAG and phosphorylcholine. The DAG that is formed has the capacity to activate PKC as described above. As PC is present in much greater abundance in cell membranes than is PIP_2, the former may serve as an important source of DAG for long-term activation of PKC. Another phospholipase, phospholipase D, has been implicated in the actions of a number of hormones that act through G protein-linked receptors. In addition to stimulating phospholipase C-mediated PIP_2 hydrolysis, the binding of vasopressin to V_1 receptors on hepatocytes and of acetylcholine to muscarinic receptors in the brain promotes the activation of phospholipase D, which catalyzes the hydrolysis of PC to form choline and phosphatidate. Phosphatidate may serve as a calcium ionophore by promoting calcium entry into cells and the mobilization of intracellular calcium from membrane stores. The phosphatidate also may be hydrolyzed by phosphatidate phosphohydrolase to form diacylglycerol, which in turn can activate protein kinase C.

The Sphingomyelin Cycle—Ceramide as a Second Messenger. Sphingomyelins are the only phospholipids in cell membranes that do not have a glycerol backbone. Rather, the backbone of sphingomyelin is sphingosine, an amino alcohol that contains an 18-carbon chain with one double bond. The amino group of sphingosine is linked to a long-chain fatty acid by an amide bond, and the primary hydroxyl group is in ester linkage with phosphocholine. Although it once was believed that sphingomyelin served merely as a structural component of plasma membranes and myelin sheaths of nerves, it recently has become apparent that sphingomyelin is actively metabolized by a cytoplasmic neutral sphingomyelinase and serves as a reservoir of second messengers in the action of a number of hormones and cytokines. Sphingomyelinase-induced hydrolysis of sphingomyelin to form ceramide and phosphocholine mediates the action of tumor necrosis factor-α (TNF-α) to stimulate apoptosis (programmed cell death) of lymphoid and myeloid cells. The ceramide that is formed causes the activation of a ceramide-activated protein phosphatase (CAPP), a serine-threonine phosphatase related to protein phosphatases 2A. Ceramide action also may be mediated in part by ceramide-activated protein kinases; however, the role of these kinases in mediating the biological effects of ceramide is unclear.

Signal Transduction through Guanylyl Cyclase Receptors. Cyclic GMP is formed from GTP in a reaction that is catalyzed by guanylyl cyclase. In contrast to adenylyl cyclase, which is exclusively localized to the plasma membrane, two forms of guanylyl cyclase have been well characterized. One is a heme-containing soluble enzyme comprised of two subunits and the other is a plasma membrane-associated protein. A third form of guanylyl cyclase, which is associated with structural elements, is present in retinal rod cells and is involved in the synthesis of cyclic GMP involved in the visual cycle. The plasma membrane-associated form was intensively studied as atrial natriuretic peptides were found to activate guanylyl cyclase and promote increased synthesis of cyclic GMP in target cells. The actions of ANP, which include vasodilation, natriuresis, and diuresis (see also Chapter 7), appear to be mediated either entirely or in part by the binding to and activation of the ANP receptor, a membrane-bound guanylyl cyclase (Fig. 3-3) resulting in increased production of the second messenger, cyclic GMP. Oligomerization of the receptor appears to be required for guanylyl cyclase activation, as is binding of ATP to the protein kinase homology domain. The mechanism(s) whereby cyclic GMP acts to mediate the actions of ANP have yet to be elucidated; however, it is apparent from studies in retinal rod cells that cyclic GMP serves to maintain cation channels in an open conformation. This action may, in part, explain the natriuretic action of ANP.

Alternatively, this natriuretic action of ANP may be mediated by its effect to inhibit aldosterone biosynthesis by glomerulosa cells of the adrenal cortex. In addition, cyclic GMP may function to activate a phosphodiesterase, which, in turn, lowers cyclic AMP levels. In this manner, cyclic GMP may act to antagonize the actions of cyclic AMP in a number of cell types.

Signal Transduction by Receptors That Contain Tyrosine Kinase Domains. As discussed above, cell surface receptors for insulin and other growth factors are transmembrane proteins that contain a cytoplasmic domain that is a tyrosine kinase. More than 50 receptor tyrosine kinases have been identified that belong to 14 different families. Binding of ligands to these receptors and subsequent activation of the tyrosine kinases result in changes in cell proliferation, differentiation, shape, and migration. Listed below are four of the families of receptor tyrosine kinases.

1. *The EGF, HER-2/*neu *family:* The structure of the EGF receptor has already been described. HER-2/*neu,* which is homologous to the EGF receptor and to the *neu* oncogene, has been found to be amplified in many adenocarcinomas and is overexpressed in breast tumors of a significant number of breast cancer patients. The identification of a ligand for this receptor, produced by human breast cancer cells in culture, suggests a role of HER-2/*neu* in autocrine growth regulation of breast tumors.

2. *The insulin/IGF-I receptor family:* Like the insulin receptor, discussed above, the IGF-I receptor is a tetramer consisting of two disulfide-linked heterodimers $(\alpha\beta)_2$. The IGF-I receptor differs from the insulin receptor in its extracellular cysteine-rich region, which is believed to be responsible for ligand binding, and in the C-terminus downstream of the tyrosine kinase domain.

3. *The PDGF, CSF-1, and c-*kit *receptor family:* PDGF is released from platelets when they adhere to injured vessels and acts to stimulate proliferation of mesenchymal cells. CSF-1 acts on hematopoietic precursor cells and promotes their differentiation into monocytes and macrophages. The c-*kit* proto-oncogene appears to encode a receptor for a mast cell growth factor. The extracellular regions of these receptors contain five repeats of an immunoglobulin-like domain containing cysteine residues. In contrast to the

EGF and insulin receptors, the tyrosine kinase domains of this group of receptors contain a 70–100 amino acid insertion (Fig. 3-3). Both PDGF and CSF-1 are disulfide-linked heterodimers. PDGF-induced activation of its receptor involves receptor dimerization and interaction with specific cytoplasmic effector molecules.

4. *The FGF receptor family:* There are as many as 18 different FGFs that mediate cell proliferation, migration, and differentiation. Certain FGFs play an important role in organogenesis during embryonic development. The FGFs also appear to serve an important role in wound healing and angiogenesis. The extracellular domain of these receptors contains three immunoglobulin-like domains with two cysteines in each, like the PDGF receptor family. The tyrosine kinase domain also is divided into two regions by an inserted stretch of only 14 amino acids.

Most, if not all, of the actions of the tyrosine kinase family of receptors are mediated by ligand-induced receptor dimerization/oligomerization, tyrosine kinase activation, and autophosphorylation. With the exception of the insulin receptor (which already exists as a dimer of two disulfide-linked α,β-heterodimers [see above]), all receptor tyrosine kinases undergo dimerization upon ligand binding. Receptor dimerization serves an essential role in tyrosine kinase activation, autophosphorylation, and transmembrane signaling. The tyrosine kinase of one receptor polypeptide chain catalyzes the phosphorylation of tyrosines on the other receptor chain in the dimer. Autophosphorylation of the receptor on tyrosine residues increases tyrosine kinase activity and enhances its capacity to phosphorylate other cellular target proteins. This occurs because the phosphorylated tyrosines on the receptor serve as binding or docking sites for target proteins that contain a sequence of amino acids referred to as a *src-homology 2* (SH2) domain. The SH2 domain is so named because of its similarity to a region present in *src*, a cellular protooncogene product involved in cell growth control. The *src*, which lacks an extracellular ligand-binding domain, is activated by binding to receptor tyrosine kinases via its SH2 region. The binding of *src* or other cellular target proteins to activated receptor tyrosine kinases through their SH2 domains orients these proteins for phosphorylation by the activated receptor tyrosine kinase.

Many of the SH2-containing cellular proteins that bind to activated receptor tyrosine kinases are components of downstream signaling pathways which involve other second-messenger systems. In this manner, the tyrosine kinase receptor family interacts with other signal transduction systems. As an example, PDGF binding to its receptor results in an increase in phosphatidylinositol turnover and in cytosolic calcium. This action of PDGF appears to be mediated in part by the association and activation of a specific isoform of phospholipase C, PLC-γ, which interacts via its SH2 domain with the phosphotyrosines in the cytoplasmic domain of the activated PDGF receptor and, consequently, is phosphorylated on tyrosine residues. The activated phospholipase C, in turn, catalyzes the hydrolysis of PIP_2, resulting in the elaboration of IP_3 with associated increase in cytoplasmic calcium. The PDGF activation of phospholipase C also catalyzes the hydrolysis of PC. It has been postulated that increased DAG formed through PC hydrolysis and the associated protein kinase C activation provides an important component of the mitogenic action of

PDGF. Autophosphorylation sites of the activated PDGF receptor also interact with the adaptor protein—growth factor receptor-bound protein 2 (Grb2)—which then recruits guanine nucleotide exchange factors that promote the binding of GTP to *Ras,* which in turn binds and activates the serine-threonine protein kinase *raf.* This ultimately results in the activation of mitogen-activated protein kinases (MAP kinases), which phosphorylate a number of cellular proteins, including the transcription factor AP-1.

It therefore is apparent that the tyrosine kinase family of cell surface receptors acts in parallel as well as in a cross-talking manner with other receptor-regulated effector systems that involve G proteins. Some of these interactions are additive or synergistic, whereas others are antagonistic. The net result is the integrated control of cellular function, homeostasis, and growth.

Signal Transduction by Members of the Cytokine Receptor Family. Receptors for growth hormone, prolactin, and other members of the cytokine receptor superfamily do not have kinase domains. Furthermore, the cytoplasmic domains of superfamily members have only limited sequence similarity; this is confined to a membrane proximal region, which is functionally required for mitogenic responses. Despite the absence of a kinase domain, ligand binding results in the rapid phosphorylation of cellular proteins, as well as the receptor itself, on tyrosine residues. The membrane proximal region of the receptor is required for coupling of ligand binding to tyrosine phosphorylation. Tyrosine phosphorylation is mediated by a family of cytoplasmic tyrosine kinases, the Janus (JAK) kinases. These kinases physically associate with the membrane proximal region of the ligand-bound receptor, resulting in autophosphorylation of tyrosine residues and further activation of the JAK kinase, and phosphorylation of the receptor, as well as other cellular proteins that bind to the receptor-kinase complex by their SH2 domains. The major cellular targets for JAK kinases are members of a family of transcription factors called *signal transducers and activators of transcription* (STATs), which bind to phosphorylated tyrosines on the activated receptor via their SH2 domains. Phosphorylation of STATs on tyrosine residues results in their dimerization and activation and subsequent binding to specific response elements within the regulatory regions of genes. It is apparent that receptor dimerization, which occurs as a result of ligand binding, is essential to initiation of the signal transduction cascade. The receptor dimerization causes an increased affinity for JAKs and facilitates cross-phosphorylation of their phosphorylation sites. A hypothetical model of the signal transduction pathway mediated by the binding of growth hormone to its receptor is represented in schematic form in Figure 3-7.

Four JAK kinase family members have been identified: JAK1, JAK2, JAK3, and tyk2; these have specificity for different ligand-receptor complexes. For example, JAK2 has been found associated with activated growth hormone, prolactin, and erythropoietin receptors; activated interferon-α/β receptors associate with JAK1 and tyk2; interferon-γ receptors associate with JAK1 and JAK2; and activated interleukin-2 receptors associate with JAK3. Further complexity results from the identification of at least four different STAT proteins, which appear to be substrates for the different JAKs. It should also be noted that binding of EGF and PDGF to their receptors, which have intrinsic tyrosine kinase activity and are autophosphorylated,

Fig. 3-7 Signal transduction mechanisms associated with binding of growth hormone (GH) to its receptor. The binding of a single molecule of GH promotes receptor dimerization. This in turn results in an increased affinity of the membrane-proximal region of the cytoplasmic domain of the receptor for the cytoplasmic tyrosine kinase, JAK2, a member of the Janus kinase family, which undergoes autophosphorylation and further activation. The activated JAK2 catalyzes phosphorylation of the receptor. The phosphorylated tyrosines on the receptor now serve as docking sites for STAT (signal transducers and activators of transcription) transcription factors, which bind via an SH2 domain and are phosphorylated on tyrosine residues. The phosphorylated STATs form dimers and bind as a dimeric complex to a specific enhancer element in the regulatory region of a GH-inducible gene (i.e., IGF-I), resulting in increased transcription initiation.

promotes tyrosine phosphorylation of JAK1 and activation of a STAT1 transcription factor that binds as part of a complex to an enhancer in the *c-fos* promoter.

STEROID HORMONES

Steroid hormones exert long-term effects on their target cells; they stimulate cell growth and differentiation and regulate the synthesis of specific proteins. Steroid hormones exert these actions on target cells after binding to specific receptors, which are ligand-inducible transcription factors localized primarily within the nucleus. The steroid–receptor complex regulates the synthesis of specific proteins primarily by altering the rate of transcription of specific genes.

The first clear indication that steroid hormones could interact with specific genes and alter their activity was the finding in 1960 that the insect steroid *ecdysone* rapidly induced the formation of puffs in specific regions of the salivary gland polytene chromosomes of the midge *Chironomus*. It has subsequently been shown that the puffs correspond to active genes; several of these genes have been found to encode salivary proteins. Although the ecdysteroids were the first of the steroid hormones shown to regulate gene activity, studies of the receptors and mechanisms of action of steroid hormones in vertebrates rapidly progressed and outpaced those concerning the ecdysteroids. This was primarily due to the synthesis of radiolabeled vertebrate steroid hormones of high specific activity and the subsequent discovery of receptor proteins in cells of vertebrates.

Over the past two decades, studies from a large number of laboratories have led to a generally accepted hypothesis for the mechanism of action of steroid hormones (Fig. 3-8). Steroids travel in the circulation predominantly bound to several classes of serum proteins. Estrogens and androgens are transported in the circulation bound to sex hormone-binding globulin (SHBG), which binds estradiol-17β and testosterone with relatively high affinity ($K_d \approx 10^{-9}\ M$). These steroids are also weakly bound to serum albumin. Glucocorticoids and progesterone are bound in the circulation to corticosteroid-binding globulin (CBG), also referred to as *transcortin.*

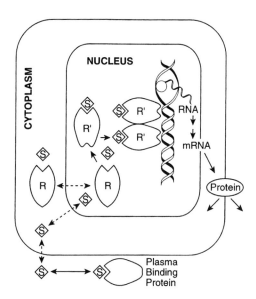

Fig. 3-8 Schematic representation of a steroid hormone responsive cell. Steroid hormones (S) in the circulation are predominantly bound to specific proteins. Only a small proportion of the circulating steroid is free; it is the unbound steroid that has the capacity to enter cells by free diffusion. Within target cells, the steroids bind with high affinity to specific receptors that are primarily localized within the nucleus. After binding steroid, the receptor (R) undergoes a process of "activation," which involves dissociation from heat shock proteins and formation of a receptor dimer. The receptor dimer binds to specific sequences of DNA proximate to steroid-regulated genes. The binding of the receptor as a dimer to these genomic regions can result in increases or decreases in the rates of gene expression. The steroid–receptor complex is believed to increase the rate of transcription of specific genes by causing the formation of a stable preinitiation complex and facilitating the binding of RNA polymerase II to the promoter regions of such genes. This results in the synthesis of RNA molecules that are processed within the nucleus to mRNAs that enter the cytoplasm and are translated into specific proteins.

It is generally believed that only the free steroid can enter cells (see Chapter 5). Presumably, steroids can freely diffuse across the plasma membranes of all cells but are sequestered only within cells that contain specific intracellular receptors. The steroid binds to its receptor with an affinity ($K_d \approx 10^{-10}$ M) that is at least 10-fold greater than the affinity with which it binds to the serum globulins.

Steroid Hormone Receptors

Cellular Localization

An issue that has been a source of controversy over the years is the subcellular localization of the unoccupied or so-called free steroid receptor. There has always been general agreement that the occupied or "bound" steroid receptor has increased affinity for chromatin and is localized to the nucleus. It was believed for some time, however, that the free steroid receptor was a cytoplasmic protein that moved to the nucleus only after binding hormone and undergoing an undefined process termed *transformation* or *activation*. This concept was derived from studies in which cells not previously exposed to a given steroid were homogenized and cytosolic and nuclear fractions were prepared by differential centrifugation. When these fractions were incubated with the radiolabeled steroid, the receptor was usually found to be present predominantly in the cytosol.

Conversely, if the cells were first incubated with the steroid hormone and then homogenized and subcellular fractions prepared, the receptor was found to be present almost exclusively in the nuclear fraction. With the availability of monoclonal antibodies specific for a number of steroid receptors and the technique of immunocytochemistry, it has generally been found that both the free and occupied steroid receptors are localized to the nucleus. Receptors for thyroid hormones, retinoic acid, and 1,25-dihydroxyvitamin D_3 are present within the nucleus, bound to their respective *hormone response elements* (HREs) in the absence or presence of bound hormone. By contrast, receptors for glucocorticoids (GR), progesterone (PR), estrogen (ER), androgens (AR), and mineralocorticoids (MR) in the absence of hormone binding are not bound to their respective HREs. Rather, these "free" receptors are present within the nucleus (PR, ER, AR, MR) or cytoplasm (GR) bound to a complex of *heat shock proteins* (hsps). Upon hormone binding, these receptors are released from the hsp complex and are activated to a DNA-binding, transcription-modulating state (see below). These activated receptors are now found within the nucleus bound to their respective HREs, which usually lie upstream of target genes.

Receptor Structure

The steroid hormone receptors belong to a superfamily of so-called *nuclear receptors* that also includes the receptor for 1,25-dihydroxyvitamin D_3, several tissue-specific forms of receptors for thyroid hormones and retinoic acid, as well as a large number of nuclear proteins for which ligands have not as yet been identified (so-called *orphan receptors*). As discussed, these molecules are members of a large superfamily of ligand-activated transcription factors that bind to specific sequences of DNA as dimers and regulate the transcriptional activity of specific genes. Through the use of recombinant DNA technology, >100 different types of nuclear receptors have been identified, making the nuclear receptor superfamily the largest family of metazoan transcription factors. By phylogenetic analysis, the superfamily can be divided into three subfamilies: Type I receptors bind the steroid hormones. These include the glucocorticoid receptor (GR), mineralocorticoid receptor (MR), androgen receptor (AR), and estrogen receptor (ER). Type II receptors bind thyroid hormones (TR), all-*trans* retinoic acid (RAR), 9-*cis* retinoic acid (RXR), and 1,25 dihydroxy-vitamin D_3 (VDR). Type III receptors, the orphan receptors, have no known ligands.

All these receptors have not only the same general structure (Fig. 3-9) but also a high degree of homology in their hormone-binding and DNA-binding regions. By comparison of the nucleotide sequences of the mRNAs as well as the deduced amino acid sequences of the receptor proteins, it has been found that there are specific domains that are highly conserved structurally and functionally among all members of this superfamily. The region of greatest homology is the DNA-binding domain (DBD), which is composed of 66–68 amino acids and contains nine perfectly conserved cysteine residues. This domain contains two repeated units enriched in the amino acids Cys, Lys, and Arg. Such repeated units have been identified in a number of nucleic acid-binding proteins. Each of these units is folded into a finger-like structure containing four cysteines that coordinate one zinc ion. The loop of the so-called zinc finger is made up of 12–13 amino acids; a spacer region of 15–17 amino acids is present between the two fingers (Fig. 3-9). These DNA-binding "fingers" have the capacity to insert into a half-turn of DNA. Such repeated units have been identified in a number of nuclear proteins that are known to act as transcription factors.

Near the carboxy-terminal end of the receptor molecules are two conserved regions (HBD$_1$ and HBD$_2$) of 42 and 22 hydrophobic amino acids, respectively, which comprise the *hormone-binding domain*. The HBD also contains a transcription activation domain, termed *activation function 2* (AF-2), which is essential for ligand-dependent activation of transcription by nuclear receptors. The carboxy-terminal regions of the members of this superfamily of receptors have a high degree of sequence similarity with the *v-erb-A* protein of the oncogenic avian erythroblastosis virus. The *v-erb-A* protein, which is not oncogenic by itself, increases the oncogenic potential of another viral protein, *v-erb-B* (which has a high degree of sequence homology with the tyrosine kinase domain of the EGF receptor, as previously discussed). Estrogens stimulate the growth of estrogen receptor-positive mammary tumors, and have been implicated as contributory factors in the pathogenesis of human breast cancer. These effects could be mediated through the induction of synthesis of growth factors or through a direct action on growth factor receptors. It has been postulated that the estrogen receptor may potentiate the action of an oncogene in breast cancer in much the same way as *v-erb-A* potentiates the oncogenic potential of *v-erb-B*.

Fig. 3-9 *Upper panel:* Schematic representation of the zinc finger–containing DNA-binding domain of the glucocorticoid receptor. Amino acids in the P-box (important in recognition of the sequence of the DNA half-site) and the D-box (important in receptor dimerization and recognition of the spacing of the two half-sites in the response element) are highlighted. The amino acids of the P-box, which are important for half-site recognition of three different groups of receptors and the sequences of the half-sites to which they bind, are indicated. *Lower panel:* Domain structures of members of the nuclear receptor superfamily, including human receptors for glucocorticoid (hGR), mineralocorticoid (hMR), androgen (hAR), progesterone (hPR), estrogen (hER), retinoic acid (hRAR), thyroid hormone (hTR), 1,25-dihydroxyvitamin D$_3$ (hVDR), and the orphan receptor, hCOUP. Three highly conserved regions are indicated, the DNA-binding domain (DBD) and two regions involved in hormone binding (HBD$_1$ and HBD$_2$). The numbers within these regions indicate the percent amino acid similarity with hGR. The hypervariable region of the receptors extends from the amino terminus (indicated by the number 1) to the DBD. The number at the right end of each schematic indicates the number of amino acids in each receptor protein. The nuclear receptors can be divided into three subfamilies based on phylogenetic analysis, structure, and function: Type I—the classical steroid receptors; Type II—TR, RAR, VDR; Type III—COUP and other "orphan" receptors.

The region of these receptors between the aminoterminus and the DNA-binding domain is hypervariable (HV) both in size and in amino acid sequence (Fig. 3-9). For example, the HV region of the glucocorticoid receptor is 421 amino acids in size, whereas the HV region of the receptor for 1,25-dihydroxyvitamin D_3 consists of only 24 amino acids. This region contains a ligand-independent transcriptional activation domain (AF-1). The transcription factor COUP, which is involved in the transcriptional activation of a number of genes, including those for chicken ovalbumin, mammalian insulin, and pro-opiomelanocortin, is a member of the nuclear receptor superfamily of proteins based on structural homology. Like the thyroid hormone (TR), retinoic acid (RAR), and 1,25-dihydroxyvitamin D_3 (VDR) receptors, COUP binds to DNA as a heterodimer with the retinoid-X-receptor (RXR); however, the existence of a ligand for COUP remains to be determined. The finding that the carboxyterminal region of COUP has significant sequence similarity to other members of the steroid receptor superfamily, and that this region of COUP is evolutionarily conserved, is suggestive of the existence of such a ligand. It has been argued that COUP may be activated by a ligand produced within the same cell in which it is synthesized. It is postulated that the steroid receptor superfamily originated from a primordial receptor gene in primitive organisms in which it may have served as a receptor for environmental nutrients and other factors. The different classes of receptors for steroids and other regulatory molecules within the present superfamily of receptors and related molecules evolved in response to the increasing regulatory requirements imposed by cellular specialization of higher eukaryotes.

Molecular Forms and Receptor Transformation (Activation)

"Free" glucocorticoid, mineralocorticoid, androgen, progesterone, and estrogen receptors are believed to exist in the cell as monomers associated with a complex of proteins that includes two molecules of a 90,000-Da phosphoprotein, hsp90, one molecule of hsp70, and a number of other proteins (Fig. 3-10). In this conforma-

Fig. 3-10 Proposed mechanism for hormone-induced activation of the glucocorticoid receptor. The inactive "free" glucocorticoid receptor (R) exists in the cytoplasm as a monomer in association with a protein complex comprised of two molecules of heat shock protein (hsp)90, one molecule of hsp70, and a number of other proteins. After hormone (H) binding, the receptor dissociates from the hsp complex and forms a homodimer with another molecule of glucocorticoid receptor. This process is required for transformation of the receptor to a DNA-binding, transcription-modulating state.

tion the receptor is incapable of binding DNA or regulating gene transcription. The binding of hormone to the receptor results in the dissociation of receptor from this complex, which forms a homodimer with another receptor molecule. This receptor homodimer has a greatly increased affinity for binding to HREs in DNA. Upon binding to DNA, the receptor homodimer recruits proteins termed *co-activators,* which facilitate transcription initiation by mechanisms to be described below.

By contrast, "free" receptors for thyroid hormone, retinoic acid, and 1,25-dihydroxyvitamin D_3 are not bound to hsps. Rather, they are bound to their HREs either as homodimers or as heterodimers with a molecule of a member of the retinoic acid receptor subfamily, termed *retinoid-X receptor* (RXR). In their "free" state, receptors in this subgroup recruit proteins termed *co-repressors* and inhibit transcription of their respective target genes by mechanisms to be described below. Upon hormone binding, the co-repressors are released and replaced by *co-activators,* which facilitate transcription initiation, as discussed above.

Regulation of Gene Expression by Members of the Nuclear Receptor Superfamily

The primary action of steroid, retinoid, and thyroid hormones is to regulate the rate of transcription of specific genes and thus to alter the synthesis of specific proteins. As discussed above, certain members of the nuclear receptor superfamily (Types I and II) are ligand-activated transcription factors that increase gene transcription upon hormone binding. This group of transcription factors interacts with specific genomic sequences, the so-called HREs, which are predominantly localized in the 5'-flanking regions of target genes, usually within several hundred base pairs upstream of the transcription initiation sites. The activated forms of these receptors bind to their HREs as homodimers (GR, MR, AR, PR, ER) or as heterodimers with RXR (TR, VDR, RAR).

Hormone-Response Elements and Regulation of Gene Transcription
After hormone binding and receptor activation, the GR, PR, MR, AR, and ER bind as homodimers to their respective HREs. The GR, PR, MR, and AR bind to an identical core HRE, which consists of a double-stranded inverted repeat or palindrome of 6 nucleotides (half-site) separated by a 3-nucleotide spacer:

AGAACAnnnTGTTCT

TCTTGTnnnACAAGA

The fact that more than one hormone receptor binds to the same sequence of DNA implies that specificity is dependent upon the type of hormone receptor(s) present in the target cell. Additionally, DNA sequences outside of the core HRE, as well as interaction with other transcription factors bound to other *cis*-acting enhancer elements, may be responsible for differential activation of target genes by structurally related hormone receptors.

The ER does not bind to HRE recognized by GR, MR, AR, and PR. Rather, the ER binds specifically to a HRE that consists of a double-stranded inverted repeat of similar sequence, also with a three nucleotide spacer:

AGGTCAnnnTGACCT

TCCAGTnnnACTGGA

Specificity for the primary sequence of the DNA half-site (e.g., AGAACA vs. AGGTCA) is determined by three amino acids in the shoulder of the first zinc finger of the receptors, the so-called P-box (Fig. 3-9). In the GR, MR, PR, and AR, these amino acids are glycine, serine, and valine. By contrast, in the estrogen receptor, these amino acids are glutamate, glycine, and alanine. Within the shoulder of the second zinc finger is the D-box or "dimerization" box (Fig. 3-9). This region of the receptor is important for dimerization of the two receptor monomers and establishes orientation of the monomers for appropriate binding to differentially spaced half-sites.

Receptors for thyroid hormones, retinoids, and 1,25-dihydroxyvitamin D_3 usually bind as heterodimers with RXR to a double-stranded, direct hexameric repeat separated by a spacer of 1–5 nucleotides. Although the sequence of the half-site is the same as that of the estrogen-responsive element ([ERE] AGGTCA/TGACCT), binding specificity is determined by the presence of a direct repeat, rather than a palindrome (as is the case for the ERE), and by the number of nucleotides in the spacer. As an example, the VDR-RXR heterodimer preferentially binds to a direct repeat with a 3-nucleotide spacer, the TR-RXR heterodimer binds preferentially to a direct repeat with a 4-nucleotide spacer, and the RAR-RXR heterodimer binds preferentially to a direct repeat with a 5-nucleotide spacer, as shown below.

AGGTCAn$_{1-5}$AGGTCA

TCCAGTn$_{1-5}$TCCAGT

Glucocorticoid, Mineralocorticoid, Progesterone, and Androgen Receptor Regulation of Gene Expression. A model of the proposed mechanism whereby steroid hormones such as glucocorticoids, mineralocorticoids, progesterone, and androgens regulate eukaryotic gene expression is shown in Figure 3-11. After binding a molecule of hormone, the receptor undergoes a conformational change, is released from the complex with hsp90 and other heat shock proteins, and forms a homodimer with another receptor molecule. The receptor dimer now binds with high affinity to an HRE, which usually exists several hundred base pairs upstream of the target gene. The receptor dimer, which may be phosphorylated, can now recruit a complex of co-activators containing histone acetyltransferase (histone acetylase) activities. Histone acetylation causes destabilization of the nucleosomal structure and a local opening of chromatin into a transcriptionally permissive state. This results in recruitment of general (i.e., basal) transcription factors to form a stable preinitiation complex at the TATA box. Co-activators (which do not bind to DNA directly) also serve to bridge transcription factors with the basal transcription complex, resulting in further stabilization, the recruitment of RNA polymerase II (Pol II), and initiation of gene transcription. The formation of the preinitiation complex may be a sequential process; the binding of transcription factor IIB (TFIIB) is the rate-limiting step. It recently has been found that a number of receptors in the nuclear receptor superfamily can bind directly to TFIIB. This suggests that the nuclear receptors also may facilitate the interaction of TFIIB with the preinitiation complex.

Fig. 3-11 Proposed mechanism for regulation of gene transcription by glucocorticoid, progesterone, mineralocorticoid, and androgen receptors. After binding hormone (H), the receptor dissociates from a complex with heat shock protein 90 (hsp90) and other proteins, and binds to its hormone response element upstream of the target gene as a homodimer. The activated receptor dimer can now recruit a complex of co-activators containing histone acetyltransferase activity. This results in an opening of chromatin structure, which facilitates assembly of the preinitiation complex, the binding of RNA polymerase II, and activation of transcription initiation.

Thyroid, Retinoid, and Vitamin D_3 Receptor Regulation of Gene Expression. As discussed above, receptors for retinoids, thyroid hormones, and 1,25-dihydroxyvitamin D_3, when bound to their HREs in the absence of ligand binding, cause silencing of their target genes. The proposed mechanism whereby the active thyroid hormone triiodothyronine (T_3) regulates gene expression is shown in Figure 3-12. In the absence of hormone binding, the thyroid hormone receptor (T_3R) is bound to its response element (a direct repeat of the sequence AGGTCA with a 4-nucleotide spacer) as a homodimer or heterodimer with RXR. The "free" receptor dimer interacts with a co-repressor complex containing histone deacetylases, which keep chromatin in a "closed" conformation and silence transcription. The binding of T_3 to T_3R stabilizes formation of a heterodimer with RXR, causes dissociation of the co-repressor complex and recruitment of a co-activator complex containing histone acetyltransferases. As described above, histone acetylation causes destabilization of the nucleosomal structure, resulting in an opening of the local chromatin structure into a transcriptionally permissive state that allows assembly of the preinitiation complex. Co-activators also facilitate interaction of transcription factors with the basal transcription complex, resulting in its stabilization, the recruitment of Pol II, and initiation of transcription of thyroid hormone-responsive genes.

Fig. 3-12 Proposed mechanism for regulation of gene transcription by thyroid hormones, retinoids, and 1,25-dihydroxyvitamin D_3. In its "free" state, the thyroid hormone receptor (T_3R) binds to its hormone response element as homodimer (shown), or as a heterodimer with a molecule of retinoid-X receptor (RXR). The free T_3R interacts with a complex of co-repressors containing histone deacetylase activity, which silence transcription by promoting a closed chromation structure and preventing formation of a stable preinitiation complex. Upon binding of triiodothyronine (T_3), the receptor undergoes a conformational change resulting in the dissociation of the co-repressor and association of a complex of co-activators containing histone acetyltransferase. This in turn facilitates transcription initiation by mechanisms described in the legend to Figure 3-11.

Tissue-Specific Expression of Hormonally Regulated Genes

The phenotype of a given cell is the result of the complement of genes that are expressed; the expression of a number of these cellular genes will be subject to hormonal regulation. A hormone acting through its cellular receptors can regulate the expression of different genes in different tissues. For example, estrogen regulates the expression of the ovalbumin gene in the chick oviduct and the vitellogenin gene in chick liver. As the estrogen receptors in oviduct and liver tissues are apparently identical, and because the DNA sequences within and surrounding eukaryotic genes should be essentially the same in all cell types of a given organism, there must be other structural features that determine which genes are expressible and available to hormonal regulation. The complement of genes that are expressed in a given cell type is determined at the time of cellular differentiation. It is apparent that such expressible genes exist in so-called DNase I-sensitive regions; that is, they reside in regions of the chromatin that are more readily digested *in vitro* by DNase I than is the bulk of chromosomal DNA. The DNase I-sensitive regions define the structural framework in a given cell for the genes that are available for expression. Most of the cellular genes are not expressed and are tightly packaged with histone proteins in higher-order chromosomal structures, rendering them DNase I resistant.

ENDOCRINE DISORDERS DUE TO ALTERATIONS IN RECEPTOR NUMBER AND FUNCTION

As discussed above, changes in the concentration of cellular receptors for a specific hormone can markedly alter the sensitivity of the target cell to that hormone; a *decrease* in the concentration of receptors can decrease sensitivity to the hormone, whereas an *increase* in receptor concentration can increase the sensitivity of the target cell to the hormone. It is apparent that the concentration of cellular receptors for a specific hormone can vary considerably with the physiologic state and that the concentration of the hormone itself can regulate the concentration of its own receptors on target cells. Most commonly, an increase in the level of a specific hormone will cause a decrease in the available number of its cellular receptors. This decrease in available receptors can be due either to receptor phosphorylation by a specific kinase and sequestration of receptors away from the cell surface, or to an actual disappearance or loss of receptors from the cell. This hormonally induced negative regulation of receptors is termed *homologous down-regulation* or *desensitization*. Studies of the down-regulation of receptors for insulin and EGF by the homologous hormones indicate that down-regulation is caused, at least in part, by a clustering of hormone-receptor complexes in coated pits on the cell surface, internalization within coated vesicles, and degradation by lysosomal enzymes. Coated pits and coated vesicles are so named because they contain a single protein, clathrin, that forms a "coat" on their cytoplasmic surfaces. There is little doubt that receptor internalization provides an important homeostatic mechanism that serves to protect the organism from the potential toxic effects of hormone excess.

Desensitization is defined as a decrease in the responsiveness of a cell to a constant level of hormone or factor upon prolonged exposure. Homologous desensitization also can result from a hormone-induced alteration in the receptor, which uncouples it from some component of the signal transduction pathway. Another form of desensitization, *heterologous desensitization,* occurs when incubation with one agonist reduces the responsiveness of a cell to a number of other agonists that act through different receptors. This phenomenon is most commonly observed with receptors that act through the adenylyl cyclase system. Heterologous desensitization reflects a broad pattern of refractoriness that has a slower onset than does homologous desensitization.

In certain instances, endocrine dysfunction arises from pathologic alterations in receptor levels and/or function. Specific examples of such endocrine dysfunction are discussed below.

Endocrine Dysfunction Caused by Homologous and Heterologous Receptor Regulation

The process of homologous down-regulation of receptors might be a contributing factor to a number of clinical states. Probably the most common receptor defect in man is the down-regulation of insulin receptors caused by chronic hyperinsulinemia of obesity. Obesity is generally characterized by hyperinsulinemia, variable degrees of glucose intolerance, and resistance to both endogenous and exogenously administered insulin. Insulin resistance associated with obesity is caused, at least in part, by a decrease in the concentration of available insulin receptors on target cells because of increased insulin-receptor endocytosis and degradation; postreceptor defects may play some role in the reduced sensitivity to insulin. When obese individuals are maintained on calorie-restricted diets for several weeks, there is a marked reduction in the circulating insulin concentration, an increase in the concentration of insulin receptors on target cells, and a decline in insulin resistance.

Another example of endocrine dysfunction resulting from homologous desensitization is the reduced sensitivity to both endogenous and exogenous catecholamines resulting from the use of β-adrenergic agonists as bronchodilators in the treatment of asthma. This reduced sensitivity to catecholamines is caused by β-adrenergic agonist-induced reduction in the concentration of β-adrenergic receptors on the cell surface and to a reduced coupling of receptors to adenylyl cyclase. Homologous desensitization of β-adrenergic receptors is associated with phosphorylation of the receptors by a β-adrenergic receptor kinase (BARK). The phosphorylation of the receptors either promotes the sequestration of receptor away from the cell surface or renders it less effective in activating adenylyl cyclase, or both. The sequestered receptors are then either recycled to the cell surface or targeted for degradation within lysosomes.

There are a number of examples of one hormone acting through its own receptors to alter the sensitivity of target cells to another hormone. Thyroid hormones can enhance the sensitivity of cardiac muscle cells to catecholamines by increasing the number of β-adrenergic receptors. This can result in an increased heart rate, atrial fibrillation, and congestive heart failure. Frequently, an alteration in cardiac function is the only manifestation of an otherwise masked hyperthyroidism.

Endocrine Dysfunction Caused by Autoimmune Disease Involving Antireceptor Antibodies

The presence of antibodies to receptors appears to be of central importance in several disease states.

Acetylcholine Receptors
In myasthenia gravis, a disease characterized by muscle weakness and flaccid paralysis, circulating antibodies to the nicotinic acetylcholine receptors are localized in the neuromuscular junctions. These antibodies do not block the binding of acetylcholine to the receptor; however, they enhance the rate of receptor degradation and thus render the skeletal muscle cells less sensitive to endogenous acetylcholine.

Thyroid-Stimulating Hormone (Thyrotropin, TSH)
Individuals with hyperthyroidism associated with diffuse goiter (Graves' disease) have circulating antibodies to the receptor for TSH, a polypeptide hormone produced by the anterior pituitary that acts on the thyroid gland to stimulate the production of the thyroid hormones (see Chapter 13). One of the effects of the thyroid

hormones is to act on the hypothalamus and pituitary to inhibit the production of TSH. These autoantibodies bind to TSH receptors on thyroid cells and mimic the actions of TSH itself. Because such antibodies are not regulated by negative feedback of the thyroid hormones as is TSH, the thyroid gland is persistently stimulated to produce elevated levels of circulating thyroid hormones (see Chapter 13).

Insulin Receptors

In patients who have an unusual form of diabetes associated with insulin resistance, there are circulating autoantibodies to the insulin receptor. The antibodies bind to insulin receptors, block insulin binding, and mimic insulin action. This usually results in desensitization to endogenous insulin with associated hyperinsulinemia and extreme insulin resistance. In rare instances, receptor desensitization does not occur and the patient manifests severe hypoglycemia.

Disorders Due to Receptor and Postreceptor Defects

Disorders Due to Defects in G Protein–Coupled Signal Transduction

As previously mentioned, the family of guanine nucleotide-binding (G) proteins mediate the actions of a wide variety of hormones and factors in tissues throughout the body. The massive secretory diarrhea associated with *Vibrio cholerae* infection was the first disorder found to be caused by the modification of a G protein. As discussed above, the cholera exotoxin catalyzes ADP-ribosylation of arginine 201 of α_s in intestinal epithelial cells. This causes a marked inactivation of the GTPase activity associated with this subunit, resulting in persistent activation of adenylyl cyclase and of cyclic AMP formation. It now is apparent that various somatic mutations of G proteins result in their activation or inactivation. Two endocrine disorders associated with activation and inhibition of G_s function are described next.

McCune-Albright Syndrome. This disorder is caused by a missense mutation of arginine 201 of α_s resulting in decreased GTPase activity and constitutive activation of adenylyl cyclase in one or more endocrine glands, including the adrenal cortex, gonads, thyroid, and pituitary thyrotrophs. This results in elevated levels of cyclic AMP formation, abnormal cell proliferation, and hyperfunction of the affected endocrine tissues. The symptoms can include acromegaly, precocious puberty, hyperthyroidism, hyperparathyroidism, Cushing's syndrome, fibrous dysplasia of bone that is polyostotic (involving more than one bone), and café au lait skin pigmentation.

Parathyroid Hormone-Resistant Hypoparathyroidism. Subjects with this disorder manifest a variety of missense mutations in the gene encoding α_s, which include loss of function mutations, and mutations that prevent coupling of α_s with activating receptors. Most affected individuals manifest a 50% decrease in α_s activity. This results in pseudohypoparathyroidism (see Chapter 15) accompanied by variable resistance to a variety of hormones that act through adenylyl cyclase activation, including thyroid-stimulating hormone, gonadotropins, and other hormones that act through G_s-coupled receptors.

Endocrine Tumors: Multiple Endocrine Neoplasia Type 1 (MEN1)

This collection of hereditary endocrinopathies involves benign and occasionally malignant neoplasms of endocrine glands, including the parathyroids, anterior pituitary, and enteropancreatic neuroendocrine tissues that result from a somatic mutation of the MEN1 gene. Tumor recurrence postoperatively is a common sequelae. The MEN1 gene, which was recently localized and identified by positional cloning and sequencing, appears to be a tumor suppressor gene. As found for other tumor suppressor genes, in the case of MEN1, one copy of the mutated gene is inherited from one parent. Tumors arise when the second gene copy is subsequently mutated by a so-called second hit. Acquired mutations of the MEN1 gene also appear to be involved in sporadic parathyroid adenomas, insulinomas, gastrinomas, and bronchial carcinoids.

Androgen Resistance

Testosterone, the major steroid product of the Leydig cells of the testis and the principal circulating androgen, serves as a prohormone in most androgen target tissues for dihydrotestosterone (DHT), which is formed from testosterone in these tissues by the action of the enzyme 5α-reductase (see Chapter 10). During embryogenesis, androgens produced by the fetal testis play a critical role in the differentiation of the male internal and external genitalia (see Chapter 8).

Androgen resistance can be caused by (a) complete absence, diminished amounts, or qualitative abnormalities of androgen receptors in target tissues, or (b) defects in the signal transduction pathway despite apparently normal androgen binding. The gene that encodes the androgen receptor is X linked; therefore, mutations are expressed in the hemizygous 46,XY state. A syndrome of complete androgen resistance in humans, termed testicular feminization (see Chapter 8) is commonly due to decreased amounts of functional androgen receptor. Testicular feminization has been found to be associated with a variety of point mutations scattered throughout the androgen receptor gene. Such mutations can result either in the insertion of a premature translational "stop codon" so that a truncated nonfunctional protein is synthesized, or in a loss of functional activity of the hormone-binding or DNA-binding domains. Affected genotypic males are born with female external genitalia and a blind vaginal pouch. Wolffian duct structures are absent or vestigial; Müllerian duct structures are absent and the external genitalia are female. Testes are present in the labia, inguinal canals, or abdomen. At puberty, these individuals develop female secondary sex characteristics. Because the negative feedback of testosterone at the hypothalamic–pituitary level is defective, circulating levels of luteinizing hormone and testosterone are elevated. Increased levels of luteinizing hormone cause enhanced secretion of estrogen by the testis, and the increased estrogen production contributes to the development of female secondary sex characteristics at puberty.

Vitamin D Resistance

Vitamin D–dependent rickets type I and type II are inherited disorders in the pathway of vitamin D action. Both are inherited as autosomal recessive traits and are associated with childhood rickets and adult abnormalities of bone mineralization termed *osteomalacia*. Vitamin D–dependent rickets type I appears to arise from a deficiency in the activity of renal 1α-hydroxylase, the enzyme that converts 25-(OH)D$_3$ into 1,25-(OH)$_2$D$_3$, the active form of the vitamin. The defect can be treated by administering physiologic amounts of 1,25-(OH)$_2$D$_3$. Conversely, vitamin D–dependent rickets type II appears to be due to a defect in the vitamin D receptor, or at the postreceptor level. In two unrelated families, children suffering from vitamin D–dependent rickets type II were found to have single point mutations in the tip of one of the zinc fingers of the DNA-binding domain of the vitamin D receptor. These mutant receptors are apparently defective in their ability to interact with and transcriptionally regulate vitamin D–responsive genes. Almost all individuals afflicted with this disorder present within the first year of life with hypocalcemia, osteomalacia, or rickets, and secondary hyperparathyroidism. An unexplained feature that is frequently associated with this disorder is total alopecia. Almost all afflicted individuals are resistant to pharmacologic doses of vitamin D and its metabolites in the healing of bone lesions and normalization of serum calcium levels.

SUGGESTED READING

Benovic JL, Bouvier M, Caron MG, and Lefkowitz RJ: Regulation of adenylyl cyclase–coupled β-adrenergic receptors. Annu Rev Cell Biol 4:405–428, 1988.

Berridge MJ: Inositol trisphosphate and calcium signalling. Nature 361:315–325, 1993.

Clapham DE, and Neer EJ: G protein $\beta\gamma$ subunits. Annu Rev Pharmacol Toxicol 167–203, 1997.

Cobb MH, and Goldsmith EJ: How MAP kinases are regulated. J Biol Chem 270:14843–14846, 1995.

Cohen P: Signal integration at the level of protein kinases, protein phosphatases and their substrates. Trends Biochem Sci 17:408–413, 1992.

Davis RJ: The mitogen-activated protein kinase signal transduction pathway. J Biol Chem 268:14553–14556, 1993.

Exton JH: Signalling through phosphatidylcholine breakdown. J Biol Chem 265:1–4, 1990.

Exton JH: New developments in phospholipase D. J Biol Chem 272:15579–15582, 1997.

Garbers DL, and Lowe DG: Guanylyl cyclase receptors. J Biol Chem 269:30741–30744, 1994.

Gether U, and Kobilka BK: G protein-coupled receptors. II. Mechanism of agonist activation. J Biol Chem 273:17979–17982, 1998.

Gilman AG: G proteins and the regulation of adenylyl cyclase. JAMA 262:1819–1825, 1989.

Glass CK: Differential recognition of target genes by nuclear receptor monomers, dimers, and heterodimers. Endocr Rev 15:391–407, 1994.

Griffin JE, McPhaul MJ, Russell DW, and Wilson JD: The androgen resistance syndromes: Steroid 5α-reductase-2 deficiency, testicular feminization, and related disorders. In: *The Metabolic and Molecular Bases of Inherited Disease,* 7th ed., Vol. 2, CR Scriver, AL Beaudet, WS Sly, and D Valle, eds., McGraw-Hill, New York, Chap. 95, pp. 2967–2998, 1995.

Hannun YA: The sphingomyelin cycle and the second messenger function of ceramide. J Biol Chem 269:3125–3128, 1994.

Ihle JN, Witthuhn BA, Quelle FW, Yamamoto K, Thierfelder WE, Kreider B, and Silvennoinen O: Signaling by the cytokine receptor superfamily: JAKs and STATs. Trends Biochem Sci 19:222–227, 1994.

Kitamura T, Ogorochi T, and Miyajima A: Multimeric cytokine receptors. Trends Endocrinol Metab 5:8–14, 1994.

Lefkowitz RJ: G protein-coupled receptors. III. New roles for receptor kinases and (β-arrestins in receptor signaling and desensitization. J Biol Chem 273:18677–18680, 1998.

Lemmon MA, and Schlessinger J: Regulation of signal transduction and signal diversity by receptor oligomerization. Trends Biochem Sci 19:459–464, 1994.

Linder ME, and Gilman AG: G proteins. Sci Am 267:56–65, 1992.

Marx S, Spiegel AM, Skarulis MC, Doppman JL, Collins FS, and Liotta LA: Multiple endocrine neoplasia type 1: Clinical and genetic topics. Ann Intern Med 129:484–494, 1998.

Meyer TE, and Habener JF: Cyclic adenosine 3′,5′-monophosphate response element binding protein (CREB) and related transcription-activating deoxyribonucleic acid-binding proteins. Endocr Rev 14:269–290, 1993.

McKenna NJ, Lanz R, and O'Malley BW: Nuclear receptor coregulators: Cellular and molecular biology. Endocr Rev 20:321–344, 1999.

Nishizuka Y: Intracellular signaling by hydrolysis of phospholipids and activation of protein kinase C. Science 258:607–614, 1992.

O'Malley BW: The steroid receptor superfamily: More excitement predicted for the future. Mol Endocrinol 4:363–369, 1990.

Pratt WB: Interaction of hsp90 with steroid receptors: Organizing some diverse observations and presenting the newest concepts. Mol Cell Endocrinol 74:C69–C76, 1990.

Pratt WB: The role of heat shock proteins in regulating the function, folding, and trafficking of the glucocorticoid receptor. J Biol Chem 268:21455–21458, 1993.

Quigley CA, De Bellis A, Marschke KB, El-Awady MK, Wilson EM, and French F: Androgen receptor defects: Historical, clinical and molecular perspectives. Endocr Rev 16:271–321, 1995.

Rhee SG, and Choi KD: Regulation of inositol phospholipid-specific phospholipase C enzymes. J Biol Chem 267:12393–12396, 1992.

Schlessinger J: How receptor tyrosine kinases activate Ras. Trends Biochem Sci 18:273–275, 1993.

Spiegel AM, Weinstein LS, and Shenker A: Abnormalities in G-protein–coupled signal transduction pathways in human disease. J Clin Invest 92:1119–1125, 1993.

Strader CD, Sigal IS, and Dixon RAF: Structural basis of β-adrenergic receptor function. FASEB J 3:1825–1832, 1989.

Stroud RM, and Finer-Moore J: Acetylcholine receptor structure, function, and evolution. Annu Rev Cell Biol 1:317–351, 1985.

Tsai M-J, and O'Malley BW: Molecular mechanisms of action of steroid/thyroid receptor superfamily members. Annu Rev Biochem 63:451–486, 1994.

Ullrich A, and Schlessinger J: Signal transduction by receptors with tyrosine kinase activity. Cell 61:203–212, 1990.

4

Cytokines and Immune–Endocrine Interactions

M. LINETTE CASEY

A close interaction between the endocrine and immune systems was first recognized near the end of the nineteenth century when it was observed that thymic size increased in response to prepubertal castration of male rabbits. Later, challenges that evoked an inflammatory response were found to produce changes in the endocrine system as well. These include a striking increase in the rate of secretion of cortisol by the adrenal cortex. Various stressful challenges lead to alterations in the production of steroid hormones by the adrenal cortex. With severe thermal injuries, for example, there is an increase in the rate of cortisol formation and, paradoxically, an equally dramatic reduction in the rate of formation of adrenal C_{19}-steroids, most notably dehydroepiandrosterone and dehydroepiandrosterone sulfate.

Several other observations support the concept of interaction between the endocrine and immune systems: (*1*) the dimorphic nature of the immune response of the two genders; (*2*) alterations in the immune response after gonadectomy or sex-steroid hormone treatment; (*3*) modification of the immune response during pregnancy; and (*4*) the identification of steroid hormone receptors in cells of the immune system. It is now clear that hormones affect cells of the immune system and that cytokines (the mediators of the immune response) affect the neuroendocrine system and the actions of hormones. During the past two decades, cytokines have been identified in appreciable numbers, and their structure, function, and mechanism(s) of action have been defined in large part.

CYTOKINES: DEFINITIONS AND CATEGORIZATION

The term *cytokine* was originally coined, by Stanley Cohen in 1974 to refer to a soluble product produced by nonimmune or immune cells that mediated an immune response. With time, the definition was broadened to include a variety of growth factors and other regulatory proteins that affect the function of immune or nonimmune cells. (The term *immune cells* refers to cells of bone marrow origin that have a central role in the immune response, namely lymphocytes, granulocytes, monocytes, macrophages, neutrophils, eosinophils, and mast cells.) *Cytokine* is used to describe proteins produced by various cell types in response to stimuli arising from various physiologic and pathophysiological states. Cytokines act in target cells through plasma membrane receptors to provoke intracellular signals that eventuate in biological effects (Fig. 4-1).

The range of biological processes affected by cytokines is broad and, in recent years, has been expanded to include nonimmune processes. Cytokines are very potent agents that can elicit massive alterations in molecular and biochemical processes, which in turn profoundly affect cellular and tissue characteristics, including differentiation and function. Various mechanisms have evolved to modulate these actions, including the presence of naturally occurring antagonists (Fig. 4-1).

The cytokine family of proteins includes the interleukins (presently, interleukin-1α and $-\beta$ through interleukin-16); tumor necrosis factor-α and $-\beta$; the hematopoietic colony–stimulating factors (CSF) (macrophage CSF, granulocyte CSF, granulocyte-macrophage CSF); the interferons ($-\alpha$s, $-\beta$, and $-\gamma$); transforming growth factors-β (TGF-β) (and the related proteins anti-müllerian hormone, activin, and inhibin; Chapters 8 through 10); chemokines (which include interleukin-6, interleukin-8, interleukin-11, monocyte chemoattractant proteins, oncostatin-M, leukemia-inhibitory factor, and others); and a number of growth factors (including epidermal growth factor and transforming growth factor-α, insulin-like growth factors; Chapter 12), and platelet-derived growth factor. Several classification systems have been used to categorize cytokines on the basis of cell type of origin, function, or structure. The usefulness of these classification systems is limited by the overlapping and multifunctional nature of many cytokines. For example, the terms *lymphokine* and *monokine* were coined to denote classes of cytokines produced by lymphocytes (especially T cells) or monocytes, respectively. Since the discovery that the origin of some cytokines placed in these categories is not restricted to lymphocytes or monocytes, the terms *lymphokine* and *monokine* are used less frequently. In another classification scheme, cytokines are categorized as inflammatory cytokines, immunomodulatory cytokines, chemokines, and growth factors (Table 4-1). *Chemokine* denotes a class of cytokines that attract specific cells of the immune system.

Cytokines act in a variety of cell types through autocrine, paracrine, endocrine, and juxtacrine mechanisms (Fig. 4-2). *Autocrine* refers to a mechanism by which a cytokine (or other agent) acts in the same cell from which it was produced and se-

Fig. 4-1 Cells of many types respond to a stimulus, such as bacterial or viral toxin, stress, or inflammatory cytokines, to produce an intracellular signal that leads to the synthesis and secretion of cytokines. These potent proteinaceous agents act in nearby cells (or in some cases, enter blood, Fig. 4-2) through specific plasma membrane–bound receptors to create a myriad of profound biological effects. Naturally occurring cytokine receptor antagonists may be present to limit the effects of cytokines by blocking interaction of the cytokine with the specific receptor.

Table 4-1 Functional Categorization of Cytokines

Function	Cytokine
Inflammatory cytokines	Interleukin (IL)-1β Tumor necrosis factor (TNF)-α IL-6
Immunomodulatory cytokines	IL-2 IL-9 IL-15 IL-3 IL-10 IL-4 IL-12 IL-5 IL-13 IL-7 IL-14

	Colony stimulating factors (CSF)
	   M-CSF macrophage CSF
	   G-CSF granulocyte CSF
	   GM-CSF granulocyte-macrophage CSF

	Monocyte chemotactic proteins (MCPs)
	   MCP-1
	   MCP-2
	   MCP-3

	Interferons (IFN)
	   IFN-α
	   IFN-β
	   IFN-γ

Chemokines	IL-6 IL-8 IL-11 MCP-1 Oncostatin M RANTES Leukemia inhibitory factor (LIF) Ciliary neurotrophic factor (CNTF)
Growth factors and other mediators	Transforming growth factor-β (TGF-β) Platelet-derived growth factor (PDGF) Epidermal growth factor (EGF) Insulin-like growth factors (IGFs) Interferons IL-6 IL-1α

creted. *Paracrine* refers to a mechanism by which a cytokine (or other agent) produced in one cell acts on a neighboring cell, access to which is by diffusion through the intercellular spaces rather than through the blood. Paracrine mechanisms are quantitatively the most important mechanisms of cytokine action. *Endocrine* refers to a mechanism by which a cytokine (or hormone) enters blood and reaches a target cell through the circulation. *Juxtacrine* refers to a mechanism whereby a cytokine that is embedded in, bound to, or associated with the plasma membrane of one cell interacts with a specific receptor in a juxtaposed cell. Cells of many different types and in all tissues have specific receptors for multiple cytokines.

Cytokines effect multiple diverse functions, both physiologically and pathophysiologically: (1) inflammatory cytokines are produced in response to infection

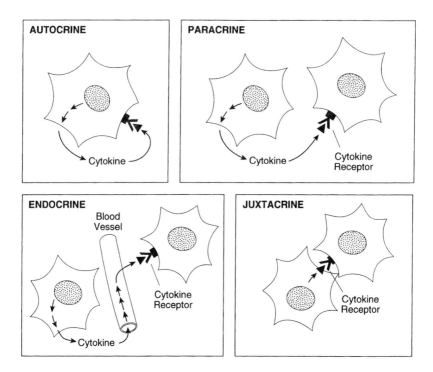

Fig. 4-2 Mechanisms of intercellular communication and action of cytokines, hormones, and other agents. Specific illustrations are given for cytokines. *Autocrine* refers to a mechanism by which a cytokine acts in its cell of origin. *Paracrine* refers to a mechanism by which a cytokine produced in one cell acts on a neighboring cell, access to which is by diffusion through the intercellular spaces rather than through the blood. Paracrine mechanisms are quantitatively the most important mechanisms of cytokine action. *Endocrine* refers to a mechanism by which a cytokine (or hormone) enters the blood and reaches a target cell through the circulation. *Juxtacrine* refers to a mechanism whereby a cytokine that is embedded in, bound to, or associated with the plasma membrane of one cell, interacts with a specific receptor in a juxtaposed cell.

and immunologic challenge; (2) some cytokines serve as normal growth or regulatory factors; and (3) some cytokines act to facilitate the maintenance of normal immune function. Each of these may modulate the secretions and function of the neuroendocrine system and each may be modulated by the actions of hormones.

CYTOKINES AND NEUROENDOCRINE FUNCTION

Cytokines modulate endocrine function in a number of ways. They act in the hypothalamus to modify the formation of releasing hormones and in the anterior pituitary to modulate the formation of hypophyseal hormones, for example, corticotropin (ACTH), gonadotropins, thyroid-stimulating hormone (TSH), prolactin, and growth hormone (GH). They also act in endocrine glands to modify responsiveness to trophic hormones or else to regulate the rate of synthesis of hormones (steroid or

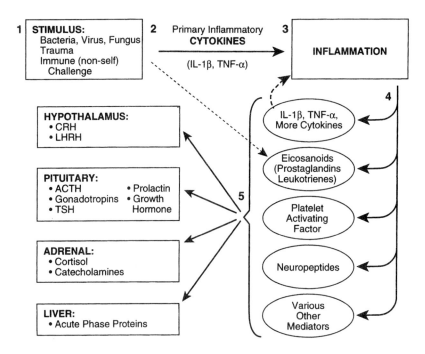

Fig. 4-3 The inflammatory response and consequences thereof. Some of the effects of the inflammatory response on the neuroendocrine system are illustrated. 1: A stimulus such as trauma, stress, immune challenge, or bacterial, viral, or fungal toxin acts to provoke the inflammatory response in mononuclear phagocytes. 2: Monocytes (mononuclear phagocytes in blood) respond rapidly with a massive outpouring of primary inflammatory cytokines, namely, IL-1β and TNF-α. 3: A profound process of inflammation ensues and propagates itself with the autoinduction of IL-1β by IL-1β. 4: Inflammation includes the production of IL-1β as well as TNF-α, IL-6, MCP-1, and many other cytokines (chemoattractants, mitogens, and hemopoietic factors), and the formation of eicosanoids, platelet-activating factor, nitric oxide, neuropeptides (by immune cells), and other bioactive agents. 5: These agents, in particular, the inflammatory cytokines IL-1β, TNF-α, and IL-6, act either directly or indirectly to increase the production of releasing hormones in the hypothalamus, pituitary hormones, cortisol, and catecholamines. In addition, the liver is stimulated to produce acute-phase proteins.

protein) by the target endocrine gland. These actions of cytokines are illustrated in Figure 4-3. In addition, cytokines are produced by and act in hormonally responsive tissues in hormonally modulated fashions.

CYTOKINE PRODUCTION IN RESPONSE TO IMMUNE CHALLENGE OR INFECTION

The production of cytokines is a dynamic process that is critical for normal function and well-being. The influence of cytokines on the neuroendocrine system can be appreciated by considering first the central role of interleukin-1β in the immune response.

The term *interleukin* (IL) was coined to describe proteins that are produced by and act on leukocytes. Since that time it has been discovered that some interleukins also are produced by nonimmune cells and that many interleukins act in cells other than leukocytes. At the time of writing this chapter, 17 interleukins have been identified in the human: IL-1α, IL-1β, and IL-2 through IL-16, numbered consecutively. In addition, a naturally occurring IL-1 receptor antagonist, which is a member of the IL-1 family, acts to block the actions of IL-1α and IL-1β.

Interleukin-1β: The Primary Cytokine

Interleukin-1β (IL-1β) is referred to as the *primary* cytokine. It is synthesized and secreted by mononuclear phagocytes in response to inflammatory stimuli such as infection or immunological challenge. It is primary because (a) it is produced very rapidly (Fig. 4-4) in response to challenge, and (b) it stimulates the production of many other cytokines.

IL-1β Synthesis, Processing, and Secretion

Bioactive IL-1β is a 17,000-Da protein that is produced by proteolytic processing of pro-IL-1β, a 34,000-Da precursor. Although pro-IL-1β is synthesized by many cell types, monocytes and macrophages are by far the principal source of bioactive IL-1β. This is because pro-IL-1β must be processed intracellularly by proteolytic cleavage to the active 17,000-Da form before it can be secreted. The proteolytic cleavage of pro-IL-1β is catalyzed by a specific enzyme called *IL-1β converting enzyme* (ICE) (Fig. 4-5), which is found in high amounts in a very few cell types, namely mononuclear phagocytes (monocytes and macrophages) and neutrophils, and

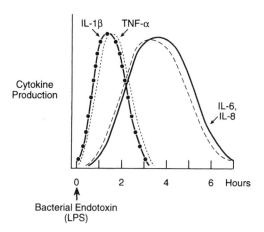

Fig. 4-4 Production of selected cytokines by monocytes in response to bacterial endotoxin (lipopolysaccharide, LPS). IL-1β, the primary cytokine, and TNF-α are produced rapidly and transiently. These cytokines stimulate the production of IL-6 and IL-8 by a variety of cell types.

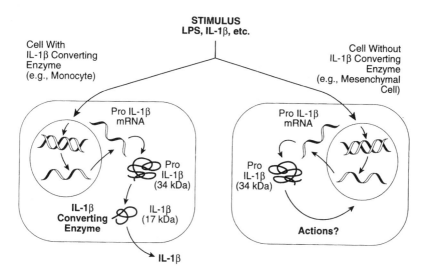

Fig. 4-5 Cell specificity of pro-IL-1β processing and active IL-1β secretion. The secretion of active IL-1β (17 kDa) in response to a stimulus is dependent on the processing of the precursor pro-IL-1β (34 kDa) by IL-1β–converting enzyme. This enzyme is expressed in a limited number of cell types, notable among which are monocytes, macrophages, and neutrophils. Other cell types that do not express IL-1β–converting enzyme respond to similar stimuli with an increase in pro-IL-1β synthesis as well. But the pro-IL-1β is not processed and, therefore, cannot be secreted. Rather, it accumulates in the cell and may exert other, yet undefined actions. LPS, lipopolysaccharide.

possibly placental trophoblasts. Many other cell types respond to immune challenge by a rapid, transient increase in the transcription of the IL-1β gene, an increase in the level of pro-IL-1β mRNA, and an increase in the synthesis of pro-IL-1β. But in cells that lack IL-1β-converting enzyme, the pro-IL-1β accumulates intracellularly and is not secreted. It is postulated that the accumulated pro-IL-1β has a specific, but yet undefined, function in these cells. In addition, the pro-IL-1β converting enzyme is believed to forestall apoptosis. Mechanisms other than ICE also exist in some cell types to facilitate the activation of pro-IL-1β.

IL-1β Action

The secreted, bioactive form of IL-1β (17,000 Da) acts locally in a paracrine or autocrine manner to stimulate the generation of IL-1β itself (a process called *autoinduction*), which serves to propagate the immune response. Also, IL-1β acts to stimulate the production of other interleukins, tumor necrosis factors, colony-stimulating factors, and interferons; IL-1β acts through two specific receptors to trigger many biological responses. The effects of IL-1β are amplified by actions of each of these cytokines through specific receptors to cause the production of yet other potent agents. These include prostaglandins and other arachidonic acid metabolites, platelet-activating factor (PAF), nitric oxide, and other potent substances. For example, IL-1β acts in a variety of cells (commonly the mesenchymal cells of a given tissue) to increase the production of IL-6. Acting in an endocrine fashion by circulating to the liver, IL-6 stimulates the synthesis and secretion of *acute-phase proteins*. These proteins include gammaglobulin and C-reactive protein and others, all of which function to protect the host and repair wounds. This is one component of the *acute phase response* to infection or antigenic and immune challenge. In addition, IL-6 acts in the liver to inhibit the synthesis of albumin and transferrin; IL-1β promotes hematopoiesis and stimulates the production of IL-2, which is a potent mitogen for T cells. It also stimulates replication of fibroblasts, a process that facilitates wound repair.

Generally, IL-1β does not enter blood in a bioactive form. Rather, IL-1β in plasma is bound to α2-macroglobulin, an abundant plasma protein. When bound to α2-macroglobulin, IL-1β is inactive. Therefore, it is unlikely that IL-1β can act in an endocrine fashion; rather, IL-1β acts principally in a paracrine or autocrine manner.

IL-1α

Interleukin-1α acts by way of the same receptors as IL-1β, yet the amino acid sequences of IL-1α and IL-1β are only 26% homologous. Whereas the actions of IL-1α and IL-1β are virtually indistinguishable, the amount of IL-1β secreted exceeds that of IL-1α by a factor of 10 under most circumstances.

The Inflammatory Response

The response of mononuclear phagocytes to infection and immunological challenges is extraordinarily rapid. It involves the local activation and chemoattraction of immune cells and the stimulation of antibody production by lymphocytes.

Tumor necrosis factor (TNF)-α, like IL-1β, is produced very rapidly in vastly increased amounts in response to antigenic challenge or infection. For example, in response to bacterial endotoxin (lipopolysaccharide), IL-1β and TNF-α are produced rapidly by mononuclear phagocytes (Fig. 4-4). The maximal production of IL-1β and TNF-α by mononuclear phagocytes occurs within approximately 2 hours of exposure to bacterial endotoxin (Fig. 4-4). The production of IL-6, IL-8, and other cytokines, which is stimulated by IL-1β and TNF-α, occurs later. Also, IL-1β further promotes the formation and secretion of TNF-α. Additionally, IL-1β autoinduction leads to the production of more IL-1β. Thus, the immune response is propagated in this manner. The cytokines IL-1β, TNF-α, and IL-6 are generally referred to collectively as *inflammatory cytokines;* IL-8, MCP-1, and IFN-γ are sometimes included in the group of inflammatory cytokines.

Although the rapid and massive response of the cytokine system to infection and other challenges is essential to the successful containment of infection, the profound effects of this system, if left unchecked, are lethal. Thus, because of the potency of cytokines and the wide-ranging actions, a necessary, indeed crucial, component of the cytokine response is self-containment, involving mechanisms for limiting or even curtailing the potent actions of the inflammatory cytokines.

By way of an example, consider these effects of bacterial infection in blood. Bacterial endotoxin (lipopolysaccharide) acts to increase the production of IL-1β and TNF-α by monocytes (Fig. 4-3). The autoinduction of IL-1β leads to more IL-1β and, thus, more TNF-α. IL-1β acts to promote the production of chemokines (such as IL-8, MCP-1, and others), which in turn act to recruit additional immune cells, including monocytes, neutrophils, and lymphocytes, to the site of infection. Both IL-1β and TNF-α stimulate the formation of IL-6, which circulates to the liver and elicits the production of acute-phase proteins (Fig. 4-3). In the hypothalamus, TNF-α and IL-1β act to stimulate the production of prostaglandins, especially PGE$_2$, which causes an increase in body temperature. Also, TNF-α acts on endothelial cells of blood vessels to promote the formation of prostacylin, a potent vasodilator (Fig. 4-3). The rapid, excessive formation of prostacylin leads to vasodilatation, which is characteristic of the vascular collapse of endotoxic shock with infections by gram-negative microorganisms.

A number of mechanisms can inhibit the continued stimulation of the cytokine system and the action of selected cytokines once the inflammatory response has been initiated. Among them are the rapid degradation of cytokine mRNAs and the production of cytokine inhibitory factors, such as cytokine receptor antagonists (Fig. 4-1), for example, the IL-1 receptor antagonist and proteins that bind cytokines with high affinity. The latter include a family of "soluble" receptors for cytokines (such as TNF-α soluble receptors). These proteins are partial or truncated forms of the plasma membrane–bound cytokine receptors that are present in plasma and bind the cognate receptors with high affinity. Two forms of TNF-α soluble receptors that correspond to the extracellular portions of each of two TNF-α plasma membrane receptors have been identified. These soluble receptors limit the effectiveness of cytokines in tissues that are removed from the site of infection, wound, or antigenic challenge. In addition, the production of IL-10, an inhibitory cytokine, is stimulated by IL-1β; IL-10 acts to limit the inflammatory response to infection by decreasing the activity and replication of T cells.

EFFECTS OF CYTOKINES ON THE HYPOTHALAMIC–PITUITARY–ADRENAL AXIS

The most familiar relationship between the immune and endocrine systems is the potent immunosuppressive action of glucocorticoids. That there are bidirectional responses between the endocrine and immune systems was a more recent observation. Cytokines, as mediators of the immune response, occupy a central role in these bidirectional responses. In fact, cytokines modulate functions of the hypothalamic–pituitary–adrenal axis, the hypothalamic–pituitary–gonadal axis (in women and men), the hypothalamic–pituitary–thyroid axis, and in other functions of the pituitary gland also, including the production of prolactin, GH, and pro-opiomelanocortin (POMC)-derived proteins (for example, β-endorphin, α-melanocyte-stimulating hormone [MSH], in addition to ACTH). These relationships between the immune and endocrine systems are summarized below.

The Origin of Cytokines That Act in the Hypothalamus

There is clear-cut evidence that cytokines, in particular IL-1β, IL-6, and TNF-α, act in the hypothalamus to increase the production of releasing hormones, including corticotropin-releasing hormone (CRH), thyrotropin-releasing hormone (TRH), and luteinizing hormone-releasing hormone (LHRH). If these actions were mediated by systemic cytokines (acting in an endocrine fashion by delivery through the circulation), permeation of the blood–brain barrier by cytokines would be required. The mechanism by which this could occur is not known. It has been postulated that these cytokines may gain access to responsive areas of the brain where the blood–brain barrier is weak or nonfunctional—for example, the median eminence, the organum vasculosum of lamina terminalis of the hypothalamus, the subfornical organ, the choriod plexus, and the area postrema at the base of the fourth ventricle. In contrast, it also has been hypothesized that these cytokines may arise in cells in the brain. One mechanism by which this may occur is by transfer of a signaling agent that is permeable to the blood–brain barrier. Additionally, monocytes, lymphocytes, and macrophages traverse the blood–brain barrier and take up residence in various areas of the brain. Resident monocytes and macrophages may secrete IL-1β and TNF-α in response to bacterial toxin or antigenic challenge. Another potential source of IL-1β in the brain are microglia, which are embryologically and functionally related to macrophages and therefore might be expected to express IL-1β-converting enzyme, which would allow for the processing of pro-IL-1β and the secretion of active IL-1β. In addition, IL-2, IL-4, IL-6, and TNF-α are produced by glial cells. The IL-1 receptors, IL-1 receptor antagonists, and receptors for a number of other cytokines are present in the hypothalamus.

Cytokine Actions in the Hypothalamic–Pituitary–Adrenal Axis

Hypothalamus
Interleukin-1β acts in the hypothalamus to increase CRH production. Both TNF-α and IL-6 also increase hypothalamic CRH production; CRH, produced in increased amounts, acts in the pituitary to stimulate the production of ACTH and other POMC-derived proteins (including β-endorphin and α-MSH). The action of IL-1β to increase ACTH production appears to be dependent strictly on an increase in CRH production. Stated differently, IL-1β does not act directly in the pituitary to increase ACTH production but rather through its action to increase CRH production. In turn, ACTH acts in the adrenal cortex to stimulate the production of cortisol, the principal glucocorticoid in the human.

Pituitary
Pleiotrophic cytokines including IL-6, leukemia-inhibitory factor (LIF), and oncostatin-M act on the anterior pituitary in a paracrine fashion to cause both differentiation and function of cells in this organ. Most notably, these cytokines act synergistically with CRH to stimulate the synthesis of POMC, and thence ACTH (Fig. 4-6). In turn, cortisol secretion by the adrenal is increased. Receptors for IL-6, LIF, and oncostatin M share a receptor called gp130, denoting a 130,000-Da glycoprotein, which is the signal transducing subunit in these receptors. Transmembrane spanning complexes are formed by dimerization with receptor subunits and are activated by ligand binding in the extracellular space, which in turn causes intracellular phosphorylation and cytoplasmic-nuclear signal transduction (Fig. 4-6). Signal transduction through gp130-linked receptors is mediated through the JAK-STAT pathway. The JAKs (Janus kinases) are specific tyrosine kinases that are associated with cytokine receptors. When ligands bind to gp130-linked receptors, members of

Fig. 4-6 In a corticotroph, specific binding of selected cytokines to gp130-linked transmembrane spanning receptors mediates activation of the JAK–STAT pathway, increased POMC gene transcription, and increased ACTH secretion.

the *signal transducers and activators of transcription* (STAT) family of proteins are activated through phosphorylation of a tyrosine. Cytokines that activate the JAK-STAT pathway include IL-4, IL-6, IL-13 LIF, G-CSF, and IFNs (Fig. 4-6). The JAK-STAT pathway is also involved in growth hormone signal transduction.

The CRH acts via a cAMP response element-binding protein to increase POMC expression, whereas LIF does not. Hence, it is likely the synergistic action of these two agents occurs at the level of the POMC gene and beyond the signal transduction mechanisms.

Additionally, LIF may also be important in the differentiation of corticotrophs. Whereas CRH facilitates corticotroph proliferation, LIF inhibits it. Acting synergistically with CRH to facilitate POMC expression, LIF thereby facilitates the differentiation of corticotrophs to a secretory phenotype. Moreover, gp130-dependent signaling also is believed to be important in the fetal pituitary, where these processes may amplify the responsiveness to CRH.

Effects of Cortisol on the Immune System

The increase in cortisol secretion by the adrenal cortex in response to the actions of IL-1β, IL-6, and TNF-α on the hypothalamus and pituitary provokes many profound effects on multiple organ systems. These changes also are caused by the administration of synthetic glucocorticoids such as dexamethasone and betamethasone. In the immune system, cortisol has profound suppressive effects on immune cell trafficking and function. Cortisol inhibits the chemoattraction and accumulation of immune cells at the site of infection or inflammation. Cortisol acts to decrease the production of IL-1β, IL-6, and TNF-α by immune cells and other cells. These actions of cortisol are triggered by a decrease in the transcription of the genes for these cytokines and several chemokines (including a neutrophil chemoattractant protein, IL-8) as well. Cortisol also promotes instability of mRNAs for some cytokines, thereby limiting the levels of cytokines that are attained.

The effects of cytokines also are limited by cortisol because it inhibits the expression of plasma membrane receptors for cytokines and membrane-associated adhesion molecules that are critical for the actions of several cytokines. The effects of inflammatory cytokines to stimulate the production of other mediators of the inflammatory response, such as prostaglandins, platelet-activating factor, nitric oxide, and others, are markedly attenuated by cortisol.

Cortisol also acts to inhibit the production and action of several growth factors that stimulate the proliferation of selected immune cell populations. Cortisol is a potent immunosuppressor of Th1 cells, a subset of T cells called *type 1 helper cells.* Some T cells and eosinophils respond to cortisol by apoptosis (a sequence of specific events in the life of a cell that eventuates in cell death). Cortisol acts to decrease the production of antibodies by B lymphocytes.

The mechanism(s) by which inflammatory responses and immunity are regulated by glucocorticoids have been evaluated in detail. McKay and Cidlowski recently reviewed the current state of extensive knowledge on this important subject. Glucocorticoid-mediated signal transduction is mediated by the glucocorticoid receptor (GR)—a classic steroid nuclear receptor—transcription factor. Another important mediator of inflammatory and immune processes is *nuclear factor-κB* (NF-κb), also an inducible transcription factor. NF-κB stimulates the transcriptional activation of a host of cytokines and other cytokine-induced genes involved in immune and inflammatory processes. These include IL-1, IL-2, IL-6, IL-8, TNF-α, IFN-β, IFN-γ, the chemokine Regulated on Activation, Normal T Cell Expressed and Secreted (RANTES), MCP-1, prostaglandin synthase type 2 (cyclooxygenase-2), and GM-, M-, and G-CSFs. NF-κB is activated by lipopolysaccharide (bacterial endotoxin, LPS) and by activators of protein kinase C. Whereas NF-kB activates a host of genes involved in immunity and inflammation, GR acts to inhibit the expression of many of these same genes, notably inflammatory cytokines and cell adhesion molecules. It now is clear that the mechanism by which GR inhibits immune and inflammatory processes is by inhibition of NF-κB action rather than by a direct action of GR in modulating gene expression. The mechanism by which GR interferes with NF-κB action is through direct, physical interaction, and hence antagonism of NF-κB action at the level of the gene. It is highly likely that the antagonism between these two transcription factors is the principal mechanism whereby homeostasis of host defense mechanisms is maintained. Stated differently, in response to immune challenge, the host defense reaction is profound, exemplified by the presence of a very potent primary cytokine (IL-1), which acts to induce other interleukins and other cytokines. The GR-mediated suppression of NF-κB transcriptional activity limits the production and actions of cytokines and thereby limits cellular damage in the host.

It is likely that other nuclear steroid receptors also interact with NF-kB in an antagonistic fashion. These include the androgen receptor, the estrogen receptor, and the progesterone receptor. The physiological importance of these interactions is not yet well-defined.

Other Effects of Inflammatory Cytokines on Adrenal Steroidogenesis

Whereas TNF-α, together with IL-1 and IL-6, acts to increase cortisol secretion by the adrenal cortex, it also acts to inhibit angiotensin II–induced aldosterone synthesis.

IL1-β Stimulates the Production of POMC-Derived Proteins

In addition to ACTH, the levels of other POMC-derived proteins and peptides are increased in response to IL-1β. Notable among these are β-endorphin and α-MSH. β-Endorphin, an endogenous opioid, effects analgesia. α-MSH has antipyretic and anti-inflammatory actions. Both α-MSH and ACTH act to oppose the effects of inflammatory cytokines by inhibiting the release of CRH in response to IL-6.

Physiologic and Pathophysiologic Importance of Interactions between the Immune System and the Hypothalamic–Pituitary–Adrenal Axis

Interactions between the immune system and the hypothalamic–pituitary–adrenal axis comprise an important negative feedback mechanism. Specifically, the cytokine-mediated stimulation of the hypothalamic–pituitary–adrenal axis leads to the production of glucocorticoid (cortisol in the human) in large amounts, which in turn suppresses the inflammatory response and most components of the immune system. An intriguing model system illustrates these relationships clearly. The Lewis rat is characterized by failure of CRH production in response to antigenic challenge or infection. As a result, these rats do not produce glucocorticoid (corticosterone in the rat) in response to infection or immune challenge. Acute arthritis develops in Lewis rats that are treated with bacterial toxins. This inflammatory disease is suppressed by the administration of synthetic glucocorticoids (such as dexamethasone or betamethasone). These observations are indicative of the physiologic and pathologic responses of the adrenal to the action of cytokines and the ability to recapitulate these relationships by administration of exogenous glucocorticoid.

The normal Fischer rat, in contrast, responds to the administration of bacterial toxin by the development of a normal inflammatory response. Adrenalectomy of the Fischer rat or suppression of adrenal function by the administration of a glucocorticoid antagonist leads to the development of an enhanced susceptibility to inflammatory disease, analogous to that in the Lewis rat. It is postulated that the development of rheumatoid arthritis in humans may be related to decreased cortisol production (or abnormal diurnal rhythm of cortisol secretion), which may be a consequence of an inappropriate response of the hypothalamus to infection or immune challenge.

IMMUNE CELL PRODUCTION OF HYPOTHALAMIC-RELEASING HORMONES AND PITUITARY HORMONES

At one time, ACTH, β-endorphin, and CRH were considered to be exclusive peptide markers of the hypothalamic–pituitary–adrenal axis. Each of these factors is now known to be produced by cells of the immune system and in the human placenta. The POMC-derived peptides (ACTH and β-endorphin) were the first neuroendocrine peptides to be identified as products of macrophages and lymphocytes.

Soon thereafter, CRH production by mononuclear phagocytes was discovered. Many skeptics were silenced by the demonstration that lymphocyte-derived and adrenal-derived POMC and ACTH have identical amino acid sequences. Similar demonstrations for lymphocyte-derived GH and LHRH had convinced even the most doubtful investigators that cells of the immune system produce these agents.

Now more than 20 different "neuroendocrine" factors have been identified as products of T or B lymphocytes, macrophages, mast cells, neutrophils, megakaryocytes, splenocytes, or thymocytes. These include CRH and LHRH, ACTH, TSH, follicle-stimulating hormone (FSH), luteinizing hormone (LH), prolactin, endorphins, met-enkephalin, arginine vasopressin (AVP), oxytocin, somatostatin, vasoactive intestinal polypeptide (VIP), substance P, and neuropeptide Y. Moreover, the regulation of neuroendocrine peptide production by immune cells is similar to that in the hypothalamus and the pituitary, as pointed out by Blalock. One similarity is that the production of trophic factors is in response to the action of releasing hormones. Another similarity is that the production of these hormones is regulated by negative feedback mechanisms similar to those observed in the hypothalamus and pituitary. But there also are several differences: Recall that the production of POMC-derived peptides in the pituitary is induced by CRH and inhibited by glucocorticoids. The same is true of lymphocyte-derived POMC-derived peptides, except that the actions of CRH and glucocorticoid in lymphocytes is indirect. CRH stimulates the production of IL-1β by macrophages; IL-1β induces B-cell production of POMC. Glucocorticoids inhibit the production of IL-1β by macrophages, thereby blocking POMC production indirectly.

The functions and regulation of secretion of these immune cell–derived releasing hormones, trophic factors, and protein hormones have been investigated. Our current understanding of the regulation of production and secretion of these factors is based in part on *in vitro* studies conducted with cells in culture. A number of different potential paracrine actions of these neuroendocrine factors have been discovered, as the following examples illustrate:

1. CRH increases natural killer (NK) cell activity, likely by stimulating POMC, and, thus, β-endorphin production in B lymphocytes.
2. TRH acts on T cells to promote the synthesis and release of TSH, which increases antibody production by B lymphocytes.
3. β-Endorphin, produced by macrophages, lymphocytes, and plasma cells, acts in a paracrine fashion on the opioid receptors on peripheral sensory neuron terminals as an analgesic.
4. T lymphocytes synthesize and release prolactin. These cells also respond to prolactin, which serves to facilitate the proliferative action of IL-2 in these cells.

The physiological and pathophysiological relevance of these findings are intriguing areas of study. Again, as stated by Blalock, who would have believed that an opiate antagonist, acting to block the action of lymphocyte-derived endorphins would be more effective in prolonging allograft survival than an immunosuppressive drug like cyclosporine? Or that a dopamine agonist that blocks prolactin release would be effective in treating experimental allergic encephalomyelitis? Or that GH would facilitate human lymphocyte reconstitution of mice with severe combined immunodeficiency? Or that the inflammatory actions of IL-1β would be attenuated markedly by α-MSH? There is little doubt that the practice of medicine will be profoundly affected as the bidirectional responses between the endocrine and immune systems are deciphered.

EFFECTS OF CYTOKINES ON THE HYPOTHALAMIC–PITUITARY–THYROID AXIS

Like hypothalamic–pituitary–adrenal function, hypothalamic–pituitary–thyroid function is suppressed by inflammatory cytokines. Both IL-1β and TNF-α act to inhibit the production of hypothalamic TRH and pituitary TSH, leading to decreases in the plasma levels of thyroxine (T_4) and triiodothyronine (T_3). Also, IL-1β stimulates the production of somatostatin by the hypothalamus, which inhibits TSH secretion by the pituitary. The principal action of IL-1β to inhibit thyroid function is in the hypothalamus, with minimal direct actions on the pituitary. Additionally, TNF-α inhibits glycosylation of TSH, which decreases its potency in the thyroid gland.

Both IL-1β and TNF-α inhibit iodide uptake by the thyroid; IL-1β also reduces the synthesis of thyroglobulin. TNF-α desensitizes the thyroid to TSH and, consequently, the production of T_4 and T_3 in response to the TSH is attenuated markedly. IFN-γ acts in the thyroid gland to block TSH action and to increase the expression of major histocompatibility complex (MHC) class I and II antigens.

Thus, IL-1β, TNF-α, and IFN-γ act to suppress thyroid function by affecting the hypothalamus, the pituitary, and the thyroid gland. It is possible, but not proven, that these direct actions of cytokines contribute to the development of *euthyroid sick syndrome,* a description of disorders characterized by decreased plasma levels of T_3 (see Chapter 13).

Cytokines, the Thyroid Gland, and Autoimmune Disease

Another postulated action of cytokines in the thyroid relates to the development of autoimmune disorders that affect this gland. Thyroid autoimmune disease, caused by the production of antibodies against self antigens expressed on cells of the thyroid gland, is characterized by impaired thyroid function. Normally, only non–self-antigens are recognized by T cells as targets for immune response. The production of anti-thyroid autoantibodies is induced in response to thyroid infiltration of T lymphocytes, which produce IFN-γ. The expression of MHC class II antigens is induced by IFN-γ. Because the expression of MHC antigens in the thyroid is usually rather low, the high level of expression in response to IFN-γ is believed to cause a breakdown in recognition of and distinction between self and non-self. Additional lymphocytes are recruited to the site and commence antibody production against antigens presented in association with these MHC molecules.

CYTOKINES AND THE HYPOTHALAMIC–PITUITARY–OVARIAN AXIS

In women with acute or chronic severe illness or infection, delays in ovulation and even chronic anovulation resulting in amenorrhea or oligoamenorrhea are common.

This process is associated in part with decreased gonadotropin secretion and, thus, hypogonadotropic hypogonadism. The involvement of cytokines in this process also is implied from the observation that the altered state of ovarian function is temporary; namely, cyclic ovulation returns once the illness is resolved. Various studies conducted in experimental animals indicate that cytokines may modulate the normal function of the anterior pituitary by way of a direct action of the cytokine on pituitary function. Ovarian estradiol-17β, secreted in large amounts by the mature graffian follicle, serves as the stimulus for the release of LH (the LH surge) that eventuates in the induction of ovulation by the mature follicle. IL-1β acts to inhibit the estrogen-induced surge in LH release, thereby supporting the hypothesis that cytokines are involved in causing the anovulation observed in women with severe illness.

Effects of Cytokines on Hypophyseal LH and FSH

In pituitary cells in culture, IL-1β induces the release of luteinizing hormone (LH) and follicle-stimulating hormone (FSH), although this finding is not readily reproducible *in vivo*. Pituitary cells also produce cytokines, notably IL-6. This observation has led to the suggestion that IL-6 may serve as an intrapituitary-releasing factor. IL-1β acts upon pituitary cells to cause increased synthesis and release of IL-6; and acting directly upon pituitary cells, IL-1β and IL-6 promote the release of FSH and LH in amounts similar to those evoked in response to gonadotropin-releasing hormone (GnRH). Other cytokines, namely activin and inhibin (members of the TGF-β family) of gonadal origin, act to modulate the release of FSH from the pituitary (for details see Chapter 9).

Cytokine Action in the Ovary

Appreciable evidence shows that cytokines may modify gonadal function in a physiologic and pathophysiologic sense. Pro-IL-β mRNA levels increase in the macrophage-enriched ovarian theca interna at about the time of ovulation; this response appears to be specific because an increase in the level of this mRNA is not identified in peripheral blood monocytes during the same time of the ovarian cycle. Granulosa cells of the ovary also produce IL-6, and the production of IL-6 by granulosa cells can be increased by treatment of these cells with IL-1β. A growing body of evidence indicates that IL-6 and other chemokines modulate the rate of formation of steroid hormones in the gonads and adrenal cortex and in extraglandular tissues as well (see p. 110). For example, the rate of estrogen formation by aromatization of C_{19}-steroids in adipose tissue stromal cells is increased strikingly by IL-11 and oncostatin-M and by inflammatory cytokines and other mediators of inflammation.

Interleukin-6 inhibits the gonadotropin-dependent formation of progesterone in granulosa cells. Both TGF-β1 and TGF-β2 are produced by the granulosa cells, and the rate of formation of TGF-β2 is increased specifically by treatment with FSH. In addition, it has been shown that TGF-β acts in a number of steroid-producing endocrine cells (including the adrenal cortex) to inhibit steroidogenesis. This action of TGF-β is attributable in part to inhibition of the transcription of the gene that encodes steroid 17α-hydroxylase/17,20-desmolase.

It has been stated often that there is a delicate endocrine balance involving the brain, pituitary, and ovary that is essential for optimal ovarian function, which culminates in the rupture of a single mature follicle with ovulation. This premise, however, is almost certainly incorrect. The regularity of cyclic ovulation in women, despite rather wide differences in the peripheral levels of gonadotropins and ovarian steroids, is testimony to the fact that a delicate endocrine balance is not essential to normalcy of ovarian function. Moreover, a variety of environmental, psychological, and pathophysiological processes may come to bear without affecting the regular cyclic ovarian function of most women. These observations suggest that there is, in addition to the brain–pituitary–ovarian axis, an intraovarian control system that modulates external stimuli in such a manner as to favor normal ovarian function with ovulation despite wide variations in the environment and in bodily function. It is quite possible that the cytokines, produced in the ovary *in situ,* contribute to this intraovarian control. But in addition to this, the formation of cytokines in response to acute or severe illness may act at the level of the brain or pituitary to forestall ovulation and thereby prevent pregnancy during times of environmental or physical danger. Thus, it can be envisioned that the cytokine family of proteins acts in a manner that modulates ovarian function—normalizing ovarian steroidogenesis and ovulation during mild fluctuations in external forces, but temporarily halting ovulation during times of impending disaster.

Cytokine Action in the Testis

Infection and illness also are associated with impaired testicular function. As in the ovary, IL-1β acts to inhibit steroidogenesis in the Leydig cells of the testis. TNF-α potentiates this inhibitory action of IL-1β. IL-6 is produced in the Sertoli cells in response to FSH. Interferons (IFNs), which are produced in the gonads, also act in an autocrine and paracrine manner to inhibit steroidogenesis.

CYTOKINES AND A STEROID-RESPONSIVE TISSUE: THE ENDOMETRIUM

The *endometrium* is a tissue that serves an essential role in reproduction and it is a classic example of sex steroid hormone responsiveness (Chapter 9). Normal function of the hypothalamic–pituitary–gonadal axes in women and men, sperm fertilization of oocyte, and blastocyst development are futile in the absence of the endometrium. Under the influence of estradiol-17β, the endometrium grows at a very rapid rate that is characterized primarily by an increase in volume due to a rapid increase in the glandular epithelium of this tissue. After ovulation, with the formation of progesterone by the corpus luteum, the endometrium is modified to a "secretory"' type that also is associated with very specific changes in the stromal component of this tissue. The stromal changes include an increase in the extracellular fluid and extracellular matrix. The mesenchymal cells of the endometrium, those that form the stroma, are modified in a process referred to as *decidualization.* Presumably, the decidualized endometrium is ideal for blastocyst implantation and placentation.

Among all human tissues, the endometrium is one of the most distinctive. It is the only tissue that undergoes rapid growth at cyclic intervals, only to be purposefully targeted for death by hypoxia and necrosis at the time of menstruation and endometrial shedding during nonfertile cycles.

The endometrium is shed in most women no fewer than 450 times, (i.e., with each nonfertile cycle). The process of endometrial growth and desquamation is unique to only a few primates, namely humans, Old World monkeys, and the great apes. This is the case because these are the only species in which the endometrium is supplied with blood by a peculiar set of arteries referred to as the *spiral* or *curling arteries*. The response of these vessels to the endocrine events of the ovarian cycle and to modifications in the volume of the endometrium gives rise to a series of vascular changes that support endometrial growth, endometrial tissue modifications for blastocyst implantation, and (in the absence of implantation) tissue hypoxia, necrosis, and desquamation with hemorrhage.

Bone Marrow–Derived Cells of the Endometrium

During the course of each endometrial cycle, there is a modification in the cellular components of the endometrium due to striking, but predictable, changes in the number and type of bone marrow–derived cells.

One of the more intriguing cells of the endometrium is the so-called large granular lymphocyte, which is present in secretory endometrium and in decidua in very large numbers. These cells are a very particular type of lymphocyte and are present in peripheral blood in very small numbers. It is postulated, therefore, that these cells originated in bone marrow, but in response to the endocrine changes of the ovarian cycle, replicate *in situ* in the endometrium and decidua. A role for prolactin in the modulation of function of these cells is especially attractive. These cells, in turn, are believed to serve as regulating trophoblast invasion into the endometrium during the time of blastocyst implantation and placentation. The cytotrophoblasts of the invading placenta do not express MHC-type II antigens; thus, it is believed that this is one mechanism whereby the invading allogeneic tissue of the fetus is accepted. But in human pregnancy with the formation of the hemochorioendothelial type of placenta, the invasiveness of the trophoblasts is extensive, involving penetration of the endometrial epithelium, stroma, and the direct invasion and destruction of the walls of the spiral arteries that supply the endometrium with blood. Therefore, some mechanism must be in place to halt the trophoblastic invasion; otherwise, each pregnancy would constitute a case of choriocarcinoma, or malignancy of the trophoblast. It is believed that the large granular cells act to permit and thus inhibit the invasiveness of the trophoblast by way of the expression of an MHC-type I antigen, called *HLA-G*, that is monomeric (i.e., it is identical in all persons). It has been established that the immune cells recognize not only foreign antigens (non–self-antigens) but also recognize the lack of self (or "missing self") in an adjacent cell.

Cytokines, Hormones, and Blastocyst Implantation

In humans and other catarrhine primates (specifically, great apes and Old World monkeys), blastocyst implantation includes trophoblastic invasion of the endometrium and endometrial blood vessels to establish a hemochorioendothelial type of placentation. With this type of placental formation, maternal blood comes into direct contact with the trophoblasts, which are of fetal origin. Thus, the maternal blood is in direct contact with an allogeneic tissue graft since paternal genes are expressed in fetal tissues. Immunologists and reproductive biologists alike have been fascinated by the fact that the foreign tissue graft of the fetus is accepted by the maternal tissues without evidence of immunological rejection. The involvement of cytokines in this process of maternal acceptance of the fetal graft is almost certain.

Moreover, the action of cytokines, produced by one of several cells of the potential implantation site, is virtually assured in the regulation of this process. It has been demonstrated that a host of cytokines are produced by the endometrium and the decidua. Some of these cytokines are produced primarily, if not exclusively, by the bone marrow–derived cells normally present in the endometrium and decidua, and others are formed by the decidual cells per se. Of interest is a potential role for LIF in endometrial and decidual differentiation and function. There is evidence that LIF gene expression and action in human endometrium is controlled by progesterone, directly or indirectly through effects on the expression of other cytokines, and it is speculated that LIF acts on the blastocyst to facilitate implantation (Fig. 4-7).

Cytokines, Hormones, and Endometrium as an Endocrine Target Organ

In addition to the responsiveness of the endometrium to sex steroid hormones, the decidua (the specialized endometrium of pregnancy) also is a source of endocrine secretions: the decidua produces prolactin in enormous quantities. The prolactin produced by the decidua does not enter the peripheral circulation of the mother but rather is transported exclusively to amniotic fluid. Moreover, factors regulating the release of prolactin by the anterior pituitary (dopamine, TRH) are not operative in the decidual cell to modulate the rate of prolactin formation in this tissue. The role

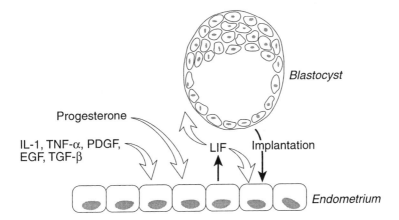

Fig. 4-7 The production of leukemia inhibitor factor (LIF) by endometrial surface epithelial cells may be stimulated by progesterone, directly or indirectly through cytokine and growth factors. In turn, LIF may facilitate implantation of the blastocyst. (Redrawn from *Cytokine Bulletin,* R&D Systems, Spring 1997.)

of the prolactin produced in the endometrium has not been defined, but several proposals have been made. The most common is that prolactin acts on the fetal membranes, which are physically contiguous with the decidua during pregnancy, to modulate the rate of water and solute transport to and from the amniotic fluid. Direct evidence for this proposition has not been presented, however. The intriguing relationship between prolactin and lymphocytes may be important in the maintenance of pregnancy and the development of the fetus. Prolactin acts on lymphocytes to increase immunological responsiveness; the formation of prolactin by lymphocytes has been demonstrated.

TGF-β, Steroid Hormones, Vasoactive Peptides, and Endometrial Function

It is also suspected that TGF-β serves an important role in the modulation of immune and endocrine functions in the endometrium. Menstruation is ultimately the result of the withdrawal of steroid hormones produced by the corpus luteum, namely, progesterone and estradiol-17β. This process comes about as follows: the endometrium, as stated above, undergoes rapid growth during the follicular phase of the ovarian cycle—this is referred to as the *proliferative phase* of the endometrial cycle. The spiral arteries, which are so named because of an extraordinary propensity of these vessels to curl and twist, also grow; indeed, these vessels lengthen at a rate far greater than the rate of increase in endometrial tissue volume. This disparity in growth between the two tissues results in even greater curling and spiraling. It has been suggested that the rate of blood flow to the endometrium may be regulated in a paracrine manner by vasoactive peptides produced in the endometrial stromal cells: parathyroid hormone–related protein (PTH-rP; Chapter 15), a potent vasodilator, is produced in the endometrial stromal cells, as is endothelin-1 (ET-1; Chapter 7), a potent vasoconstrictor. Formation of PTH-rP is increased in response to progesterone treatment of the endometrial stromal cell, whereas the expression of prepro-ET-1 is inhibited by progesterone treatment. TGF-β acts in the stromal cells to counteract the action of progesterone. Thus, TGF-β acts as an antiprogestin by way of a progesterone receptor–independent process in a gene-specific manner to modulate the function of endometrial cells.

The expression of TGF-β in the endometrium increases at the time of decidualization and at the time of blastocyst implantation. Possibly, the increase in TGF-β expression first observed in the endometrium is the result of the early stages of hypoxia, which come about because of the further coiling of the spiral vessels as progesterone levels begin to decline during the late secretory phase of the endometrial cycle. This happens as follows: with the great lengthening of the endometrial spiral arteries that accompanies endometrial tissue growth, there is even greater curling of the vessels. With progesterone withdrawal, there is a reduction in endometrial tissue volume without a reduction in the spiral artery length. This creates further coiling of these vessels, which becomes so severe as to impede blood flow. With the reduction in blood flow, hypoxia begins. As the volume of the endometrium is reduced even further, the coiling of the spiral arteries becomes so severe that blood flow is almost completely impeded. Hypoxia becomes severe, resulting in necrosis of this tissue. Just prior to the onset of bleeding that accompanies menstruation, however, the spiral arteries enter into a phase of severe vasoconstriction. This vaso-constrictive phenomenon is believed to be the consequence of ET-1 action via the adventitial surface of the spiral arteries; the ET-1 originates in the contiguous stromal cells of the endometrium, which also is the site of TGF-β formation. Until recently, it was believed that progesterone withdrawal was the cause of the onset of menstruation. It is now clear that this concept was an overly simplistic view of the physiological processes involved.

In retrospect, it is easy to understand that a process as physiologically important as menstruation and preparation for a renewed opportunity for pregnancy could not be left to the uncertainties of progesterone withdrawal. Rather, the regulation of endometrial blood flow by locally produced vasoactive peptides is a much more reasonable explanation for the lack of excessive blood loss in most women with menstruation; namely that ET-1 acts as the tourniquet of the endometrium. By promoting severe vasoconstriction of these vessels at the time of menstruation, blood loss is limited.

In the endometrium, as in other tissues, TGF-β is a potent inducer of ET-1 formation. Thus, TGF-β is poised to participate in the process of implantation by promoting decidualization of the endometrium or in the process of menstruation by promoting the formation of the vasoconstrictor, ET-1. TGF-β acts to promote its own formation (i.e., autoinduction). In this manner, TGF-β can be produced in the endometrium in response to generalized changes in the endometrial environment (for example, sex steroid hormone modifications or hypoxia) or to the secretions of the implanting blastocyst, which includes the trophoblastic formation of TGF-β. Indeed, with implantation there is a wave-like propagation of the TGF-β immunoreactivity in the endometrium that begins at the site of implantation and proceeds outward to involve the entire endometrium in a decidual response. The molecular mechanism by which TGF-β acts through receptor-mediated activation of kinases in a variety of cell types has been reviewed recently by Hu and colleagues.

Interestingly, PTH-rP is produced in many normal, nonmalignant tissues, and there appears to be an especially high production of PTH-rP in tissues of reproduction. Very large amounts of PTH-rP are produced in the mammary tissue of lactating women and experimental animals, and PTH-rP enters the milk in very large quantities. Additionally, PTH-rP is also produced in the myometrium during pregnancy and in the decidua of women; it is also produced in the placenta and in other fetal organs including the kidney and parathyroid gland. In fact, it is now believed that PTH-rP is the parathormone of the fetus. It is envisioned that the formation of PTH-rP in the endometrium serves not only to increase vasodilatation and endometrial and decidual blood flow but also to facilitate the transfer of calcium across the trophoblast after implantation of the blastocyst. TGF-β also acts to increase the rate of formation of PTH-rP in the endometrium and particularly in the endometrial stromal cell, the progenitor cell of the decidua. PTH-rP, but not PTH, will cause a transfer of calcium across the trophoblast from mother to fetus.

The endometrium, therefore, is virtually a prototype tissue for an examination of the relationships between immune and endocrine functions. The endometrium also acts to control its own cytokine destiny; it has been demonstrated that chemoattractant proteins are produced by the mesenchymal cells of the endometrium. IL-8, which is a potent chemoattractant for neutrophils and T lymphocytes as well as monocyte chemoattractant protein-1 (MCP-1), is produced in the endometrial stromal cells, and the rate of formation of these chemoattractants is modulated by the sex steroid hormones of the ovarian cycle. It is likely, therefore, that the endometrium, in response to the changing sex steroid hormone milieu of the cycle, is able to attract the proper bone marrow–derived cells into this tissue to further modulate the function of the endometrium. At the same time, the endometrium is poised to respond rapidly to infection. As a consequence of the anatomic reality of the female genital tract, the endometrium is potentially accessible to the outside environment via the patent cervical and vaginal canals. Infection in the endometrium during pregnancy would represent a great risk for septic abortion or preterm labor. The containment of infection by the efficient immune system of the endometrium undoubtedly contributes to the high success rate of pregnancies, despite the finding of microorganisms in large quantities in the vaginal fluid of all women.

There is increasing evidence that sex steroid hormones and cytokines act in concert to modulate the differentiation and function of the human endometrium. For example, it is likely that the process of menstruation involves the actions of matrix metalloproteinases (MMPs), which affect the degradation of basement membrane and extracellular matrix components. The production of these enzymes is regulated hormonally, and the specific tissue/cell localization in the endometrium is supportive of local regulation. Definitive evidence from *in vitro* studies shows that a number cytokines, including IL-1, TNF-α, IL-8, MCP-1, and TGF-β, arising either in endometrial stromal or epithelial cells or from macrophages, neutrophils, or mast cells, may modulate the expression of selected MMPs in this tissue (Fig. 4-8).

EFFECTS OF CYTOKINES ON EXTRAGLANDULAR ESTROGEN BIOSYNTHESIS: IMPLICATIONS IN TUMOR GROWTH

Estrogen is synthesized principally in the ovary of reproductive-age women. In postmenopausal women, estrogen is derived principally by extraglandular conversion of C_{19}-steroids to estrone in peripheral tissues including skin, muscle, fat and bone, by the enzyme complex referred to as *aromatase* (Chapter 9). Thereafter, estrone is converted to the bioactive estrogen, estradiol-17β, by 17β-hydroxysteroid dehydrogenase type 1 (Chapter 9). Estrogen is believed to increase the rate of growth of some breast cancers. This action appears to be distinct from that in endometrial cancer, where estrogen seems to have a causative role. Aromatase is expressed in stromal cells of the breast adipose tissue. In breast cancer, the levels of aromatase are increased in stromal cells near the site of the tumor. Investigators in the laboratories of Simpson and Mendelson found that inflammatory mediators including prostaglandin E_2, IL-1, IL-6, and TNF-α caused marked increases in the expression of aromatase in adipose stromal cells. Interestingly, the effectiveness of IL-1 and IL-6 in stimulating aromatase expression is enhanced greatly in the presence of a glucocorticosteroid. Possible sources of these cytokines and PGE_2 include macrophages (PGE_2, TNF-α, and IL-1), infiltrating lymphocytes (IL-6), and adipose stromal cells per se (IL-6). The stimulatory action of IL-6 on aromatase expression is markedly enhanced by IL-6 soluble receptor, which may be derived from malignant epithelial cells. In addition, the stimulatory effects of TNF-α might be a consequence

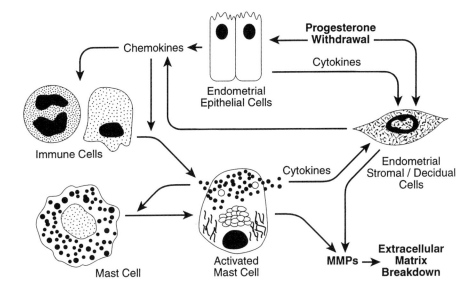

Fig. 4-8 A decline in the plasma level of progesterone (progesterone withdrawal), as occurs near the end of the ovarian cycle when progesterone production by the corpus luteum decreases, affects epithelial and stromal cells of the endometrium directly. In addition, progesterone withdrawal is associated with a change in the tissue distribution and population of immune cells, including mast cells, macrophages, and other migratory immune cells. These cells may be modulated by factors, including chemokines and cytokines, produced by endometrial epithelial and stromal cells in response to progesterone. The production of matrix metalloproteinases by mast cells and immune cells will, in response to this progesterone-regulated series of events, facilitate breakdown of the extracellular matrix and cellular basement membranes in the endometrium, thereby promoting the process of menstruation. (Redrawn from Salamonson, Trends Endocrinol Metab 9:308, 1998.)

of an increase in gp130 expression, which is important for IL-6 and IL-6 soluble receptor-mediated signaling (Fig. 4-6).

SUGGESTED READING

Blalock JE: The syntax of immune–neuroendocrine communication. Immunol Today 15: 504–511, 1994.

Chrousos GP: The hypothalamic–pituitary–adrenal axis and immune-related inflammation. N Engl J Med 332:1351–1362, 1995.

Clemens MJ: *Cytokines.* Information Press, Oxford, UK, pp. 1–121, 1991.

Fukata J, Imura H, and Nakao K: Cytokines as mediators in the regulation of the hypothalamic–pituitary–adrenocortical function. J Clin Invest 16:141–155, 1993.

Gaillard RC: Neuroendocrine–immune system interactions: The immune–hypothalamo–pituitary–adrenal axis. Trends Endocrinol Metab 5:303–309, 1994.

Hamblin AS: *Cytokines and Cytokine Receptors,* IRL Press, Oxford University Press, New York, 1993.

Hu PP-C, Datto MB, and Wang X-F: Molecular mechanisms of transforming growth factor-β signaling. Endocr Rev 19:349–363, 1998.

McKay LI, and Cidlowski: Molecular control of immune/inflammatory responses: Interactions between nuclear factor-κB and steroid receptor-signaling pathways. Endocr Rev 20:435–459, 1999.

Melmed S: gp130-Related cytokines and their receptors in the pituitary. Trends Endocrinol Metab 9:155–161, 1998.

Reed MJ, and Purohit A: Breast cancer and the role of cytokines in regulating estrogen synthesis: An emerging hypothesis. Endocr Rev 18:701–715, 1997.

Reichlin S: Neuroendocrine–immune interactions. N Engl J Med 329:1246–1253, 1993.

Salamonsen, LA: Current concepts of the mechanisms of menstruation: A normal process of tissue destruction. Trends Endocrinol Metab 9:305–309, 1998.

Sasano H, and Harada N: Intratumoral aromatase in human breast, endometrial and ovarian malignancies. Endocr Rev 19:593–607, 1998.

Tabibzadeh S: Cytokines and the hypothalamic–pituitary–ovarian–endometrial axis. Hum Reprod Update 9:947–967, 1994.

5

Assessment of Endocrine Function

JAMES E. GRIFFIN

The first step in the laboratory assessment of endocrine function is usually to measure hormone levels. The ability to measure hormone concentrations accurately in plasma and urine has greatly enhanced our understanding of normal endocrine function. Perhaps the single most important factor in the development of modern endocrinology has been the discovery and use of the radioimmunoassay to measure the small quantities of hormones that circulate in the blood. Because static hormone measurements may not provide sufficient insight into the status of a given endocrine system, various dynamic endocrine tests have been developed. These dynamic endocrine tests usually take advantage of a known action of a hormone or of the mechanisms that control its secretion in order to probe for evidence of an abnormality of endocrine function. And as we have gained understanding of the receptor mechanisms of hormone action, assessing the number and binding affinity of a hormone's receptors in certain target tissues has become increasingly important. This chapter deals with these various ways of assessing endocrine function.

PLASMA HORMONE LEVELS

Types of Assays

Hormones circulating in the plasma were first detected by *in vivo* bioassays in which plasma or extracts of plasma were injected into animals and a biological response was measured. Unfortunately, most *in vivo* bioassays lack the precision, sensitivity, and specificity to measure the low concentrations in plasma and are inconvenient to perform. Real progress in measuring plasma hormone levels came almost 40 years ago with the use of competitive binding and subsequently the development of the radioimmunoassay. In both these assays the unknown concentration of a hormone in plasma is estimated by the ability of the hormone to compete for binding to a specific binding protein (antibody in the case of radioimmunoassays) with a labeled hormone. By comparing the competition of a known amount of hormone in a reference standard with the plasma or plasma extract, the amount of hormone in the plasma can be estimated. The observation that almost any hormone could be used as an antigen to develop a specific antibody meant that the technique could be applied to hormones without known binding proteins. In many such immunoassays, the hormone is labeled with an isotope (radioimmunoassay); however, nonisotopic immunoassays have become common in which an enzyme or fluorescent tag is used instead of an isotope. In some instances, these nonisotopic assays are quite sensitive and readily automated. Because assays that do not involve radioactivity result in less equipment costs and no potential risk of exposing personnel to radioactivity, they are preferable. Immunoassays have been developed for all polypeptide, steroid, and thyroid hormones.

For many hormones, the traditional competitive immunoassay is being replaced by another form of immunoassay termed the *immunometric assay*. These immunometric assays often have better sensitivity and specificity than the competitive immunoassay and can be accomplished in a shorter period of time (see below).

While radioimmunoassays provide information about immunoreactive hormone in the plasma, they do not necessarily correlate with biological activity of the measured hormone. The site in the molecule to which the antibody is directed may not be the site involved in receptor binding (see Chapter 3). Thus, an attempt was made to utilize the interaction of the hormone with its specific receptor in radioreceptor assays and in certain *in vitro* bioassays. In a radioreceptor assay the specific receptor sites on cells or cellular components are substituted for the antibody as a binding protein for the hormone (or ligand). Thus, the specificity of binding is determined not by the antibody determinants but by the biological receptor that mediates hormone action. Such radioreceptor assays can add to the information obtained from radioimmunoassays by assessing in some sense "bioactive" hormone, as when there is heterogeneity of a polypeptide hormone (e.g., insulin or growth hormone) in plasma. The radioreceptor assay may also be useful in assessing total activity in plasma related to a class of compounds interacting with one type of receptor, such as competition for a labeled glucocorticoid binding to the glucocorticoid receptor. Likewise, potential drug interference with androgen receptor binding has been assessed by competition of such compounds with labeled androgen for binding to the androgen receptor. Radioreceptor assays are also useful in assessing the presence of autoantibodies to hormone receptors in the plasma of some subjects with endocrine disorders—for example, antibodies to the thyrotropin or insulin receptors.

Although radioreceptor assays give some clue to the biological activity of a hormone, they measure only the first step in hormone action, the binding of hormone to its receptor. They do not assess the effects of hormone–receptor interactions in generating second messenger(s) or in stimulating a specific response. Thus, the assessment of plasma hormone levels has come full circle with the development of *in vitro* bioassays. These assays involve the incubation of plasma or plasma extracts with endocrine tissues, membrane preparations, or cultured cells. Perhaps the most extensively used of these *in vitro* bioassays is the dispersed rat Leydig cell assay for luteinizing hormone (LH) and human chorionic gonadotropin (hCG) in which the testosterone response to gonadotropic stimulation is measured. This assay has greater sensitivity than the radioimmunoassay or radioreceptor assays. It permits the detection of bioactive LH when immunoreactive LH is unmeasurable, and has made it possible to demonstrate physiological regulation of the qualitative aspects of LH secretion in the form of changing bioactive to immunoactive ratios of LH in the plasma. The exact chemical nature of these qualitative differences in circulating LH is not fully understood.

One way to assess for potential qualitative differences in a circulating hormone is Western analysis of the protein migration in a gel followed by the molecular biology techniques to assess the gene as described in Chapter 2.

Principles of Radioimmunoassay

The principle underlying radioimmunoassay of hormones is the competitive inhibition of binding of a radiolabeled antigen (Ag*) (hormone) to antibody (Ab) by unlabeled antigen (Ag) present in a reference hormone standard or in a plasma sample (the unknown):

$$Ag^* + Ab \underset{K_d}{\overset{K_a}{\rightleftharpoons}} Ag^* - Ab$$

$$Ag + Ab \underset{K_d}{\overset{K_a}{\rightleftharpoons}} Ag - Ab$$

The antigen–antibody reaction is reversible, as shown by the arrows, with an association rate constant of K_a and dissociation rate constant of K_d. The rate of dissociation is slower than the rate of association, and at equilibrium the observed amount of antigen bound to antibody is a result of the combined rates of association and dissociation. Following an appropriate period of incubation the antibody-bound antigen (B) is separated from the unbound or free antigen (F) by one of several different methods. Because a fixed amount of antibody is present in each assay tube, the amount of labeled hormone bound to antibody (the measured radioactivity) is a function of the concentration of unlabeled hormone in either the standard or the unknown sample. The higher the concentration of unlabeled hormone, the lower the quantity of radioactive hormone bound to the fixed amount of antibody. The results of a radioimmunoassay can be plotted several different ways. The plot of the ratio of B/F labeled hormone, or the ratio of the amount bound in the presence of standard (B) to the amount bound in the absence of any unlabeled hormone (B_0), as a function of amount of standard, is curvilinear (Fig. 5-1). To facilitate automated calculation of results, logarithmic transformation of the data expressed as B/B_0 that usually results in a straight line is often used. However, one should keep in mind that there are limitations to linear transformation of radioimmunoassay curves in that they obscure the lack of sensitivity at both ends of the standard curve. As shown in the curvilinear plot of Figure 5-1, the ability to determine reliably the unknown hormone concentration when the B/B_0 ratio falls on the portions of the curve with the least slope (e.g., 5–10 ng and 500–1000 ng) is quite limited despite the ability of logarithmic transformation of the data to give calculated values. A requirement for validation of a radioimmunoassay is that a dilution curve of the reference standard and the hormone to be measured must exhibit parallel dose–response lines as evidence of similar interaction with the antibody.

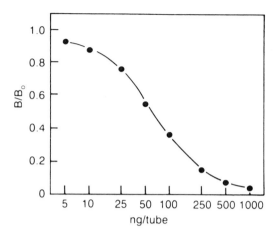

Fig. 5-1 Standard curve for radioimmunoassay of plasma testosterone. The ratio of the amount of radioactive testosterone bound in the presence of standard (*B*) to the amount bound in the absence of any unlabeled hormone (*B_0*) is plotted as a function of the amount of standard (unlabeled hormone) in each assay tube. Note that it is a semilogarithmic plot and that assay sensitivity is low at both extremes of hormone concentration.

Antibodies suitable for radioimmunoassays are usually of the IgG class of immunoglobulins. Partially purified hormones are injected into laboratory animals to induce synthesis of immunoglobulins with sufficiently high sensitivity and specificity. If the hormone has a molecular size less than 1000 Da, it may be necessary to couple it to a carrier protein such as albumin to make it sufficiently immunogenic. In general, small peptides, steroids, and thyroid hormones need to be coupled to carrier proteins. Antibodies produced in this manner are polyclonal. It is also possible to produce monoclonal antibodies to hormones. For routine use, however, these monoclonal antibodies have not proved superior to traditional polyclonal antibodies because in general they are not of the highest affinity that might be found in a population of polyclonal antibodies.

Peptide and thyroid hormones are labeled with ^{125}I. For peptide hormones iodination is performed using $Na^{125}I$ to incorporate the label into tyrosyl or histidyl residues in the hormone. With small polypeptides lacking tyrosine or histidine in their structure, it is necessary to add a tyrosyl residue or substitute it for another acid in a manner to minimally alter the conformation of the polypeptide. For optimal stability and immunoreactivity, only one atom of ^{125}I is incorporated per mole of hormone. With steroid hormones, ^{3}H is incorporated into the structure with a variable number of ^{3}H atoms per molecule to achieve the desired specific activity. The presence of ^{3}H in the structure does not result in any difference in immunoreactivity compared with unlabeled hormone.

Antibody-bound and free hormone can be separated by several different methods. The most widely used method for polypeptide hormone assays is the precipitation of the antigen–antibody complex with a second antibody. Thus, if the first antibody (to the hormone) was generated in a rabbit, an antibody to rabbit γ-globulin generated in another species is used to precipitate the original antigen–antibody complex. The most common means of separating antibody-bound and free hormone in steroid radioimmunoassays is by using dextran-coated charcoal. The unbound steroid is adsorbed to the surface of the charcoal and centrifuged to the bottom of the tube. The soluble antigen–antibody complex remains in the supernatant.

Problems in the Interpretation of Radioimmunoassays

In selecting an antisera for use in a given assay one must consider its specificity to avoid problems in the interpretation of assay results. The glycoprotein hormones LH, follicle-stimulating hormone (FSH), thyroid-stimulating hormone (thyrotropin, TSH), and hCG are examples of a group of related hormones that may present problems in assay specificity. Because they contain a common α-subunit, antisera generated to the intact hormone may cross-react with other members of the group. As it is the β-subunit of each of these hormones that confers immunological and biological specificity, it is necessary to select antisera that recognize this component of the molecule if the assay is to have appropriate specificity.

Furthermore, problems may arise in assay specificity due to heterogeneity in the forms of a given peptide hormone that circulates in the blood. Many peptide hormones have glandular precursors (see Chapter 2) with different biological activities that circulate to a greater or lesser extent depending on the clinical situation. Likewise, some peptide hormones have inactive metabolites that normally circulate but may be present in greater concentrations in given disease states. Thus, proinsulin may at times be present in the circulation with full immunoreactivity but less biological activity than insulin itself. And in the case of hormone metabolites, it is now recognized that a C-terminal portion of the parathyroid hormone (PTH) molecule is a metabolite that has a longer half-life than the intact hormone and is measured with some antisera in addition to intact PTH. The increased levels of the C-terminal fragment that accumulate in states of diminished renal function can result in inaccurate assessments of PTH. Fortunately, other antisera are available that recognize the intact molecule primarily by being directed to determinants on the N-terminal portion of the molecule (see Chapter 15).

Some peptide hormones are quite sensitive to proteases present in serum. The degradation of hormone before assay may result in artifactually low levels of hormone being measured as the degraded hormone may not react with antibody if its structure is sufficiently altered. In such instances, protease inhibitors may be added to the tube before the blood sample is collected, or the blood may be quickly refrigerated to inhibit enzyme activity. Corticotropin (ACTH), for example, requires such special attention to avoid degradation.

Circulating endogenous antibodies to hormones provide an additional problem in the interpretation of radioimmunoassays. Fortunately, such antibodies rarely occur spontaneously; however, antibodies to insulin are common in diabetic patients who are receiving exogenous insulin. The effect of a circulating antibody to the hormone on the usual double antibody radioimmunoassay is a spuriously high estimated concentration of the hormone in the plasma sample. The human circulating antibody will bind labeled hormone in addition to the assay antibody obtained from an animal species. However, the addition of a second antibody will only precipitate the labeled hormone bound to the animal antibody, resulting in apparently low bound radioactivity that is interpreted as high concentrations of unlabeled hormone in the unknown sample. When circulating antihormone antibodies are suspected, their presence can be detected by omitting the assay antibody and incubating the labeled hormone with the patient's plasma and then using agents such as ammonium sulfate to precipitate the hormone–antibody complex.

Characteristics and Advantages of Immunometric Assays

To achieve optimal sensitivity in the classical radioimmunoassay, the concentration of the labeled ligand must be critically adjusted, the antibody must be quite dilute, and the incubation must often be conducted for more than 24 hours. The immunometric assay method differs from the radioimmunoassay in several ways and does not have the requirements listed above for achieving high sensitivity. First, there is no labeled hormone or ligand in the assay. Instead, one of two monoclonal antibodies, each offering high specificity, is either labeled with radioiodine or another detection system. The second antibody is usually directed at another antigenic site on the hormone of interest and is coupled to a solid phase (e.g., a bead) for separation. Either antibody may be reacted with the ligand first. However, typically the labeled antibody is involved in the first incubation, and a "sandwich" reaction results when the second antibody is added (i.e., the ligand forms a bridge between the two antibody molecules).

Second, because the sensitivity is not dependent on competition of hormone with labeled ligand for antibody, the antibodies are generally used in excess to allow all the hormone in a sample to be bound by the antibodies. This condition of antibody excess allows the binding reactions (and the assay) to be completed in only a few hours. Third, in the absence of the competition for antibody binding inherent in radioimmunoassays, the working range of assays is not so limited and may actually span all anticipated values without requiring repeat assays with dilution. Finally, because there is no labeled ligand in the assays, the problem of circulating endogenous antibodies to hormones (see above) is eliminated.

Immunometric assays have a variety of names based on the detection method or label attached to one of the antibodies. The label may be ^{125}I as in immunoradiometric assays, or a nonradioactive molecule may serve as signal such as a fluorophor in immunofluorometric assays, an enzyme in immunoenzymometric assays, or a chemiluminescent molecule in immunochemiluminometric assays. As discussed in Chapter 13, TSH is one of the hormones for which the development of immunometric assays has changed clinical assessment dramatically. There are different immunometric assays with each of the above signal systems developed for TSH. The chemiluminescent detection system may be the most sensitive because of a high signal-to-noise ratio. Immunometric assays are now standard for parathyroid hormone, gonadotropins, and many other hormones.

Immunometric assays have greatly enhanced the sensitivity of hormone assays, leading to a variety of terms such as "sensitive" and "ultrasensitive." The lower limit of detection of commonly measured peptide hormones such as TSH has been decreased one or two orders of magnitude (see Chapter 13). In comparing the reported sensitivities of immunometric assays it is important to distinguish functional from analytical sensitivity. The analytical sensitivity limit is defined as the theoretically lowest value that can be statistically distinguished from zero in the intra-assay mode. A more practical sensitivity limit is the 20% interassay coefficient of variation or functional sensitivity. For example, manufacturers of several immunometric TSH assays may report an analytical sensitivity of 0.03 μU/ml. However, only those assays with a functional sensitivity of $\leq$0.2 μU/ml may be able to reliably distinguish the suppressed TSH values of hyperthyroid patients from normal subjects (see Chapter 13).

With the development of immunometric assays using an excess of monoclonal murine and other species antibodies, the potential of confounding heterophilic antibodies became apparent. Some patients were found to have nonspecific antibodies in their serum that were species specific for the antibodies used in the immunoassays. For example, in assays using murine-derived signal and capture molecules, human anti-mouse antibodies (HAMA) in a patient's serum could result in the anti-mouse antibody providing a link between signal and capture molecule and cause a spuriously high value. A little over 3% of unselected patient serum samples contain sufficient HAMA to give falsely elevated readings in the TSH assay. As a result, manufacturers have added small quantities of serum or immunoglobulin from animals of the same species as the immunoglobulin used in the assays to absorb potential human antibodies that could interfere. Even with these additions of animal immunoglobulin, rare patient sera have such elevated HAMA or other similar antibodies to result in falsely high readings in the assay.

Sampling the Plasma

The best way to sample the plasma to measure a hormone concentration depends on the given hormone. In the case of hormones whose plasma levels are relatively constant (e.g., thyroxine), the use of an isolated plasma sample provides a reliable estimate of hormonal status under usual circumstances. To assess hormone levels accurately for those hormones with pulsatile secretion (e.g., LH, testosterone), a single plasma sample may or may not be representative of mean plasma levels. With these hormones it is necessary to draw three or more samples at 20- to 30-minute intervals and pool aliquots of each for a single determination. For hormones with significant diurnal or sleep-related secretion the time of sampling may also be important. Because of the circadian rhythm of the ACTH–cortisol axis, for example, one expects higher plasma levels in the early morning hours. And the characteristic timing of an episode of growth hormone secretion soon after an individual falls asleep may be used to guide sampling for diagnostic purposes. In addition, one must recognize that sleep-related secretion may occur only during a certain period of life, as in LH secretion during mid-puberty. In women the plasma levels of gonadotropins, estradiol, and progesterone must be interpreted in light of the phase of the menstrual cycle.

Effect of Plasma-Binding Proteins

Whereas polypeptide hormones circulate in the plasma unbound to other plasma constituents, steroid and thyroid hormones circulate largely bound to albumin and specific binding proteins. Less than 1% of thyroxine (T_4) and triiodothyroxine (T_3) and only about 1%–3% of androgens, estrogens, and glucocorticoids in the plasma are in the unbound or free form. The free hormone concentration of these hormones can be determined *in vitro* by a tedious procedure termed *equilibrium dialysis*. For some time, the free fraction was regarded as the biologically active portion of the circulating hormone concentration as it was thought to be the only fraction available for entry into cells and interaction with receptors.

It is now clear that the transport of steroid and thyroid hormones into cells is more complicated that free fraction estimated *in vitro* as being the only component of the hormone in the circulation available to enter cells. Dissociation of protein-bound hormone can occur within a capillary bed so that the active fraction can be larger than the free fraction measured under equilibrium conditions *in vitro. In vivo* methods (Fig. 5-2) are needed to estimate the capillary exchangeable hormone because interaction of binding proteins, such as albumin, thyroid hormone–binding globulin (TBG), or sex hormone–binding globulin (SHBG), with the components on the microcirculation surface (e.g., endothelial glycocalyx) may lead to conformational changes at the hormone-binding site on the plasma protein. Such conformational changes may result in markedly increased rates of hormone dissociation

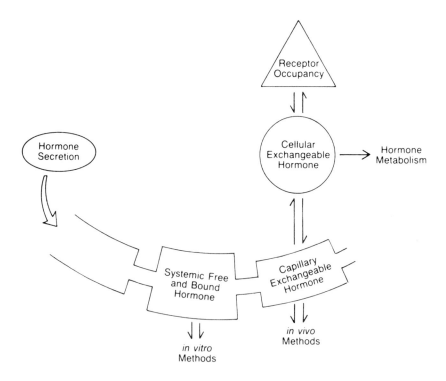

Fig. 5-2 Diagram depicting the concept of the difference between "free" hormone in the circulation as assessed by *in vitro* methods (e.g., equilibrium dialysis) and capillary exchangeable (or tissue available) hormone as assessed by *in vivo* methods. The capillary exchangeable fraction is usually much greater than the systemic free fraction. (Redrawn from Pardridge WM, unpublished.)

from albumin and/or SHBG in the microcirculation that are not measured *in vitro*. Such *in vivo* methods have been developed using arterial injection of animals. Although there are differences for specific hormones, in general it now appears that it is the free *plus* the albumin-bound hormone that is available for entry into most tissues. In the case of plasma testosterone, this free plus albumin-bound component is about half of the total circulating hormone. The delivery of the free plus albumin-bound hormone to target tissues results in an amount of hormone in the tissue that would be necessary for half-saturation of steroid and thyroid hormone receptors at normal plasma concentrations of total hormone.

The laboratory measurement of free plus albumin-bound steroid and thyroid hormones is technically easier than the measurement of free hormone. The free plus albumin-bound fraction can be measured with the ammonium sulfate precipitation technique. This is not widely done at present; instead, total steroid and thyroid hormone concentrations are usually measured. When the level of specific binding proteins is likely to be increased (TBG and SHBG in pregnancy) or decreased (TBG in debilitating illness), some assessment of the amount of binding protein is important in interpreting the total hormone concentrations. Both TBG and SHBG may be quantitated directly, and the amount of thyroid hormone–binding sites may be inferred by the T_3 resin uptake test (see Chapter 13).

Interpretation of "Normal Ranges"

Caution is needed in the interpretation of "normal ranges" for plasma levels of most hormones. Because the stated normal range is often quite broad, extending to a 2- to 3-fold variation (e.g., thyroxine, testosterone), it is possible for the level in an individual to be halved or doubled and still be within the so-called normal range (although abnormal for that individual). As almost all hormone systems are under some regulatory feedback control, measuring both members of a "hormone pair" (e.g., thyroxine and TSH, testosterone and LH) may provide insights not available from individual values (Fig. 5-3). Although this is classically thought of in relation to the pituitary trophic hormones and the hormones secreted by their target endocrine glands (Fig. 5-3), the concept is broader and applies to such hormone pairs as calcium and PTH, insulin and glucose, and plasma osmolality and vasopressin.

This paradigm is central to the assessment of endocrine status. For example, because the normal range of plasma thyroxine is broad, a low-normal T_4 coupled with an elevated TSH indicates early, compensated thyroid failure. Likewise, a high-normal PTH in a patient with a simultaneously elevated serum calcium has a completely different implication from the same PTH value in a patient with a low serum calcium. Basically, the measurement of hormone pairs allows assessment of the effects of a hormone upon its regulatory control mechanism. Other possible outcomes of measuring both members of a hormone pair are also indicated in Figure 5-3.

In the context of the pituitary and its target endocrine glands, finding low levels of both members of the hormone pair indicates the primary problem to be trophic hormone deficiency or pituitary failure (e.g., low TSH and T_4) (Fig. 5-3). High levels of target gland hormone coupled with low levels of trophic hormone suggest autonomous secretion of the target endocrine organ (i.e., typical hyperthyroidism results in suppression of TSH secretion). The finding of elevated levels of both mem-

Fig. 5-3   Diagram depicting the possible interpretations of alterations in trophic and target gland hormone pairs (e.g., thyroxine and thyrotropin). (Redrawn with modification from Griffin JE: In: *Williams Textbook of Endocrinology,* 8th ed., JD Wilson and DW Foster, eds., Saunders, Philadelphia, p. 1664, 1992.)

bers of a hormone pair is compatible with several different forms of deranged endocrine physiology (Fig. 5-3). Autonomous secretion of a trophic hormone can arise either at the normal site or at an ectopic location; for example, excess cortisol production may be due to the secretion of pituitary ACTH or from secretion of ACTH by lung tumors. Alternatively, the combined elevation of trophic and target endocrine gland hormones can result from resistance to the action of the target endocrine gland hormone (e.g., elevated LH and testosterone in androgen resistance). Insight into which of these two explanations for elevation of both members of a hormone pair is likely often derives from the clinical situation. Autonomous hypersecretion of the trophic hormone typically results in clinical evidence of target gland hormone excess, whereas target gland hormone resistance is usually associated with evidence of hormone deficiency. Knowledge of the relative frequency of autonomous trophic hormone secretion versus resistance to target gland hormone action is also helpful. Thus, because glucocorticoid resistance is rare, elevation of ACTH and cortisol usually signals the presence of autonomous ACTH secretion.

URINARY HORMONE EXCRETION

Measurement of urinary excretion of a hormone or hormone metabolite may reflect overall hormone secretion or mean plasma levels. Thus, the 24-hour urinary 17-hydroxycorticoids and/or the urinary free cortisol may be a better estimate of glucocorticoid secretion throughout the day than an isolated plasma cortisol. The 17-hydroxycorticoids represent a summation of glucocorticoid metabolites, whereas the urinary free cortisol "sums" the plasma levels of cortisol above the saturation of binding proteins. Likewise, measurement of urinary metabolites of catecholamines may provide a useful clue to their episodic excess in the plasma.

Urinary hormone measurements have been used less since the development of reliable plasma immunoassays. Not only are reliable timed urine collections difficult to obtain, but urinary hormone measurements have some inherent limitations. To ensure completeness of urine collection, total creatinine should be measured on all specimens. Men excrete about 1.5 g of creatinine each day, and women excrete about 1.0 g. Some calculations of normal values for urinary hormone excretion try to account for variably complete collections by expressing the value per gram of urinary creatinine. Because many urinary hormone measurements involve determination of a metabolite rather than the hormone itself, drugs or disease states that alter hormone metabolism may thus alter the urinary measurement without an abnormality of hormone secretion. In addition, some urinary hormone metabolite measurements include hormones from more than one source and, thus, are of little value in assessing specific glandular secretion. Because urinary 17-ketosteroids are a measure of both adrenal and gonadal androgens, for example, they are a poor index of testicular function (see Chapter 10). Finally, because some hormones are not primarily excreted either intact or in metabolite form in the urine, measurement of the small amounts of these hormones present in the urine is obviously of little value. The thyroid hormones are examples of this latter category (see Chapter 13).

HORMONE PRODUCTION RATES

Measuring the actual secretion or production rate of a hormone may overcome most of the problems inherent in plasma hormone levels and urinary hormone excretion in assessing endocrine function. However, such measurements are technically difficult and usually involve the administration of radioisotopes. The production rate can be measured directly by the dilution of an infused radioisotope with endogenous nonradioactive hormone over a period of time. Alternatively, the metabolic clearance rate (MCR) of a hormone may be determined and together with mean plasma concentration (PC) used to estimate production rate (PR) by the formula PR = MCR $\times$ PC. In either case, the measurement of hormone production rates remains primarily a research procedure.

DYNAMIC TESTS OF ENDOCRINE FUNCTION

Dynamic endocrine tests provide information about endocrine function beyond that which is obtained from measurements of single hormones or even of hormone pairs. These tests are based on either the stimulation or the suppression of endogenous hormone production. The ultimate functional test of endocrine function is to demonstrate a normal response in target tissues to physiological or stressful stimuli *in vivo*. Thus, for example, if the urine can be maximally concentrated in response to water deprivation one can infer that the osmolality-sensing mechanisms in the hypothalamus, the secretion of vasopressin, the receptor for vasopressin, and postreceptor events in vasopressin action in the kidney are all normal (see Chapter 7). However, such *in vivo* tests of tissue effects are not available for most endocrine systems; and even when they are available, failure of the final expected response does not identify the level of the defect. Other functional tests of endocrine status are therefore necessary.

Stimulation Tests

Stimulation tests are usually used when hypofunction of an endocrine organ is suspected. They are designed to take advantage of known endogenous control mechanisms to assess reserve capacity to produce hormone. A trophic hormone can be administered to test the capacity of the target gland to increase hormone production. The trophic hormone can be a hypothalamic releasing factor such as thyrotropin-releasing hormone (TRH) or a substitute for a pituitary hormone (cortrosyn for ACTH or hCG for LH). The capacity of the target gland to respond is measured by the increase in the plasma level of the appropriate hormone (TSH, cortisol, and testosterone in these examples). Alternatively, a stimulatory test may be performed by producing an increase in the secretion of an endogenous trophic hormone and measuring the effect on a target gland hormone level. For instance, metyrapone is given to block a late step in cortisol synthesis, and the ability of the pituitary to respond is assessed by the increase in ACTH as well as its subsequent effect on a plasma cortisol precursor (see Chapter 14). Stimulation tests in which endogenous trophic hormone secretion is altered actually assess the overall capacity of the hypothalamic–pituitary–target organ axis to respond to challenge.

Some stimulation tests are useful in suspected hyperfunction of endocrine glands. For example, the presence of an exaggerated calcitonin response to pentagastrin or calcium administration may indicate a premalignant change called thyroid C-cell hyperplasia. Another stimulation test useful in deranged physiology associated with endocrine hyperfunction is the TRH test in suspected hyperthyroidism. In hyperthyroid states the response of TSH following TRH injection is blunted, so that in this case a failure of response is a positive test.

One stimulation test is useful in assessing potential hormone resistance. The increase in urinary cyclic AMP and phosphate following PTH administration is blunted or absent in patients with PTH resistance (pseudohypoparathyroidism) but normal in patients with hypoparathyroidism due to PTH deficiency. Tests to assess resistance to other hormones would be helpful in endocrine diagnosis.

Suppression Tests

Suppression tests are used when endocrine hyperfunction is suspected. They are designed to determine whether negative feedback control mechanisms are intact. A hormone or other regulatory substance is administered, and the inhibition of endogenous hormone secretion is assessed. For example, glucocorticoid (dexamethasone) is given to persons with suspected hypercortisolism to assess its capacity to inhibit ACTH secretion and thus cortisol production by the adrenal. In this type of test, failure to suppress indicates the presence of autonomous secretion either of the target endocrine gland hormone or of the trophic hormone. Other suppression tests use glucose in evaluation of suspected growth hormone excess and saline in assessment of excess aldosterone secretion.

Problems in Interpreting Dynamic Tests

Several factors influence the response to stimulation and suppression tests. Change in response to a test with age, the need for repeated stimulation to elicit a normal response, the inherent rhythmicity in the secretion of some hormones, and the response characteristics of deranged physiologic processes are important considerations in the interpretation of test results. For example, the TSH response to TRH stimulation is decreased in older men (but not in older women). In subjects with long-standing ACTH deficiency, repetitive stimulation may be required to bring out a normal glucocorticoid response to ACTH stimulation. Similarly, men presumed to have severe hypothalamic disease may show a subnormal LH response to an initial bolus of luteinizing hormone-releasing hormone (LHRH) but respond normally to acute stimulation following a week of daily infusions of LHRH. Apparently, the normal pituitary requires the priming effect of the repeated infusions of the hypothalamic hormone to demonstrate its ability to respond to a bolus. Such a protocol may help distinguish between hypothalamic and pituitary hypogonadism (Fig. 5-4). Some usually reliable dynamic tests of endocrine function are occasionally misleading owing to the unusual patterns of response of the specific endocrinopathy. An uncommon pattern of pituitary-dependent hypercortisolism is associated with periodic hormonogenesis resulting in seemingly paradoxical stimulation of cortisol levels in response to dexamethasone suppression testing.

Other disease states may pose difficulties in interpreting dynamic endocrine tests. For instance, hypothyroidism, hyperthyroidism, and hypercortisolism all may cause impaired growth hormone responsiveness to the usual stimuli. The response of growth hormone to insulin-induced hypoglycemia and other stimuli may also be

Fig. 5-4   Mean serum LH responses of 10 men with hypogonadotropic hypogonadism to a 250-μg intravenous bolus dose of luteinizing hormone–releasing hormone (LHRH) before and after daily infusions (500 μg over 4 hours) of LHRH for 1 week. Five men had presumed hypothalamic disease and five had presumed pituitary disease. (From Snyder PJ, et al: Repetitive infusion of gonadotropin-releasing hormone distinguishes hypothalamic from pituitary hypogonadism. J Clin Endocrinol Metab 48:864–868, 1979; © 1979, The Endocrine Society.)

blunted in the presence of obesity. In contrast, patients with severe malnutrition or chronic kidney or liver disease tend to have elevated basal levels of growth hormone with either lack of suppression or paradoxical increase following a glucose load. In addition, a number of psychiatric disorders are associated with abnormal dynamic endocrine tests in the absence of a specific endocrine disorder. Depression is the psychiatric disorder most often associated with aberrant dynamic endocrine tests. Quite commonly, patients with severe primary depression have an impaired suppression of plasma cortisol following dexamethasone administration, and the cortisol response may return to normal after treatment of the depression. In about one-fourth of all patients with acute psychiatric illness, the response of TSH to TRH is blunted or absent without thyroid disease.

Drugs may interfere with dynamic endocrine tests in several ways. Some drugs, such as high doses of glucocorticoids and L-dopa administration, directly impair pituitary function testing in regard to stimulation of secretion of growth hormone and TSH, respectively. A commonly used anticonvulsant medication, phenytoin, impairs testing of both the reserve of the pituitary–adrenal axis as described above with metyrapone and its suppressibility with dexamethasone by stimulating the hepatic metabolism of both test substances.

MEASUREMENT OF HORMONE RECEPTORS

With continued increase in our knowledge about the receptor mechanisms of hormone action (see Chapter 3), the measurement of receptor number and affinity is becoming more commonplace in the overall evaluation of endocrine function. The major form of endocrine pathophysiology in which receptor measurements are useful is hormone resistance. Diseases due to resistance to hormone action have now been described for most hormones. In general, the characteristic of such states is the lack or incompleteness of the expected hormone's effects in the presence of normal or increased circulating levels of the hormone. The types of tissues used for hormone–receptor measurements vary with the hormone and receptor of interest and include lymphocytes, red blood cells, tissue biopsies, and cultured skin fibroblasts. Examples of the types of receptor and postreceptor abnormalities detected by such studies include the reversible effects of obesity on insulin receptor number, the abnormalities of the GTP-binding protein in some subjects with PTH resistance, and impaired induction of the enzyme 25-hydroxyvitamin D 24-hydroxylase in one form of resistance to vitamin D.

Recently, mutations in cell surface receptors and their associated postreceptor proteins have been shown to result in hormone excess. Thus, point mutations in TSH and LH receptors cause hyperthyroidism and Leydig cell hyperplasia, respectively. Activating mutations in the α_s component of the GTP-binding protein have been associated with variable hyperfunction of multiple endocrine glands in the same individual.

Hormone–receptor measurements have proved informative in another way with regard to at least one form of hormone-responsive malignancy, cancer of the breast. Measurements in breast biopsies of the estrogen receptor and of a protein made in breast tissue in response to estrogen acting through its receptor, that is, the progesterone receptor, have been useful in predicting the response of such tumors to hormonal manipulation.

SUGGESTED READING

Gorden P, and Weintraub BD: Radioreceptor and other functional hormone assays. In: *Williams Textbook of Endocrinology,* 8th ed., JD Wilson and DW Foster, eds., Saunders, Philadelphia, pp. 1647–1661, 1992.

Griffin JE: Dynamic tests of endocrine function. In: *Williams Textbook of Endocrinology,* 8th ed., JD Wilson and DW Foster, eds., Saunders, Philadelphia, pp. 1663–1670, 1992.

Lefkowitz RJ: Clinical implications of basic research. N Engl J Med 332:186–187, 1995.

Pardridge WM: Transport of protein-bound hormones into tissues in vivo. Endocr Rev 2:103–123, 1981.

Pardridge WM: Serum bioavailability of sex steroid hormones. Clin Endocrinol Metab 15: 259–278, 1986.

Price CP, and Newman DJ, eds: *Principles and Practice of Immunoassay,* 2nd ed., Stockton, New York, 1997.

Segre GV, and Brown EN: Measurement of hormones. In: *Williams Textbook of Endocrinology,* 9th ed., JD Wilson, DW Foster, HM Kronenberg, and PR Larsen eds., Saunders, Philadelphia, pp. 43–54, 1998.

Spencer CA, LoPresti JS, Patel A, Guttler RB, Eigen A, Shen D, Gray D, and Nicoloff JT: Applications of a new chemiluminometric thyrotropin assay to subnormal measurement. J Clin Endocrinol Metab 70:453–460, 1990.

Spencer CA, Takeuchi M, and Kazarosyan M: Current status and performance goals for serum thyrotropin (TSH) assays. Clin Chem 42:140–145, 1996.

Spiegel AM, Weinstein LS, and Shenker A: Abnormalities in G-protein–coupled signal transduction pathways in human disease. J Clin Invest 92:1119–1125, 1993.

Verhoeven GFM, and Wilson JD: The syndromes of primary hormone resistance. Metabolism 28:253–289, 1979.

Ward G, McKinnon L, Badrick T, and Hickman PE: Heterophilic antibodies remain a problem for the immunoassay laboratory. Am J Clin Pathol 108:417–421, 1997.

6

The Anterior Pituitary and Hypothalamus

SERIO R. OJEDA
SAMUEL M. McCANN

As indicated in Chapter 1, the core of the neuroendocrine system is represented by the hypothalamic–pituitary complex. The hypothalamus is composed of a diversity of neurosecretory cells arranged in groups, which secrete their products either into the portal blood system that connects the hypothalamus to the adenohypophysis (see below) or directly into the general circulation after storage in the neurohypophysis. The hypothalamic hormones secreted by the neurohypophysis are arginine vasopressin (AVP), also called antidiuretic hormone (ADH), and oxytocin (OT). The functions and regulatory mechanisms controlling the secretion of these hormones are discussed in Chapter 7.

The hypothalamic hormones delivered to the portal blood system are transported to the adenohypophysis where they stimulate or inhibit the synthesis and secretion of different trophic hormones. In turn, these hormones regulate gonadal, thyroid, and adrenal function, in addition to lactation, bodily growth, and somatic development. Because of the nature of their actions, the hypothalamic hormones are classified as *releasing* or *inhibiting* hormones. As will be seen later in this chapter, the adenohypophysis can be divided into three parts. The bulk of the adenohypophyseal hormones is produced in two of these parts, the pars distalis or anterior pituitary and the pars intermedia, also known as the intermediate lobe. The trophic hormones produced in the anterior pituitary include adrenocorticotropic hormone (ACTH), β-endorphin, thyroid-stimulating hormone (TSH), growth hormone (GH), prolactin (PRL), and the gonadotrophins, luteinizing hormone (LH) and follicle-stimulating hormone (FSH). The pars intermedia produces several hormones that are synthesized as part of a large-molecular-weight precursor known as pro-opiomelanocortin (POMC). Tissue-specific processing of this prohormone results in the formation of β-lipotropin, β-endorphin, α-melanocyte-stimulating hormone (α-MSH), and corticotropin-like intermediate peptide (CLIP), a product composition quite different from the predominant formation of ACTH, β-lipoprotein, γ-lipotropin, and β-endorphin in the anterior pituitary.

This chapter focuses on the hypothalamic control of adenohypophyseal function, with special reference to the anterior pituitary. No attempts are made to discuss the actions of the different pituitary trophic hormones on their target glands as this is considered in detail in Chapters 9 and 10 (gonadotropins and PRL), Chapter 13 (TSH), and Chapter 14 (ACTH). An exception to this is GH. Although Chapter 12 considers some aspects of the control and actions of GH, a broader discussion of its physiological actions will be presented here because GH is the only anterior pituitary hormone that does not have a clear-cut target gland.

ANATOMY

The pituitary gland (Fig. 6-1) has two parts: one portion is of neural origin, the neurohypophysis, which will be discussed in Chapter 7; the other portion, the adenohypophysis, is ectodermal in origin and is derived from the pharynx. In embryonic development, an evagination from the roof of the pharynx pushes dorsally to reach a ventrally directed evagination from the base of the diencephalon. The dorsally projecting evagination, known as *Rathke's pouch,* forms the adenohypophysis, whereas the ventrally directed evagination of neural tissue forms the neurohypophysis. The neurohypophysis has three parts: the median eminence, the infundibular stem, and the neural lobe itself. The median eminence represents the intrahypothalamic portion, and lies just ventral to the floor of the third ventricle protruding slightly in the midline. The main part of the neurohypophysis, the infundibular process (neural lobe), is connected to the median eminence by the infundibular stem. Tissue from the adenohypophysis spreads dorsally to surround the infundibular stem and median eminence and is known as the *pars tuberalis.* The infundibular stem and surrounding pars tuberalis constitute the pituitary stalk. The adenohypophysis can be divided into the *pars distalis,* which is the ventral portion, the *pars intermedia,* which is that portion adjacent to the neural lobe and separated from the pars distalis by the residual lumen of Rathke's pouch, and the pars tuberalis. The pars intermedia is rudi-

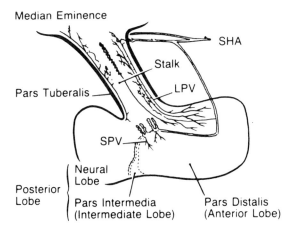

Fig. 6-1 Details of the anatomy of the pituitary gland showing the median eminence, pars tuberalis, stalk, infundibular stem and pars tuberalis, neural lobe, intermediate lobe, anterior lobe, posterior lobe, long portal vessels (LPV), superior hypophyseal arteries (SHA), and short portal vessels (SPV).

mentary in humans. The pars distalis is frequently termed the *anterior lobe* because of its anterior position in most animals. The intermediate and neural lobes constitute the posterior lobe.

There is no significant functional innervation of the adenohypophysis by way of the hypothalamus or neural lobe. Instead, a humoral pathway is provided by means of the hypophyseal portal system of veins (Fig. 6-1). These take origin from capillary loops in the median eminence of the tuber cinereum and drain blood in parallel veins down the stalk. In the anterior lobe, the portal vessels break up into the sinusoids that provide its blood supply. Venous blood drains from the gland into the cavernous sinus. There may also be an arterial supply to the gland, but the portal vessels furnish the main blood supply to the anterior lobe. In addition to the vessels just described, which are called the *long portal vessels,* there are also short portal venous vascular connections that arise in the neural lobe and pass across the intermediate lobe to the anterior lobe. These are known as the *short portal vessels.*

The pituitary is a very vascular structure, with the various pituitary cell types lining the sinusoids of the gland. By light microscopy, the pituitary cells can be classed as acidophils, basophils, and chromophobes, depending on the affinity of their cytoplasm for either acidic or basic dyes. By electron microscopy, further subdivisions of these cells can be made (based on secretory granule size and number), and cells secreting particular pituitary hormones can be characterized. For example, the stomatotrophs secrete somatotropin (GH), the lactotrophs secrete PRL, and so forth. It was the long-held view that each cell type produced a single pituitary hormone. It is now clear that certain cells are able to secrete more than one hormone. An example of this type of cell is the gonadotroph. Some of these cells secrete both FSH and LH; others may secrete one or the other of these hormones.

Uptake of hormones into and delivery of substances from the vascular system are favored by the presence of fenestrated capillaries within the gland. Because the vascular supply is primarily portal in nature, capillary pressure in the gland is very low and the permeability of these capillaries is high. The situation may be analogous to that in hepatic sinusoids with high permeability not only to pituitary protein hormones but also to the plasma proteins. Thus, a balance between hydrostatic pressure tending to produce ultrafiltration and colloid osmotic pressure tending to cause uptake of extracellular fluid is achieved at a very low sinusoidal pressure.

The *hypothalamus* is located at the base of the brain, ventral to the thalamus from which it is separated by the hypothalamic sulcus. Its anterior boundaries are provided by the optic chiasm; laterally it is separated from the temporal lobes by the hypothalamic sulci and its posterior limits are defined by the mammillary bodies. The base of the hypothalamus is the tuber cinereum, the central part of which is the median eminence. The anatomical relationships of the hypothalamic–pituitary unit to other structures of the base of the brain are shown in Figure 6-2.

ANTERIOR PITUITARY HORMONES AND
THEIR HYPOTHALAMIC CONTROL

Evidence for hypothalamic control of the anterior pituitary has come primarily from studies involving hypothalamic lesions or stimulation of animals such as the rat,

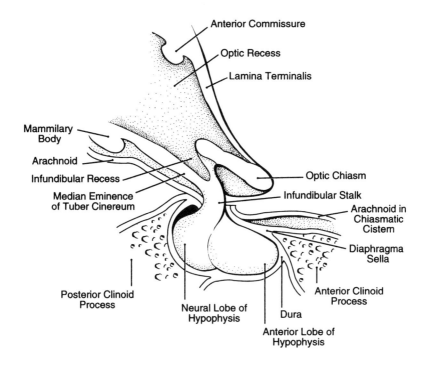

Fig. 6-2   Relationship of the hypothalamic–pituitary unit to other structures of the base of the brain. (Redrawn from Reichlin S: In: *Williams Textbook of Endocrinology,* 7th ed., JD Wilson and DW Foster, eds., Saunders, Philadelphia, p. 495, 1985.)

guinea pig, and rhesus monkey. The secretion of ACTH, GH, TSH, FSH, and LH can be increased by hypothalamic stimulation, whereas lesions that destroy the median eminence of the tuber cinereum result in decreased secretion of all of these hormones with the exception of PRL and α-MSH, which are increased. Thus, there is a net stimulatory influence of the hypothalamus on the secretion of most anterior pituitary hormones. Although these experiments clearly established that the hypothalamus controls the release of pituitary hormones, they did not provide insight into the underlying mechanism.

The Neurohumoral Hypothesis of Control of Anterior Pituitary Hormone Secretion

From the very early days of neuroendocrinology, it was clear that the anterior lobe of the pituitary gland does not receive significant secretomotor innervation. The presence of the hypophyseal portal system of veins that drain blood from capillary loops in the median eminence down the hypophyseal stalk to the adenohypophyseal sinusoids suggested that the brain might exert a neurohumoral control over the pituitary (Fig. 6-3).

Early evidence for the neurohumoral hypothesis was confusing, because experiments in which the pituitary stalk was sectioned gave variable results. This question was settled by placing an impervious plate between the cut ends of the stalk:

Fig. 6-3 Hypothalamic localization of the neurons that secrete thyrotropin-releasing hormone (TRH), growth hormone–releasing hormone (GHRH), and luteinizing hormone–releasing hormone (LHRH) based on human and animal studies. The neurons (solid dots) are shown in a coronal section through the plane of the densest cell bodies. The projection pathway of axons toward the median eminence is depicted by the solid lines forming an arrow. Arcuate nucleus, ARC; dorsomedial hypothalamic nucleus, DMH; fornix, FX; median eminence, ME; optic chiasm, OC; paraventricular nucleus, PVN; suprachiasmatic nucleus, SCN; supraoptic nucleus, SON; third ventricle, vIII; ventromedial hypothalamic nucleus, VMH. (From Riskind PN, and Martin JB: In *Endocrinology,* 2nd ed., Vol. 1, LJ De Groot, ed., Saunders, Philadelphia, p. 101, 1989.)

a permanent derangement of pituitary function was the consequence. The earlier discrepancies had resulted from variable regeneration of hypophyseal portal vessels across the cut edges of the stalk. Further evidence for the neurohumoral hypothesis came from ingenious grafting experiments in which the gland was removed from the hypophyseal capsule and then reimplanted under the median eminence so that it could be revascularized by hypophyseal portal vessels. Such grafts led to the return of normal anterior pituitary function, whereas grafts placed in other loci at a distance from the portal vessels so that they had to be revascularized by other arterial twigs led to a permanent dysfunction of the gland.

Identification of Hypothalamic Releasing and Inhibiting Hormones

The next logical step was to make extracts of the median eminence region, the area that is drained by the portal vessels, and to inject the extracts into animals to determine whether they could alter anterior pituitary function. It was soon shown that injection of extracts of the posterior pituitary released ACTH. Although synthetic vasopressin, a posterior pituitary peptide, could release ACTH, some investigators were able to separate a substance in the posterior pituitary extracts, apparently different from vasopressin, that would also release ACTH. Unfortunately, this substance occurred in trace amounts and was not uniformly present in these extracts. The controversy cleared when it was shown that extracts of median eminence tissue contained more ACTH-releasing activity than could be accounted for by the amount of vasopressin present. This finding indicated that a corticotropin-releasing factor or hormone (CRH) existed in addition to vasopressin (Table 6-1).

Table 6-1 Hypothalamic Releasing and Inhibiting Hormones[a]

Hypothalamic hormone	Purified	Synthesized	Stimulates	Inhibits	Cell bodies in
Vasopressin	Yes	Nonapeptide	ACTH	0	SO, PVN
Corticotropin-releasing hormone (CRH)	Yes	41AA peptide	ACTH	0	PVN
LH-releasing hormone (LHRH)	Yes	Decapeptide	LH, FSH	0	POA, MBH
FSH-releasing factor	Yes	No	FSH	0	PVN/POA?
Thyrotropin-releasing hormone (TRH)	Yes	Tripeptide	TSH, PRL	0	PVN
Growth hormone–releasing hormone (GHRH)	Yes	44AA peptide	GH	0	ARC
Growth hormone secretagogue(s)	No	Only a synthetic hexapeptide is available	GH	0	?
Growth hormone–inhibiting hormone (GHIH) (somatostatin)	Yes	Tetradecapeptide	0	GH, PRL, TSH, gastrin, glucagon, insulin	APR
Prolactin (PRL)-inhibiting factors					
(PIFs), dopamine,	Yes	Yes	0	PRL	ARC
peptidergic PIF	No	No	0	PRL	?
PRL-releasing factors (PRFs)					
a. Prolactin-releasing peptide	Yes	20–31AA	PRL	0	DMH, SN
b. Oxytocin	Yes	Nonapeptide	PRL	0	SO, PVN
c. TRH, VIP, PHI, AII neurotensin substance P	Yes	—	PRl	0	PVN, SO
MSH-releasing factor (MRF)	Yes	No	MSH	0	
MSH-inhibiting factor (MIF)	Yes	No	0	MSH	
Pituitary adenylate cyclase-activating peptide (PACAP)	Yes	27 and 38AA	ACTH, GH	0	SO, PVN

[a]AA, amino acid; ACTH, adenocorticotropic hormone; AAII, angiotensin II; APR, anterior periventricular region; ARC, arcuate nucleus; DMH, dorsomedial nucleus; FSH, follicle-stimulating hormone; MBH, medial basasl hypothalamus; MSH, melanocyte-stimulating hormone; PHI, peptide histidine-isoleucine; POA, preoptic area; PVN, paraventricular nucleus; SN, solitary nucleus; SO, supraoptic nucleus; TSH, thyroid-stimulating hormone; VIP, vasoactive intestinal polypeptide.

The discovery of a CRH distinct from vasopressin provoked a search for similar factors that stimulate release of other anterior pituitary hormones. In rapid succession LH-, FSH-, GH-, and TSH-releasing activities, in addition to a PRL-inhibiting activity, were found in hypothalamic extracts. Evidence was also found for PRL- and MSH-releasing activities and a MSH-inhibiting activity.

An intensive effort was made to purify these new substances, to separate them from other active substances in hypothalamic extracts, and to determine their structure so that this could be confirmed by synthesis. Because only very small amounts of the releasing hormones are present in hypothalamic tissue, this proved to be a herculean task; isolation and determination of their structure required the processing of hundreds of thousands of hypothalamic fragments.

Hypothalamic Releasing and Inhibiting Hormones

Thyrotropin-Releasing Hormone (TRH)

This hormone acts on the anterior pituitary gland to release TSH as well as PRL; it is a tripeptide (pyro-Glu-His-Pro amine; Table 6-2) derived from a large precursor that has a molecular weight of about 29,000 Da. The TRH precursor contains five copies of the sequence Gln-His-Pro-Gly, which presumably originates the mature TRH molecule following glutamine cyclization and formation of the terminal amide. Within the hypothalamus, TRH is mainly synthesized in neurons of the parvocellular division of the paraventricular nucleus (Fig. 6-3 and Table 6-1) and also in some cells of the preoptic region. Axons project caudally from these regions and then project ventrally into the median eminence where the bulk of TRH is stored. TRH is also found outside the hypothalamus, even in the spinal cord, suggesting its involvement in other central nervous system functions.

Prolactin-Releasing Hormone (PRH)

Although it has been known for years that hypothalamic extracts are capable of stimulating PRL release from the anterior pituitary, the identity of the factors that might contribute to this activity was only partially known. Several neuropeptides, including TRH, oxytocin, and vasoactive intestinal polypeptide (VIP) can elicit PRL release, but their physiological relevance as specific PRL-releasing factors is questionable. Recently, a novel hypothalamic PRL–releasing peptide (termed *PRP*) and its cognate pituitary receptor were identified by molecular cloning. The PRP preproprotein generates two bioactive peptides by proteolytic cleavage, one peptide of

---

Table 6-2 Structure of Three Hypothalamic Hormones: LHRH, TRH, and Somatostatin

TRH (P-Glu-His-Pro-NH$_2$)
     1   2   3

LHRH I (P-Glu-His-Trp-Ser-Tyr-Gly-Leu-Arg-Pro-Gly-NH$_2$)
          1   2   3   4   5   6   7   8   9   10

LHRH II (P-Glu-His-Trp-Ser-His-Gly-Trp-Tyr-Pro-Gly-NH$_2$)

Somatostatin(Ala-Gly-Cys-Lys-Asn-Phe-Phe-Trp-Lys-Thr-Phe-Thr-Ser-Cys)
                1   2   3   4   5   6   7   8   9   10 11 12 13 14

31 amino acids and a shorter form of 20 amino acids. Both peptides release PRL in a specific fashion, without affecting other pituitary hormones. They are recognized by a seven-transmembrane domain receptor (see below) previously considered to be an orphan receptor (i.e., a receptor for which there is no known ligand). Although these findings strongly suggest that PRP is a true PRL-releasing hormone, immunohistochemical studies have failed to show PRP immunoreactive fibers in the external region of the medial eminence, thus making less likely the possibility that PRP, like other hypophysiotropic hormones, reaches the anterior pituitary via the portal vasculature.

Luteinizing Hormone–Releasing Hormone (LHRH)

This hormone, more commonly known as *gonadotropin hormone–releasing hormone* (GnRH) because it stimulates the release of both LH and FSH, belongs to a family of decapeptides highly conserved throughout vertebrate evolution. Thus far, nine different variants have been described in nonmammalian species. Characteristically, the LHRH peptide sequence is followed by that of an associated peptide of variable length. In fish, there are three separate genes encoding different LHRH forms. Interestingly, the sequence of one of these genes predicts the existence of two, instead of one, associated peptides. Until recently, it was thought that mammalian LHRH was encoded by a single LHRH gene. Evidence now exists for the existence of a second gene. The first LHRH gene (LHRH-I) encodes a 92-amino acid precursor protein, which upon proteolytic cleavage originates the LHRH decapeptide and a 56-amino acid–associated peptide. The second LHRH gene (LHRH-II) encodes a decapeptide that differs from LHRH-I by three amino acids (Table 6-2) and that has been found to be expressed in a variety of vertebrate species, in addition to mammals. The genomic structure of this gene is similar to LHRH-I, but the gene is located on a different chromosome (chromosome 20 instead of 8). LHRH II encodes an associated peptide that is 50% longer than the associated peptide encoded by LHRH I (84 vs. 56 amino acids). The function of LHRH II is currently unknown. Although it is expressed in the brain, its abundance is much greater in peripheral tissues such as the kidney, bone marrow and prostate.

In most mammals examined to date, LHRH-I is contained in neurons scattered throughout the anterior and medial part of the hypothalamus, and the preoptic septal areas. However, in primates—including humans—a substantial fraction of LHRH neurons is also localized to the medial basal hypothalamus and arcuate nucleus (Fig. 6-3 and Table 6-1). The LHRH nerve terminals projecting to the portal vasculature are predominantly localized to the lateral portion of the median eminence, although in humans a medial distribution is also observed. Neurons containing LHRH II are also found in the hypothalamus, but in different regions from those producing LHRH-I.

Corticotropin-Releasing Hormone (CRH)

This hormone is a 41-amino acid peptide that stimulates the secretion of ACTH and β-endorphin from the adenohypophysis. CRH derives from a 196-amino acid precursor highly conserved among mammalian species. The CRH gene contains only two exons separated by a rather short intervening sequence; the mature peptide sequence is entirely encoded by the second exon. CRH synergizes with vasopressin to stimulate ACTH release. The hypothalamic neurons that produce CRH are mostly found in the medial parvocellular portion of the paraventricular nucleus, where they frequently co-localize with other peptides, particularly vasopressin (Fig. 6-3 and Table 6-1). As in the case of TRH, CRH-containing neurons are also found in several extrahypothalamic areas, suggesting the involvement of CRH in nonendocrine functions.

Somatostatin or Growth Hormone-Inhibiting Hormone (GHIH)

This 14-amino acid peptide (Table 6-2) acts on the pituitary gland to inhibit GH secretion. It can also inhibit TSH release. GHIH has a cyclic structure that results from the formation of two intramolecular disulfide bonds between its two cysteine residues. It is now clear that the original 14-amino acid somatostatin molecule belongs to a family of related peptides, which includes a 28-amino acid peptide, a 12-amino acid fragment derived from the amino terminus of somatostatin 28, and even larger forms having molecular weights of up to 16,000 Da. The somatostatin gene contains two exons separated by a short intervening sequence; both somatostatin 14 and 28 are encoded by sequences present in the second exon. Because there appears to be only one somatostatin gene in mammals, the different somatostatin peptides are likely to derive from alternative messenger RNA processing and/or posttranslational modifications of the propeptide.

Somatostatin is widely distributed in the organism, including several regions of the brain, the gastrointestinal tract, and pancreas. Within the hypothalamus, the principal source of somatostatin fibers projecting to the median eminence is neurons of the anterior periventricular area (Fig. 6-3 and Table 6-1).

Growth Hormone-Releasing Hormone (GHRH)

GHRH is a 44-amino acid peptide derived from a 108-amino acid precursor protein encoded by a single gene. The GHRH gene contains five exons that together with the corresponding intervening sequences span 10 kb of the human genome. Judging from the structure of the GHRH precursor protein, proteolytic processing may yield two peptides of unknown function, in addition to GHRH. The GHRH stimulates GH secretion from the pituitary gland. Its location is the most restrictive of all releasing factors. The majority of the GHRH-producing neurons in the hypothalamus are found in and around the arcuate nucleus, close to the median eminence (Fig. 6-3 and Table 6-1).

Growth Hormone Secretagogues (GHS)

Almost 20 years ago, a synthetic hexapeptide was shown to stimulate growth hormone release from the anterior pituitary. Subsequent studies indicated that this compound, as well as others of the same class, acted independently from GHRH and somatostatin-mediated pathways, thereby suggesting the existence of both an endogenous compound with GH releasing activity and a specific receptor for such a compound. In 1996, the predicted receptor was identified and shown to be a seven-transmembrane domain G protein–coupled receptor. This finding made clear that synthetic GH secretagogues mimic the actions of a hormone that participates in the physiological control of GH release. The identity of this hormone remains to be established.

Anterior Pituitary Hormones

All adenohypophyseal hormones are protein or polypeptide in nature. Their names, number of amino acids, and molecular weights are presented in Table 6-3.

Growth Hormone (GH)

As discussed in Chapter 12, there are several forms of GH, but it appears that the predominant species secreted under physiological conditions is a 191-amino acid form with a molecular weight of 22,650 Da. Growth hormone is structurally related to human chorionic somatomammotropin, a peptide produced by the placenta. There are at least five GH-related genes and pseudogenes in the human genome. All of them have five exons separated by four introns; alternative splicing of exon B leads to the synthesis of a 20 kDa GH variant, instead of the predominant 22 kDa form. This variant lacks amino acid residues 32 to 46, which are present in the larger form. Growth hormone exhibits species specificity that is undoubtedly due to differences in molecular structure among the species. The hormone is stored in specific secretory granules in cells specialized for its synthesis, known as *somatotrophs,* which are acidophils. The secretory granules in humans have a diameter of approximately 300 μm. The somatotrophs are the most abundant cell type in the pituitary gland and they are filled with secretory granules. The store of GH in the pituitary is quite large and actually represents 4%–8% of the gland by dry weight. The hormone is released from the somatotrophs by exocytosis. It is extruded into the extracellular space, particularly in the vicinity of the so-called vascular pole of the cell adjacent to a pituitary sinusoid.

Table 6-3 Human Anterior Pituitary Hormones

	Amino acids	Carbohydrate (CHO)	Molecular weight
I. Corticotropin-related peptide hormones:			
Single small peptides derived from common precursor			
1. α-Melanocyte-stimulating hormone (α-MSH) (α-melanotropin)	13AA		1,823
2. Corticotropin (ACTH)	39AA		4,507
3. β-Lipotropin (β-LPH)	91AA		9,500
4. β-Endorphin, β-LPH (61–91)	31AA		3,100
II. Glycoprotein hormones:			
Composed of two dissimilar peptides. The α chain is similar in structure or identical.			
The β-chain differs with each hormone and confers specificity.			
1. Follicle-stimulating hormone (FSH) (follitropin)	α 89AA β 115AA	18% CHO 5% Sialic acid	32,000
2. Luteinizing hormone (LH) (lutropin)	α 89AA β 115AA	16% CHO 1% Sialic acid	32,000
3. Thyrotropin (TSH)	α 89AA β 112AA	16% CHO 1% Sialic acid	32,000
III. Somatomammotropin hormones:			
Single peptide chains with 2 or 3 SS[a] bonds; no carbohydrate			
1. Prolactin (PRL)	198AA		23,510
2. Growth hormone (GH) or somatotropin	191AA		22,650

[a]SS = disulfide.

The actions of GH and additional aspects of its control will be considered after the discussion of the hypothalamic hormones. Other details are provided in Chapter 12.

As indicated above, GH secretion is regulated by at least two releasing and one inhibiting hormone, namely GHRH, GHS, and somatostatin. Under normal circumstances, the rate of GH release depends on a balance between the stimulatory effect of GHRH/GHS and the inhibitory effect of somatostatin. GHRH exerts its biological actions by binding to a membrane-anchored protein shown to be a guanine nucleotide-binding regulatory protein (G protein)–coupled receptor. As such, the GHRH receptor contains seven transmembrane domains. Its activation by GHRH results in cyclic AMP formation. The GHRH receptor gene appears to be expressed only in the anterior pituitary gland, in which two mRNA transcripts of 2.5 and 4 kb can be detected.

The receptor of GHSs (termed *GH secretagogue receptor*) also belongs to the superfamily of seven-transmembrane domain G protein–coupled receptors. The GHS receptor is a 366-amino acid protein with a molecular weight of about 40 kD. A shorter form of 286 amino acids also exists, but both forms appear to be derived from a single gene by alternative splicing of the primary RNA transcript. In addition to being present in the pituitary gland, the GHS receptor is also expressed in the arcuate-ventromedial nuclei of the hypothalamus and the infundibular region of the median eminence. Patients with GHRH deficiency also fail to respond to GHSs, suggesting the existence of an additional defect of GHS receptor function.

The somatostatin receptor is another seven-transmembrane domain, G protein–coupled receptor. Thus far, five different somatostatin receptors have been described, with an overall sequence homology of 40% to 60%. Despite these large divergencies in amino acid sequence, the somatostatin receptors recognize both somatostatin 14 and 28 with high affinity; all of them are negatively coupled to adenylate cyclase. Interestingly, their tissue distribution is also divergent; some have greater expression in the brain than in peripheral tissues and vice versa.

Prolactin (PRL)

Prolactin (Table 6-3) is a 23,000 molecular-weight protein hormone that bears considerable structural resemblance to GH. In fact, both hormones appear to have evolved from gene duplication of a common ancestral gene. Despite this, the PRL and GH genes are located on different chromosomes. While in humans there appears to exist a single PRL gene, in rodents there is evidence for at least three related genes, all of which are expressed in the placenta. As in the case of GH, there are several forms of PRL. The predominant form of 199 amino acids has a molecular weight of 23,000 Da. The main function of PRL is to induce mammary gland growth and milk secretion in the properly prepared breast following delivery of the infant (see Chapter 9). In laboratory rodents, PRL affects gonadal function and helps maintain the structure and function of accessory sex organs. Whether PRL acts similarly in humans is not known. The fact that PRL receptors have been found in the ovary of primates, however, suggests a physiological role for the hormone in higher species. An important function of prolactin is to up-regulate immune function in animals and humans. It does so by stimulating lymphocyte proliferation and by providing together with GH the initial signals that prepare cells for proliferation and differentiation.

The human pituitary contains 5 times less PRL than GH. Prolactin is produced by lactotropic cells, which can constitute up to 25% of the normal population of anterior hypophyseal cells. Both the number and the size of the lactotrophs are increased by estrogen, and this becomes particularly noticeable during pregnancy. Serum PRL levels are higher in nonpregnant women than in men, reflecting the difference in estrogen production between the two sexes. However, not all changes in PRL secretion are related to sex steroids, as shown by the increase in circulating PRL levels that occurs during sleep in both males and females.

Prolactin secretion is controlled by PRL-inhibiting and PRL-releasing factors. Several neuropeptides have been shown to stimulate PRL release, including TRH, oxyocin, VIP, the VIP-related peptide, peptide histidine isoleucine (PHI), angiotensin II, substance P, and neurotensin. None of them stimulate PRL secretion in a specific fashion. The recent identification of a hypothalamic peptide able to specifically stimulate PRL release under conditions in which several other putative PRL releasing factors were ineffective provided strong evidence that this peptide, termed *PRL releasing peptide* (PRP), represents one of the long-sought-after PRL releasing factors. The PRP receptor, known as *hGR3, GPR10* or *UHR-1*, binds PRP with high affinity. Its encoding cDNA contains an open reading frame predicting a polypeptide of 370 amino acids that bears significant structural similarities with other members of the G-coupled receptor superfamily. Activation of hGR3 by PRP does not affect the release of any pituitary hormone, with the exception of PRL. A conclusive demonstration that PRP is a physiologically meaningful PRL-releasing factor will require evidence showing that PRP is released into the portal circulation and that inhibition of its expression results in PRL deficiency.

Dopamine is a major PRL-inhibiting factor. Dopamine inhibits PRL secretion by binding to a dopamine receptor of the D_2 subtype. This receptor inhibits adenylate cyclase via coupling to a G protein of the G_i type. The D_2 receptor belongs to a family that comprises at least three other members. All of them contain seven transmembrane domains, a topology characteristic of all known G protein–linked receptors. Dopamine reaches the portal vessels after being released from terminals of the tuberoinfundibular dopaminergic tract that ends in juxtaposition to the hypophyseal portal capillaries (Fig. 6-3 and Table 6-1). Receptors for the catecholamine are found in the pituitary. Blockers of dopamine action can reverse the inhibition of PRL release normally exercised by the hypothalamus, and it is estimated that the concentration of dopamine in portal blood may be sufficient to hold PRL secretion in check, except when stimulated by stress or by the suckling stimulus. The elevation in PRL that occurs under these conditions is probably related not only to withdrawal of dopaminergic inhibition but also to secretion of PRL-releasing factors.

Adrenocorticotropin (ACTH)

Adrenocorticotropin, as its name implies, is the adenohypophyseal hormone that controls the function of the adrenal cortex. It is a relatively small molecular-weight polypeptide hormone consisting of a single chain of 39 amino acids. The complete structure is known and the hormone has been synthesized (Fig. 6-4, Table 6-3). In-

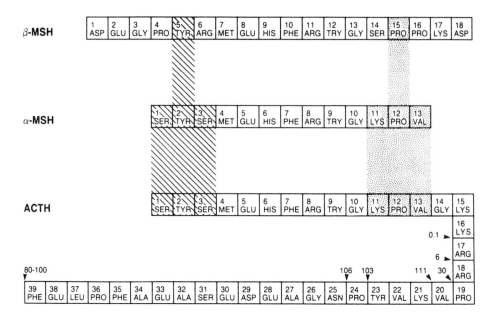

Fig. 6-4 The structure of human corticotropin (ACTH) and the melanocyte-stimulating hormones (MSHs). The shaded areas represent similarities in amino acid sequence. Figures with arrows on the ACTH molecule indicate the biological activity of peptide fragments beginning at the N-terminal amino acid to the point indicated by the arrow. (From Daughaday WH: The adenohypophysis. In: *Williams Textbook of Endocrinology*, 5th ed., RH Williams, ed., Saunders, Philadelphia, pp. 31–79, 1974.)

terestingly, the entire molecule is not needed for biological activity. The first 16 amino acids beginning with the N-terminal amino acid are all that is required for minimal biological activity. Progressive increases in activity occur as the length of the chain increases until full biological activity is present with a polypeptide consisting of the first 23 amino acids.

Recombinant DNA techniques have revealed that ACTH is part of the POMC precursor molecule. The POMC molecule and its constituents are illustrated in Figure 6-5. This large peptide is produced in certain specific loci of the brain and in the anterior and intermediate lobes of the pituitary gland. Processing of the prohormone varies depending on its cellular site. In the anterior lobe, it is processed to ACTH and β-endorphin, an endogenous opioid peptide of 31 amino acids. It has analgesic action but is not secreted in sufficient amounts to be physiologically significant in this regard. In the intermediate lobe of rodents, the processing of proopiomelanocortin is different, peptide bonds in the ACTH sequence being broken between the 13 and 18 position, resulting in the production of α-MSH (ACTH 1–13) and CLIP (ACTH 18–39). In the brain, it appears that the major products are ACTH, β-endorphin, and also α-MSH.

Evidence from light microscopic studies has suggested that in the adenohypophysis, ACTH is secreted by basophils. With the electron microscope ACTH-producing cells appear irregularly shaped and replete with secretory granules. Ra-

Fig. 6-5 Diagram of the structure of the pro-opiomelanocortin (POMC) molecule and the hormones derived from it by proteolysis. The precursor POMC protein contains a leader sequence (signal peptide) that is followed by a fragment that contains the sequence of γ-MSH (amino acids 51–62), the ACTH molecule (1–39) that contains the sequences for α-MSH (ACTH 1–13) and corticotropin-like intermediate lobe peptide CLIP (ACTH 18–39), and the β-lipotropin (1–91) molecule that contains the sequences of γ-LPH (1–58) and β-endorphin (61–91). The latter also includes the sequence for met-enkephalin (first five amino acids of β-endorphin). Potential sites for proteolytic cleavage are indicated by the presence of the basic amino acids arginine-lysine (Arg-Lys). (From Reichlin S: In: *Williams Textbook of Endocrinology,* 7th ed., JD Wilson and DW Foster, eds., Saunders, Philadelphia, p. 502, 1985.)

dioimmunoassay of plasma ACTH is the method of choice for evaluating ACTH secretion, although plasma glucocorticoid levels can also be measured as an index of ACTH secretion.

The secretion of ACTH is augmented by noxious stimuli of various sorts termed *stresses,* and this will be discussed in Chapter 14. In addition, ACTH secretion is also inhibited by glucocorticoids, an example of classic negative feedback regulation. As indicated above, the hypothalamus controls ACTH secretion via a CRH. The biological actions of CRH are initiated by the binding of the neuropeptide to a membrane protein structurally related to the calcitonin–VIP–GHRH family of G protein–coupled receptors. The CRH receptor is a 415-amino acid protein displaying seven putative transmembrane domains. It is encoded by a 2.7 kb mRNA and is positively coupled to adenylate cyclase. Two types of CRH receptors have been described. CRH_1 is mainly expressed in the pituitary and brain; CRH_2 has two forms, CRH_{2a} and CRH_{2b}, derived from alternative splicing of the mRNA primary transcript. Whereas form 2a is predominantly expressed in brain, form 2b is largely expressed in two peripheral tissues, the heart and skeletal muscle. Humans do not appear to express this receptor isoform.

Vasopressin has a physiological role in the control of ACTH release as there is a deficiency in ACTH release in animals with hereditary diabetes insipidus; such animals lack endogenous vasopressin. Another indication that vasopressin is a corticotropin-releasing factor is its direct action in stimulating ACTH release in a dose-related fashion from the pituitary incubated *in vitro.* Finally, vasopressin is present in high concentrations in portal blood collected from the pituitary stalk of monkeys and rats; at a range capable of stimulating ACTH release.

It is now apparent that vasopressin and CRH cooperate in the control of ACTH release. Vasopressin can potentiate the action of CRH at both hypothalamic and pituitary levels. Antisera against CRH given intravenously largely block the stress response, which can also be inhibited partially by vasopressin antisera. Furthermore, it appears that the vasopressin that reaches the pituitary comes predominantly from vasopressinergic neurons that extend to the median eminence to end in juxtaposition to portal vessels. Many of the vasopressinergic neurons apparently also contain CRH, so that there may be co-release of the two peptides into portal blood.

Melanocyte-Stimulating Hormone (MSH)

In lower forms such as reptiles and amphibia, MSH is clearly formed in and secreted by the intermediate lobe of the pituitary gland. Immunohistochemical analysis of adult human pituitary glands has shown that α-MSH cells are more frequently present in the anterior lobe than in the pars intermedia, which in humans is rudimentary. In both, the scattered intermediate-type cells that form the rudimentary pars intermedia and the anterior lobe, α-MSH co-localizes with ACTH. There are two forms of MSH in nearly all species. The first is known as α-MSH and contains 13 amino acids (Fig. 6-4, Table 6-3). These 13 are identical with the first 13 amino acids of ACTH. The β-MSH is a somewhat larger molecule and exhibits considerable species variation in both size and amino acid sequence. It consists of 22 amino acids. Amino acids 11–17 of β-MSH and ACTH are identical. In view of the overlap in structure between the MSHs and ACTH, it is not surprising that ACTH has MSH-like activity. The converse, however, is not true, and MSH has no ACTH-like activity, except possibly during embryonic development.

Melanocyte-stimulating hormone, as its name implies, acts on the melanocytes in lower forms such as amphibians and reptiles to stimulate the dispersion of melanin granules within these cells, which causes darkening of the skin and permits the animal to blend with its environment. Even in humans, continued administration of MSH for a period of days will produce skin darkening. Both α-MSH and related peptides have been shown to delay the extinction of learned avoidance behaviors and food-motivated behaviors in a variety of experimental models. Administered intraventricularly, α-MSH has also been shown to have antipyretic and anti-inflammatory effects. It also inhibits the release of CRH and LHRH at low concentrations (10^{-13} M) in the rat. Although for a long time these effects were considered as pharmacological, the recent cloning of a family of receptors for the melanocortin peptides in both humans and rodents and the identification of their sites of expression in the brain have provided compelling evidence for a physiological role of MSH in the regulation of mammalian brain function. To date, four types of melanocortin receptors (MC1-R to MC4-R) have been molecularly characterized, and three of them were found to bind MSH (only MC2-R binds ACTH selectively). All four receptors are functionally coupled to adenylate cyclase. Although their roles in the nervous system appear to be complex and diverse, a specific function in the inhibitory control of feeding behavior was recently assigned to one of them (MC4-R) by demonstrating that its genetic deletion or pharmacological inhibition results in hyperphagia and obesity. The secretion of MSH has been postulated to be controlled by both MSH-releasing and MSH-inhibiting factors. However, the physiologic significance of these factors is not clear, and it appears that the major hypothalamic inhibitory control over MSH secretion is exercised by dopaminergic nerves in the intermediate lobe.

Pituitary Glycoprotein Hormones

The pituitary hormones discussed above are relatively simple proteins. The adeno-hypophysis secretes other more complex hormones that have a carbohydrate moiety attached to the protein component that in turn is composed of two interconnected amino acid chains. These hormones are called *glycoproteins* because of their carbohydrate moiety. There are three pituitary glycoprotein hormones, namely thyrotropin (thyroid-stimulating hormone, TSH), follicle-stimulating hormone (FSH), and luteinizing hormone (LH), each with a molecular weight of about 30,000 Da. They consist of two subunits, an α-subunit that is identical in the three hormones, and three different β-subunits that confer biological specificity to each hormone (Table 6-2). The α- and β- chains are synthesized separately, and they are combined before joining the carbohydrate moieties. At the time of secretion, an excess of α-chains is secreted so that one can detect α-chain in the plasma by radioimmunoassay. When the secretion rate is elevated, a small amount of free β-chain may also appear in the plasma.

Thyroid-Stimulating Hormone (TSH)

As discussed in Chapter 13, this hormone stimulates secretion of the hormones thyroxine and triiodothyronine by the thyroid gland. As indicated above, the α-chain is identical to that of the gonadotropins, and the biological specificity is conferred by the β-chain, which is unique for TSH. There is a high degree of conservation in the amino acid sequence of the TSH-β subunit among different mammalian species. In all cases, the subunit appears to be encoded by a single gene, the expression of which is subjected to regulatory control by thyroid hormones. Like other glycoprotein hormones in the pituitary, TSH is secreted by basophilic cells, termed *thyrotrophs,* and these cells are characterized by the presence of abundant, relatively small secretory granules. The thyrotrophs make up to 15% of the cells of the adenohypophysis. The TSH secretion is under negative feedback control by thyroid hormones (see Chapter 13) and is stimulated by the hypothalamic peptide, TRH. Thyrotropin-releasing hormone initiates its biological actions by binding to a membrane-anchored receptor that, like the GHRH, somatostatin, and CRH receptors, belongs to a family of G protein–coupled receptors containing seven highly conserved transmembrane domains. The TRH receptor is a protein of 393–412 amino acids and appears to be the product of a single gene. Binding of TRH to the receptor results in phospholipase C activation, calcium mobilization, and cyclic AMP formation (see below).

Follicle-Stimulating Hormone (FSH)

This gonadotropin stimulates the ovarian follicles to grow. When given to a hypophysectomized animal, the only action of FSH is to stimulate growth of the follicles beyond the early antrum phase. As indicated in Chapter 9, primordial follicles are surrounded by only one layer of granulosa cells. As they grow into graafian follicles, a small, fluid-filled lumen, known as the *antrum,* eventually forms between the layers of proliferating granulosa cells. This process requires the presence of FSH. In the presence of LH, FSH increases estrogen secretion by the ovary. In the male, FSH acts to promote spermatogenesis. Further details of these actions are given in Chapters 9 and 10.

Like other glycoprotein hormones, FSH is produced in basophils. Electron microscopy and immunocytochemical methods reveal that it is secreted by cells called *gonadotrophs*. Some of these secrete only FSH, but others secrete both FSH and LH. The FSH is produced in cells that have very small secretory granules relative to those of other pituitary cells.

The synthesis and secretion of FSH is controlled by LHRH, which promotes the synthesis of the FSH β-subunit via activation of at least two signaling pathways: one mediated by protein kinase C (PKC), the other by mitogen-activated protein kinase (MAPK).

Luteinizing Hormone (LH)

Pituitary control of the gonads requires still another glycoprotein hormone, LH, also known as *interstitial cell-stimulating hormone* (ICSH) because it stimulates the interstitial cells of both ovary and testes. The function of this hormone is to induce ovulation and the formation of the corpus luteum in the female, and to stimulate steroid secretion in both the ovary and the testes (see Chapters 9 and 10). The hormone is structurally similar to FSH and again possesses the common α-chain. Its β-chain is different from that of FSH and TSH and confers specific biological activity to the molecule. Once more, LH is found in basophils. As in the case of FSH, some gonadotrophs secrete only LH, but others secrete both FSH and LH.

The secretion of LH is stimulated by LHRH. The peptide releases not only LH but, to a lesser extent, FSH as well, which has led to the concept that LHRH is sufficient to account for the hypothalamic stimulation of both FSH and LH release. Because dissociation of FSH and LH release can occur following hypothalamic lesions and stimulations and also in a variety of physiological states, an FSH-releasing factor may exist; however, this point remains controversial. Thus far only partial purifications of the putative FSH-releasing factor have been reported.

The LHRH receptor is a 327-amino acid protein with a molecular weight of 37,000 Da. The nucleotide sequence of the receptor indicates that it, as in the case of the GHRH, somatostatin, CRH, and TRH receptors, contains seven transmembrane domains characteristic of G protein–coupled receptors. Surprisingly, the LHRH receptor lacks the cytoplasmic C-terminus region, which appears to be important for the biological activity of other G protein–coupled receptors. The 5'-flanking region of the mouse LHRH receptor gene contains the regulatory elements for tissue-specific expression and for LHRH-dependent regulation.

Interestingly, transgenic mice carrying a reporter gene under the control of the LHRH receptor promoter express the reporter gene not only in the pituitary but also in the testis and brain. This latter location is consistent with previous observations demonstrating the presence of LHRH binding and LHRH receptor mRNA in several regions of the brain, and it strengthens the notion that LHRH exerts actions on the brain, in addition to stimulating gonadotropin secretion from the pituitary gland.

With the elucidation of the structures of these releasing and inhibiting hormones, it has been possible to prepare many analogs of each of the factors. In the case of LHRH, the initial aim was to obtain inhibitory analogs that might suppress fertility. However, it was accidentally found that analogs more active than the natural compound could easily be prepared if unnatural amino acids were substituted at positions likely to be subject to proteolysis. The agonist analogs have proven to be important clinically.

Actions of Releasing and Inhibiting Hormones on Other Pituitary Hormones

We have already alluded to the fact that TRH stimulates not only TSH but also PRL release. Whether the latter action has physiologic significance remains uncertain. Similarly, LHRH has FSH-releasing activity, which has resulted in LHRH being also called *gonadotropin-releasing hormone* (GnRH). It has also been reported that LHRH, under certain conditions, stimulates PRL release, but the physiological significance of this effect remains unclear. Somatostatin inhibits not only the secretion of GH but also the secretion of most other pituitary hormones if given in sufficient dosage. It also suppresses the functions of many other systems, probably because it is distributed widely throughout the body (see below).

Distribution of the Mammalian Peptides in Lower Forms

The initial clue that these hypothalamic peptides might be found in lower forms came from work on CRH, as the amphibian skin peptide sauvagine has CRH activity when tested on the pituitaries of rats. Similarly, urophysin I, a peptide obtained from the urophysis, a neurohypophysis-like organ in the caudal spinal cord of fish, has CRH activity. Subsequently, it was shown that yeast mating factor had structural homology with the mammalian LHRH and released LH from rat pituitaries, albeit with one ten-thousandth the potency of the mammalian hormone. It had previously been demonstrated that LHRH would induce mating behavior in higher forms, including mammals. Although all the evidence is not yet in, it appears that these peptides exist throughout the phylogenetic scale down to unicellular organisms. They probably have a similar function in unicellular organisms as in higher organisms. As differentiation increases up the phylogenetic scale, their localization is restricted to certain areas, but their basic functions do not change. Thus, LHRH is a reproductive peptide, whereas CRH and vasopressin are stress peptides.

Mechanism of Action of Releasing and Inhibiting Hormones

Peptide hormones act by combining with highly specific receptors on the cell membrane of target cells. The peptide–receptor interaction then activates one or more of the several possible pathways for stimulation of secretion (see Chapter 3). One pathway involves activation of adenylate cyclase with the generation of cyclic AMP. The cyclic AMP formed activates a protein kinase that may mediate most of the effects of the cyclic nucleotide on cellular function. In the case of the pituitary, it has been suggested that activation of a protein kinase by cyclic AMP results in phosphorylation of certain membrane constituents that promote exocytosis, the mechanism for secretion. The secretory granules migrate to the cell surface and fuse with the cell membrane, and the granular core containing the hormone is extruded into the extracellular space, particularly at the vascular pole of the cell. Of the various pituitary cells, it would appear that the somatotrophs utilize the cyclic AMP pathway based on the ability of cyclic AMP to activate secretion and of its augmentation by inhibition of the breakdown of cyclic AMP by phosphodiesterase inhibitors. Similarly, the stimulatory effect of CRH on ACTH release appears to be mediated by cyclic AMP. In the gonadotrophs, the cyclic AMP system seems to play a minor role, possibly only in enhancing synthesis of LH.

Calcium plays an important part in the releasing process. Extracellular calcium is required for optimal release of all pituitary hormones. It may also be mobilized from intracellular stores in the case of some of the hormones as well. For those releasing factors that operate via the cyclic AMP mechanism, a cyclic AMP–dependent protein kinase may be involved in opening calcium channels, allowing entrance of the ion and possibly mobilizing it from intracellular stores.

The products of arachidonic acid metabolism can promote exocytosis, and their relative importance varies with the pituitary cell type, just as the relative importance of cyclic AMP seems to vary with the cell type. Prostaglandins appear to be important in the release of growth hormone and ACTH, and they can activate the production of cyclic AMP. In other cells such as the gonadotrophs, it appears that metabolites of arachidonic acid different from prostaglandins, such as the leukotrienes and epoxides, may also be involved in the exocytosis process.

Arachidonic acid release from the cell membrane may result from a receptor-mediated activation of phospholipase C, a membrane-bound enzyme that catalyzes the hydrolysis of polyphosphoinositides into inositol triphosphate and diacylglycerol. The latter not only contains arachidonate, which is then made available to phospholipase A for subsequent metabolism, but also interacts with protein kinase C, a calcium-dependent, phospholipid-activated enzyme. Protein kinase C phosphorylates several proteins that then participate in the process of hormone release. Inositol triphosphate, the other product of phospholipase C activity, mobilizes intracellular calcium from the endoplasmic reticulum.

The releasing process is not completely understood, but each cell type utilizes these various pathways to varying degrees. The role of guanylate cyclase and its product, cyclic GMP, is not yet clear.

The inhibiting hormones such as somatostatin and dopamine act in part by inhibition of adenylate cyclase and in part also by other mechanisms such as decreasing the availability of calcium to the cell.

If the cell membrane is depolarized by placing pituitary tissue in a high potassium medium, release is also induced. It is not known whether depolarization of the cell membrane actually accompanies the releasing process of normally secreting pituitary cells, but when it is artificially induced by a high potassium concentration, it probably increases calcium uptake by the cells, which then mediates the releasing process.

The means by which the secretory granules migrate to the cell surface remain an enigma. It has been postulated that this might involve microtubules or microfilaments; however, colchicine, which disrupts microtubules, not only fails to block the release of several pituitary hormones but actually augments it, suggesting that the tubules might hold the granules in the interior of the cell, and that after dissolution of the tubules, the granules then migrate spontaneously to the surface, possibly because of electrostatic forces between the granule and the inside of the cell membrane.

The releasing hormones act on the cell very rapidly (within less than a minute) to either promote or inhibit release of particular pituitary hormones; however, their precise effect on the biosynthesis of these hormones has not been elucidated. With sufficient stimulation of release, synthesis is promoted, probably via an increase in the mRNA required for the synthesis of the pituitary hormone in question. Whether this is secondary to the release process or represents another primary action of the releasing hormone on the biosynthetic process itself remains to be determined.

In general, our knowledge of the intracellular signaling mechanisms that mediate the stimulatory–inhibitory effects of releasing–inhibiting hormones on pituitary hormone secretion is still incomplete. Surprisingly, releasing hormones such as TRH and LHRH have been found to utilize the same intracellular signal transduction pathways to exert their stimulatory effects on TSH–PRL and LH–FSH release. Both receptors are coupled to the same G proteins, which are insensitive to pertussis toxin and activate a phosphoinositide-PKC–mediated pathway. Activation by their respective ligands results in the stimulation of phospholipase C, enhanced phosphoinositide turnover, calcium mobilization, cAMP formation, and arachidonic acid release. This situation is not unique to releasing hormones as it has also been observed in the case of growth factors. It is possible that the specificity in these seemingly common signaling pathways is provided by binding to additional G-proteins and/or differential activation of a family of serine/threonine protein kinases known as *mitogen-activated protein kinases* (MAPKs) or *extracellular signal-related kinases* (ERKs). These kinases, which are rapidly activated by both growth factors and releasing hormones, such as LHRH, appear to play an essential role in a number of signaling cascades leading to nonproliferative changes in cell activity.

Factors Affecting Responsiveness of the Adenohypophysis to Releasing and Inhibiting Hormones

The hormonal state is very important in determining the responsiveness of the adenohypophysis to the various releasing hormones. In the case of TRH, pituitary responsiveness is enhanced by removal of the thyroid and consequent loss of negative feedback by thyroxine and triiodothyronine. Conversely, responsiveness is suppressed by the administration of thyroid hormones. In fact, the negative feedback of thyroid hormone seems to take place predominantly in the pituitary gland to modulate its responsiveness to TRH (Fig. 6-6, for other details see Chapter 13).

Negative feedback results in decreased transcription of the pro-TRH gene. At the pituitary level, thyroid hormone excess results in a decreased number of TRH receptors on thyrotrophs and decreased transcription of TSH-α and -β genes. Release of TRH is under inhibitory control via circulating thyroid hormones.

In the case of CRH, there is also good evidence that adrenal steroids feed back directly at the pituitary to inhibit the response to CRH (Fig. 6-6); however, this feedback also takes place at the hypothalamic level to inhibit release of CRH and vasopressin.

The interplay between gonadal steroids and the hypothalamic–pituitary axis is particularly complex (see Chapters 9 and 10). Following removal of the gonads and the elimination of feedback by the gonadal steroids, predominantly estrogen in the

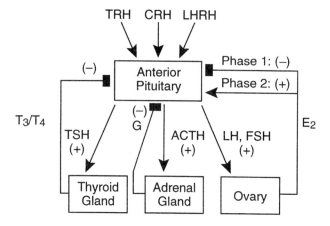

Fig. 6-6 Modulation of anterior pituitary responsiveness to hypothalamic releasing hormones. (−) Inhibits the response to the releasing hormone; (+) facilitates the response. G, glucocorticoids; E_2, estradiol; T_3, triiodothyronine; T_4, thyroxine; Phase 1, early phase; Phase 2, later phase, only in females.

female and testosterone in the male, levels of both FSH and LH are elevated. The release of these pituitary hormones is pulsatile and occurs rhythmically. The timing of the discharge varies among species and even among individual animals within a species. In the human, these pulses occur hourly and are called the *circhoral rhythm* of LH release. This rhythm is brought about by pulsatile release of LHRH.

Following removal of negative feedback, the enhanced LHRH release increases not only the discharge of gonadotropins but also their synthesis, so that the quantities stored in the gland increase. This augmented storage is associated with an increase in responsiveness to the neurohormone. Small doses of estrogen or androgen can suppress the responsiveness to LHRH, and this occurs quickly. At least in the case of estrogen administration, it can take place within 1 hour. With long-term therapy, there is suppression not only of release, but also of its synthesis, and the pituitary content of gonadotropin consequently falls. This is associated with a further decline in responsiveness to LHRH, which may be caused in part by down-regulation of LHRH receptors.

In the female, complex endocrine relationships occur during the menstrual cycle. Responsiveness to LHRH during the early follicular phase is minimal. Responsiveness increases as the follicular phase progresses and reaches its height at the time of the preovulatory discharge of LH. Treatment of women with estrogen has a biphasic effect on pituitary responsiveness to LHRH; the initial suppression is followed by an augmented responsiveness (Fig. 6-6). Thus, estrogen secreted by the preovulatory follicles is probably responsible for the enhanced responsiveness to LHRH that occurs in the late follicular phase.

In addition, the characteristics of the preovulatory discharge of LH in response to LHRH change, the response becoming much more rapid and pulse-like. This further change in responsiveness probably emanates from LHRH itself, as it can be induced by a priming injection of LHRH in the late follicular phase of the cycle. Responsiveness then declines after the ovulatory discharge.

The mechanism by which estrogen augments responsiveness to LHRH is not known. It might induce the formation of additional receptors for the neurohormone, or, alternatively, it might alter the synthesis of LH and provide a larger pool of re-leaseable LH. Similarly, the mechanism for the self-priming action (positive feed-back) of LHRH remains to be elucidated, but this could be explained by an effect on synthesis of a releasable pool of LH or, alternatively, by an effect of LHRH to induce new LHRH receptors. The ability of LHRH to up-regulate its own receptors has been demonstrated.

This remarkable increase in responsiveness to LHRH as a function of the steroid milieu undoubtedly accounts in part for the preovulatory discharge of LH, but it is believed that an enhanced release of LHRH is also involved. This is induced once again by estrogen from the preovulatory follicle (see Chapter 9). This increased re-lease of LHRH is probably responsible for bringing on the self-priming action of LHRH that characterizes the late preovulatory phase. Evidence for the increased re-lease of LHRH at the preovulatory surge of LH is provided by the detection of very high levels of LHRH in portal blood collected from the transected stalk at this stage of the cycle in animals.

It would appear, then, that the preovulatory discharge of LH is brought about by enhanced release of LHRH coupled with a marked increase in responsiveness to the neurohormone. The result is a discharge of LH far greater than that necessary to induce ovulation. Perhaps this is part of a fail-safe mechanism to ensure full ovu-lation even when follicular development is not optimal; it might serve to prolong the reproductive life of the individual.

Putative Synaptic Transmitters Involved in Controlling the Release of Releasing Hormones

The neurons that produce releasing factors are in synaptic contact with a host of pu-tative neurotransmitters. The most abundant neurotransmitter in the hypothalamus is the excitatory amino acid glutamate. The hypothalamus is also supplied with monoaminergic nerve fibers. There is a heavy input of noradrenergic fibers from neurons whose cell bodies lie in the brain stem. The distribution of these neurons has been mapped by fluorescent histochemistry. There are also terminals from epi-nephrine-containing neurons that end in the hypothalamus. These also appear to originate from neurons whose cell bodies are located in the brain stem.

Axons of serotonin-containing neurons whose cell bodies lie in the medial raphe nuclei project to the suprachiasmatic, anterior hypothalamic, and median eminence regions. Assays for choline acetyltransferase indicate the widespread distribution of cholinergic fibers within the hypothalamus as well. There is also an abundance of histamine that appears to be located in synaptosome-like structures, and this amine is concentrated particularly in the median eminence region where it may also serve as a synaptic transmitter. There is evidence as well for a γ-aminobutyric acid-containing (or GABAergic) system that is localized partially in the infundibular nu-cleus with projections to the median eminence. Other GABAergic neurons are small interneurons localized throughout the hypothalamus where they may impinge on dendrites or somata of releasing-hormone neurons to inhibit their secretory activity.

Great effort has been put into experiments with rodents and monkeys to determine the role of these possible transmitters in controlling the release of the various releasing hormones. The most extensive studies have been done on gonadotropins. As discussed in Chapter 9, it appears that among the important neurotransmitter systems involved in the control of LHRH secretion are those that employ excitatory amino acids to stimulate LHRH release and GABA to inhibit LHRH neuronal activity. In addition there are excitatory noradrenergic synapses that may contribute to inducing not only the preovulatory release of LHRH but also the increased LHRH release that follows castration. In the case of the preovulatory release of LHRH, the synapses may be in the preoptic-anterior hypothalamic region, whereas in the case of the increased release in the castrate, the synapses may be on the other population of LHRH neurons, located in the arcuate nucleus. The stimulatory effect of the noradrenergic system on LHRH release appears to be complemented by intrahypothalamic neurons that produce neuropeptide Y. This peptide has been shown to not only stimulate LHRH release at the level of the median eminence but also to synergize with LHRH in the pituitary gland following its release into the portal blood.

Dopamine has been postulated to both stimulate and inhibit LH release. The evidence is confusing, but the view held at the present time is that this catecholamine may have only a minor role.

Serotonin, when injected into the third ventricle in castrates, can inhibit LH release; this indicates that it is an inhibitory transmitter, but other evidence suggests that it may facilitate preovulatory LH release. Histamine can stimulate LH release following its intraventricular injection in large doses. It is still not clear whether this has physiological significance.

Considerable evidence shows a cholinergic link in gonadotropin release, because atropine can block gonadotropin release when it is administered systemically, microinjected into the third ventricle, or implanted within the hypothalamus.

In the case of ACTH, considerable evidence indicates that CRH is under the stimulatory control of the noradrenergic system; there is some evidence for cholinergic and serotoninergic stimulatory components as well. TRH has not been investigated extensively, but may be under adrenergic control. Growth hormone release also appears to be under adrenergic control with a stimulatory α-receptor and an inhibitory β-receptor component, but the relative importance of dopamine and norepinephrine has yet to be clearly established.

Prolactin is definitely under inhibitory control via dopamine. There is a tuberoinfundibular dopaminergic tract, the neurons of which have cell bodies lying in the arcuate nucleus and axons projecting to the external layer of the median eminence. Here they terminate in juxtaposition to hypophyseal portal capillaries. Dopamine agonists, such as bromocriptine, can lower plasma prolactin in hyperprolactinemic patients.

In addition to these classical low-molecular-weight transmitters, the hypothalamus is a repository for a veritable host of neuropeptides. Not only are there the releasing and inhibiting factors just discussed, and vasopressin and oxytocin, but brain opioid peptide systems are also present. Within the hypothalamus, infundibular neurons produce POMC. Their axons project to other parts of the hypothalamus and other brain regions and apparently establish synaptic contacts with other cells, secreting β-endorphin, ACTH, and possibly α-MSH into the synaptic cleft. Studies using opiate receptor blockers, such as naloxone, have shown that the opioid peptides are involved in stress-induced PRL release. The peptide involved appears to be β-endorphin based on studies with specific antibodies against β-endorphin that block stress-induced PRL release. β-Endorphin also appears to have a physiologically significant inhibitory role in the control of gonadotropin secretion.

Enkephalin and dynorphin neurons and even other classes of opioid peptides are also localized in neurons within the hypothalamus. The functional significance of these other opioid peptides remains to be clarified.

In addition to these brain peptides, many peptides that were originally thought to be localized exclusively in other organs have now been found in the brain. Among these are angiotensin II, which was first thought to be formed only in the circulation after release of renin from the juxtaglomerular apparatus of the kidney. There are angiotensin II-producing neurons within the hypothalamus, and they may play a stimulatory role in controlling ACTH and PRL secretion. The more recently discovered atrial natriuretic peptides, whose main locus is the atria of the heart, have now been found within neurons in the hypothalamus and may suppress ACTH as well as vasopressin secretion (see Chapter 7). Of particular interest is the peptide *pituitary adenylate cyclase activating peptide* (PACAP; Table 6-1). It is apparently released into the portal vessels and acts in the pituitary to induce cyclic AMP formation. Despite its potency in this regard, it has not been found to be an effective stimulus for hormone release. Recent experiments have shown that it may regulate POMC gene transcription.

Many gastrointestinal peptides originally thought to be localized only in the gut have been found in brain neuronal systems. An example is vasoactive intestinal polypeptide, which may play a role in controlling pituitary hormone secretion via both hypothalamic and pituitary actions. Cholecystokinin is also present in the brain and appears to have significance in the control of pituitary hormone secretion, as do neurotensin and substance P. Antagonists against these various peptides and antisera directed against them have been used to determine their physiological significance.

Short Loop Feedback of Pituitary Hormones to Alter Their Own Release

A variety of pituitary hormones exert short loop negative feedback actions to suppress their own release. In this case, the hormone inhibits its own release without reaching the general circulation (Fig. 6-7). This is in contrast to the so-called long loop feedback of pituitary target gland hormones such as gonadal steroids. It was originally thought that the short loop feedback of pituitary hormones might be mediated in the hypothalamus by reverse flow in portal vessels, which would deliver the pituitary hormones to the hypothalamus. There is some evidence for reverse flow under certain circumstances, but it appears that some pituitary hormones may actually be produced in the brain. In the case of ACTH, it is now known that the POMC molecule is synthesized in neurons in cells of the medial basal hypothalamus (arcuate nucleus). ACTH, a fragment of this molecule, may be secreted from cells producing POMC. Evidence also shows that PRL-secreting and LH-secreting neurons exist within the brain. Short loop negative feedback has been clearly established for PRL and GH. In the latter case, the feedback may be mediated not only by GH it-

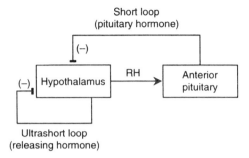

Fig. 6-7 Short and ultrashort loop feedback systems in the hypothalamic–pituitary unit. RH, releasing hormone.

self but also by IGF-I (see below), either delivered via the peripheral circulation or made directly in the brain. There is also considerable evidence of short loop feedback for LH and FSH as well as ACTH. Little work has been done on TSH, but in all probability the same mechanism applies to this hormone.

Ultrashort Loop Feedback of Releasing and Inhibiting Hormones to Modify Their Own Release

Ultrashort loop feedback is an alteration in the release of hypothalamic peptide induced by the peptide itself acting within the brain. It may occur as direct recurrent inhibition or via interaction with an interneuron that in turn alters the discharge rate of the peptidergic neuron (Fig. 6-7).

There is evidence from animal experiments for ultrashort loop negative feedback of the releasing hormone neurons to inhibit their own release in the case of somatostatin, GHRH, and LHRH.

Extrapituitary Actions of Releasing Hormones

The distribution of releasing hormones in brain regions outside the hypothalamus (e.g., brain stem, cortex) suggests that they exert extrapituitary actions. As indicated earlier, TRH is found in other brain regions and even in the spinal cord; somatostatin is distributed widely throughout the nervous system and also has been found in the delta cells of the pancreatic islets of Langerhans. Because somatostatin can inhibit the release of both insulin and glucagon, it probably acts locally to control the release of these hormones from the islets.

The clearest behavioral effect of releasing hormones is the induction of mating behavior by relatively low doses of LHRH in animals. The occurrence of LHRH in the preoptic area, the region of the brain that is known to be involved in mating behavior, plus the onset of this behavior shortly after the preovulatory discharge of LHRH, suggested this effect of LHRH. Indeed, LHRH induces mating behavior in many species including nonhuman primates and possibly humans. This is not caused by the gonadotropins released, as these hormones have no effect on mating behavior and as induction of the behavior is seen in the hypophysectomized rat. Further studies have shown that the effect can be obtained by microinjecting LHRH into the preoptic-anterior hypothalamic and arcuate median eminence regions, whereas similar injections into lateral hypothalamus or cortex are ineffective. There is a latency between the injection of LHRH either into the brain or systemically and the onset of mating behavior, suggesting that some intervening steps might be involved.

Thyrotropin-releasing hormone has effects that indicate an arousal action of the hormone—that is, it shortens the duration of pentobarbital anesthesia. The doses required are very large; however, if the hormone is present at synaptic sites in the brain, it is conceivable that these responses to high doses could be physiological. Somatostatin, in contrast, has been shown to depress animals. Thus, the concept is emerging that the releasing factors may have important extrapituitary actions. One could even envision the possibility that they may serve as peptidic neurotransmitters and that this might be a role as important as that of governing the release of anterior pituitary hormones. There is evidence that the action of releasing factors in the CNS may integrate complex hormonal and neural mechanisms—for example, blood pressure and fluid control (vasopressin) or reproductive processes (LHRH).

Another example is GHRH, which has been shown to promote sleep when administered intracerebrally. Conversely, CRH not only stimulates ACTH release, but also has a variety of other effects on the central nervous system, which mimic the response to stress. Thus, CRH induces anxiogenic effects, increases cardiovascular activity, induces anorexia, and inhibits LHRH secretion. All of these effects are independent of its stimulatory effects on glucocorticoid secretion.

PITUITARY GROWTH HORMONE, ITS ACTION AND ITS CONTROL

Now that the overall hypothalamic control of anterior pituitary hormone secretion has been considered, the actions of GH and control of its secretion will be discussed in more detail.

Actions of Growth Hormone

Growth hormone (GH) has powerful effects on growth and metabolism. Its absence is associated with dwarfism. Its excessive secretion leads to giantism or acromegaly (see below). To study the precise action of GH, it is best to utilize hypophysectomized animals or hypopituitary patients. The hormone can then be administered and its metabolic effects noted. Administration of GH produces the following effects:

1. Decrease in blood amino acid concentrations.
2. Decrease in blood urea nitrogen.
3. Positive nitrogen balance, defined as the difference between daily nitrogen intake in food and excretion in urine and feces as nitrogenous wastes.
4. Increased DNA, RNA, and protein synthesis—that is, a protein anabolic effect.
5. Elevated blood glucose via decreased utilization of carbohydrates and decreased sensitivity to the plasma glucose-lowering action of insulin.

6. Increased oxidation of fat leading to a decrease in the respiratory quotient (R_Q = CO_2 output divided by O_2 intake). The respiratory quotient for the metabolism of carbohydrates to CO_2 and water is 1.0, whereas that for the metabolism of fats is 0.7. Protein metabolism leads to an R_Q of about 0.8. The increased utilization of fats is often accompanied by an elevation of the free fatty acids in blood because of lipid mobilization from fat stores and by an increase in ketone body formation (β-hydroxybutyric acid, acetoacetic acid, acetone) associated with the increased fatty acid oxidation (see Chapter 16).
7. Growth.
8. Stimulation of the growth and calcification of cartilage.
9. High doses of GH given over a long period of time can induce diabetes mellitus in dogs and cats. The action is via an exhaustion of the insulin-secreting beta cells of the islets of Langerhans, which are overstimulated by the elevated plasma glucose as a result of GH secretion. The syndrome is called *metahypophyseal diabetes*. Whether this is the cause of the impaired glucose tolerance observed in acromegalic patients has not been determined.

Mechanism of Action of Growth Hormone

Growth hormone initiates its actions by binding to a single transmembrane-domain, membrane-anchored receptor that is a member of the cytokinine/hematopoietin receptor superfamily. Other members of this family include receptors for ciliary neurotrophic factor, erythropoietin, and interleukin-2, among others. The GH receptor is encoded by a 4.7-kb mRNA that appears to be the product of a single gene. The nucleotide sequence predicts a mature protein of 620 amino acids, with a molecular weight of 70 kDa. The difference between this estimation and the actual weight (130 kDa) determined by gel analysis appears to be due to the heavy glycosylation of the receptor's extracellular domain. The GH receptor is covalently linked to ubiquitin, a proteolytic molecule that appears to be responsible for the short half-life of the receptor.

The complex metabolic effects of GH can be viewed as a means of increasing protein synthesis and turning to fat as the main source of calories so as to spare amino acids for protein synthesis. At the same time, utilization of glucose is suppressed.

The mechanism by which growth hormone accomplishes these myriad effects is incompletely understood. The following facts are known:

1. Growth hormone stimulates the uptake of amino acids by muscle and liver cells, as demonstrated by its clear-cut enhancement of the uptake of the nonutilizable amino acid, α-aminoisobutyric acid. Administering GH leads to the accumulation of this amino acid within cells. The effect on amino acid uptake may be part of the anabolic actions of GH.
2. Although some synthesis of protein can be accomplished under the influence of GH even if RNA synthesis is blocked, it is apparent that later on increased synthesis of RNA is stimulated by GH. These effects do not appear to result from a primary action of the hormone, but due to IGF-I (insulin-like growth factor) instead (see below and Chapter 12). Ultimately, not

only RNA, but also DNA synthesis is increased and finally cell division occurs.

3. The mechanism of action of GH on fat and carbohydrate metabolism is less well understood, but the hormone appears to block the phosphorylation of glucose after carbohydrate has penetrated cells.

4. It is now clear that GH requires an intermediary in order to influence cartilage and bone metabolism. This material was initially called *sulfation factor* because of its ability to stimulate the incorporation of [^{35}S]sulfate into cartilage, but it is now called *somatomedin C* or *insulin-like growth factor I* (IGF-I). It is a small peptide produced by the liver and other tissues (see Chapter 12).

The initial evidence for the existence of IGF-I was that GH added to cartilage *in vitro* did not stimulate the incorporation of labeled sulfate, whereas plasma from animals treated with GH did so. As discussed in Chapter 12, the active peptide has been isolated and its structure determined.

Long bones grow by proliferation of cartilage cells in the epiphyseal plate, which is followed by growth due to ossification occurring in diaphyseal and epiphyseal ossification centers. In the absence of GH in hypophysectomized animals, the epiphyseal ossification center atrophies and there is a very thin epiphyseal plate of cartilage. Administration of GH causes a thickening of this cartilage plate, and this has served as a bioassay for the hormone.

Additionally, IGF-I may be involved in mediating some or even all of the other actions of GH on metabolism.

Control of Growth Hormone Secretion

Episodic GH Secretion

Growth hormone is secreted in a pulsatile fashion throughout life. The pattern of secretion has an ultradian rhythm, with a frequency of about one pulse every 2 to 3 hours, and appears to be caused by changes in the secretory activity of those hypothalamic neuroendocrine cells involved in regulating the secretion of GH from the pituitary gland (i.e., GHRH and somatostatin neurons). The bursts of secretion are caused by an increase in GHRH output, the troughs by an enhanced production of somatostatin. Studies in sheep, however, have shown that such a relationship is not always apparent.

Episodic GH secretion is influenced by sex, age, and sleep. Women secrete more GH than do men; they show a higher GH baseline, larger bursts of secretion, and an overall higher 24-hour total secretory output of the hormone. In both sexes, however, the rate of secretion is elevated during the first few days after birth, decreasing thereafter, possibly as a consequence of an enhanced IGF-I negative feedback. At puberty, GH secretion increases again in both sexes, paralleling the changes in height velocity associated with the attainment of sexual maturity. After completion of linear growth and attainment of adulthood, the rate of GH secretion returns to prepubertal levels. It remains stable throughout at least the fifth decade of life to decrease again during aging. In all these instances, the most prominent episodes of GH release occur at night. The release of the hormone increases during the onset of deep sleep (stages III and IV), and decreases during the phase of rapid eye movement (REM) sleep, which is associated with dreaming. It is not clear, however, that sleep is absolutely required for nocturnal GH secretion to increase, as nocturnal episodes of GH release may occur in the absence of slow-wave sleep. It would appear that sleep and circadian activation of GH release are independent, but coincidental events (Fig. 6-8).

Central Mechanism Controlling GH Secretion

As indicated above, GH secretion is controlled by a regulatory mechanism that involves three types of hypothalamic peptides—GHRH, somatostatin, and a still unidentified GH-releasing peptide predicted by the existence of a receptor that binds

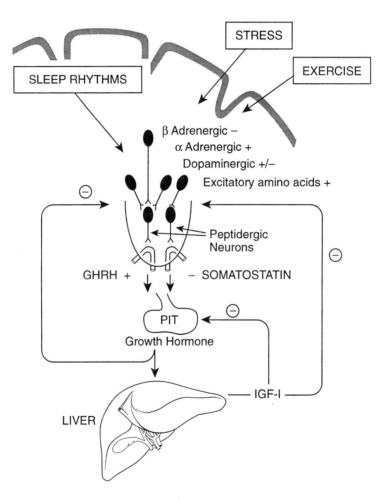

Fig. 6-8 Schematic diagram of the hypothalamic control of growth hormone secretion. For details see text. (Modified from Reichlin S: In: *Williams Textbook of Endocrinology,* 7th ed., JD Wilson and DW Foster, eds., Saunders, Philadelphia, p. 529, 1985.)

synthetic peptides with GH-releasing activity (GHSs). The neuroendocrine neurons producing GHRH are mostly located in the arcuate, ventromedial and dorsomedial nuclei of the basal hypothalamus. Lesions of this area, particularly in the ventromedial nucleus, impair GH secretion. Conversely, stimulation of this region results in GH release. Somatostatin-producing neurons are mainly located in the anterior periventricular area of the hypothalamus, but they are also present in the arcuate and ventromedial nucleus, intermingled with GHRH neurons. In fact, there is evidence that somatostatin neurons influence GHRH secretion via direct synaptic contacts.

Several neurotransmitter systems are involved in the control of GH secretion. They do so mainly via regulation of GHRH and somatostatin release from the hypothalamus. Thus, catecholamines acting via α_2-adrenergic receptors, dopamine acting via D_1 or D_2 receptors, and excitatory amino acids acting via both NMDA and nonNMDA receptors stimulate GH secretion by activating GHRH and inhibiting somatostatin release. Dopamine, however, may also have inhibitory effects, possibly mediated by a stimulation of somatostatin release. In contrast to the stimulatory effect of α-adrenoreceptor–mediated neurotransmission, activation of β-adrenergic receptors suppresses GH release, presumably by facilitating somatostatin output.

An additional central mechanism involved in the control of GH secretion is an ultrashort loop feedback effect exerted by both somatostatin and GHRH on their own secretion. These effects have been demonstrated by experiments showing that while the intraventricular administration of somatostatin increases GH secretion, injection of GHRH suppresses it.

Metabolic Signals Regulating GH Secretion

Glucose, amino acids and nonesterified fatty acids play an important role in the regulation of GH secretion. Administration of insulin to produce hypoglycemia results in a prompt increase in GH release, caused by the hypoglycemia. Because of this effect, insulin-induced hypoglycemia is used as a provocative test to stimulate GH secretion in individuals with suspected GH deficiency. Certain amino acids, particularly arginine given orally or intravenously, are extremely potent in inducing GH secretion, an effect that appears to be mediated by a concomitant increase in GHRH output and a decreased secretion of somatostatin. Some of these effects may be mediated by the conversion of arginine to nitric oxide, a gaseous neurotransmitter recently found to be involved in the hypothalamic control of anterior pituitary function. Nonesterified fatty acids reduce GH secretion, but the mechanisms underlying this effect are not well understood.

Hormones Influencing GH Secretion

Glucocorticoids exert a dual effect on GH secretion; first they stimulate and then they inhibit GH secretion. Thyroid hormones are required for a normal GH output, and the gonadal steroids, estrogen and androgens, facilitate the secretion of the hormone throughout the life span of the individual. The recently discovered lipostatic hormone *leptin* also stimulates GH secretion, likely via inhibition of NPY neurosecretion. A leptin-induced increase in GH secretion appears important for the activation of metabolic processes aimed at regulating changes in body weight and preventing obesity.

Other Factors Controlling GH Secretion

Exercise and stress are two "nonspecific" but potent stimulants of GH secretion. It is likely that they release GH as part of a preparatory "fight or flight" response that shifts metabolism from carbohydrates to fat.

CLINICAL ASSESSMENT OF ANTERIOR PITUITARY FUNCTION

Clinical assessment of anterior pituitary function to determine whether it is normal includes the history, physical examination, and usually some form of laboratory testing. Because physiological regulation of anterior pituitary hormone secretion needs to be considered in assessing pituitary function, the evaluation for possible deficiency or excess of each of the clinically relevant anterior pituitary hormones is briefly discussed in this section (but also see Chapter 5).

Growth Hormone

A random serum GH measurement is not useful for assessing adequacy of secretion as levels may be low in normal individuals. Provocative tests are necessary. Screening tests include the measurement of GH following exercise or 90 minutes after the onset of sleep. If screening tests are abnormal, more definitive tests are required. The two most commonly used definitive tests are the measurement of GH following insulin-induced hypoglycemia or the administration of L-dopa. Serum ACTH, cortisol, glucagon, and epinephrine are also increased following hypoglycemia.

As with possible GH deficiency, a random serum GH may not be reliable in assessing growth hormone excess. Because GH is secreted episodically, if the random sample is drawn at the height of a secretory episode, seemingly elevated levels may be obtained in normal individuals. Growth hormone levels are normally suppressed by the rise in glucose that occurs 30 to 90 minutes following an oral glucose load. Patients with GH excess do not suppress and often have a paradoxical increase in GH after glucose. IGF-I levels are also measured to assess the possibility of GH excess (see Chapter 12).

Prolactin

Although PRL secretion can be stimulated by a number of agents (including commercially available TRH) and inhibited by L-dopa, it is not necessary to perform such maneuvers for routine clinical assessment. A single basal serum PRL determination is usually sufficient to determine the presence of PRL excess, and PRL deficiency is not usually a clinical concern. Because PRL is the only anterior pituitary hormone with predominant negative control by the hypothalamus, it is often elevated by lesions that interfere with the hypothalamic–pituitary portal blood flow. Such elevation is less pronounced than that seen with primary overproduction of PRL by adenomas of the pituitary (see below).

Thyroid-Stimulating Hormone

Deficiency of TSH may be assessed by a single serum measurement. As with all anterior pituitary hormones that have target endocrine glands, however, the interpretation of the adequacy of TSH secretion requires measurement of the other member of the hormone pair, thyroxine. Deficiency of TSH secretion is not usually manifested by a lower than normal serum TSH value, but instead the TSH is inappropriately normal in the presence of a low serum thyroxine (see also Chapter 5).

Likewise, TSH excess may be assessed by a single serum measurement. Uncommonly, thyroid hormone excess is associated with inappropriately normal or increased levels of TSH. This is in contrast to the usual form of thyroid hormone overproduction, in which the TSH level is below normal or undetectable (see Chapter 13). Thus, TSH levels must be interpreted in light of the other member of the hormone pair, thyroxine, because excess TSH may only be manifested as an inappropriately normal level.

Gonadotropins (LH, FSH)

In a woman, the presence of normal spontaneous cyclic menses indicates that gonadotropin secretion is normal (see Chapter 9). In women who do not have evidence of normal ovarian estrogen secretion, a single serum sample for measuring LH and FSH is sufficient to determine whether primary ovarian failure is present (elevated gonadotropins) or whether hypothalamic–pituitary abnormalities exist (low or normal gonadotropins). Similarly, in a man, gonadotropins must be interpreted in light of testicular function (see Chapter 10). Because LH is secreted in pulses with resultant pulses of testosterone secretion, aliquots from three serum samples obtained at 20-minute intervals should be pooled for a more accurate estimate of basal levels of LH and testosterone. Again, elevated levels of gonadotropins with low testosterone indicate primary testicular failure, whereas low or normal gonadotropin levels signal hypothalamic or pituitary disease. Thus, LHRH testing may help distinguish hypothalamic from pituitary causes of low gonadotropins (see Chapter 10).

Gonadotropin excess unrelated to gonadal failure may occur in women or men as a result of a pituitary adenoma and may be assessed by basal plasma levels. The α-subunit common to all the glycoprotein hormones is often secreted in excess by such gonadotroph cell adenomas.

Adrenocorticotropin

The clinical assessment of ACTH secretion usually involves the measurement of a product of the target gland (e.g., cortisol). Thus, ACTH deficiency is assessed by screening for sufficiency of the pituitary–adrenal axis. This is done with the short ACTH stimulation test by measuring the serum cortisol 1 hour after ACTH injection. Basal cortisol levels alone are not sufficient for diagnostic screening. If the response to the short ACTH stimulation test is abnormal, either hypothalamic–pituitary or adrenal abnormalities may be present. Prolonged ACTH administration may then be used to identify an adrenal problem, or ACTH and glucocorticoid secretion may be stimulated by insulin-induced hypoglycemia or the drug metyrapone to identify a pituitary problem (see Chapter 14).

Excess ACTH as a possible cause of excess cortisol secretion is associated by suppression tests as basal cortisol levels are not reliable indicators of glucocorticoid excess, and plasma ACTH may not be elevated in patients with pituitary-dependent cortisol excess. Dexamethasone, a synthetic potent glucocorticoid, is given at 11:00

P.M., and the serum cortisol is measured at 8:00 A.M. the next day. If the individual is normal, ACTH and consequently cortisol will be low the morning after dexamethasone is given. Failure of the cortisol to suppress below $5\mu g/dl$ indicates the need for definitive testing with a prolonged suppression test to determine the cause of the adrenal hyperfunction (see Chapter 14).

DERANGED HYPOTHALAMIC–PITUITARY FUNCTION

Hypothalamic Disease

A variety of hypothalamic disorders including tumors, trauma, infections, congenital malformations, genetic defects, and vascular alterations can affect the secretion of different releasing hormones either selectively or collectively, depending on the location and extent of the lesion. In general, lesions of the median eminence–tuber cinereum region decrease pituitary function. An exception to this is the secretion of PRL, which increases after such lesions because of the loss of its inhibitory hypothalamic tone.

A deficit of individual hypothalamic hormones results in isolated pituitary hormone deficiency. Prominent examples of this condition are the syndromes of hypothalamic hypothyroidism caused by TRH deficiency, olfactory-genital dysplasia (Kallmann's syndrome or isolated gonadotropin deficiency) characterized by a deficit in LHRH secretion associated with hyposmia, and idiopathic dwarfism caused by GHRH deficiency. Kallmann's syndrome is particularly interesting because the deficit in LHRH secretion is related to the failure of embryonic LHRH neurons to migrate from their site of origin (the olfactory placode) to their final destination in the hypothalamus, possibly due to a defect in a neuroadhesion molecule.

Hypopituitarism

If hypopituitarism develops in a child, the defect in GH secretion leads to the development of a pituitary dwarf. In this condition there is a proportional reduction in body size, in contrast to the conspicuous shortening of the long bones in the so-called achondroplastic dwarf. If the deficiency extends to other anterior pituitary hormones, other symptoms and signs will be present. These can include weakness, fatigue, and headaches, but they are of little diagnostic significance. The development of hypopituitarism in adulthood may also produce weakness, fatigue, and headaches, plus signs and symptoms associated with decreased secretion of gonadotropins such as loss of axillary and pubic hair and breast atrophy. The reduction in GH is probably at least in part responsible for the pallor and fine wrinkling of the facial skin seen in adult hypopituitarism. In women, menstrual cycles cease, and there is genital atrophy. In men, secondary testicular failure can cause loss of libido and potency, muscle strength, beard growth, and testicular size, the latter because of the diminished gonadotropin secretion, the former because of the loss of testosterone. Hypopituitarism may be caused by hypothalamic disease or by disorders that directly affect the pituitary gland, such as tumors, infarct, and damage by radiation therapy (see also Chapter 12).

Acromegaly and Gigantism

An excess of GH release leads to the development of gigantism if the hypersecretion has been present during early life, which is a rare condition, and to acromegaly if hypersecretion occurs after body growth has stopped. In the case of gigantism, a rather symmetrical enlargement of the body results in a true giant with overgrowth of long bones, connective tissue, and visceral organs. In the case of acromegaly, the epiphysial and diaphysial centers of the long bones (i.e., femur, tibia, etc.) fuse and elongation of these bones is no longer possible. In this condition there is an overgrowth of cancellous bones, resulting in a protruding jaw, termed *prognathism,* thickening of the phalanges, overgrowth of soft tissue that thickens the skin, and over growth of the visceral organs. Acromegaly and gigantism are caused by eosinophilic adenomas consisting of somatotrophs, leading to the excessive secretion of GH.

Hyperprolactinemia

This is the most common example of pituitary hyperfunction and is brought about by microadenomas of the lactotrophs. Hyperprolactinemia can also result from treatment with the dopamine receptor blockers that are commonly prescribed for psychiatric illness. In women, hyperprolactinemia frequently leads to amenorrhea and galactorrhea. The amenorrhea is caused by the disturbance in gonadotropin secretion arising from prolactin excess. Galactorrhea is caused by the direct effect of PRL on the breast. In men, galactorrhea is not common; however, hyperprolactinemia can cause loss of libido, impotence, and decreased sperm density usually associated with a decrease in the plasma levels of LH and testosterone. The diagnosis can be made by measuring plasma PRL and then examining for the presence of micro- or macroadenomas of the pituitary by computed tomographic scanning or magnetic resonance imaging. Hyperprolactinemia can be treated with a dopamine agonist, such as bromocriptine, or by surgical removal of the adenoma.

SUGGESTED READING

Argetsinger LS, and Carter-Su C: Mechanism of signaling by growth hormone receptor. Physiol Rev 76:1089–1107, 1996.

Gershengorn MC, and Osman R: Molecular and cellular biology of thyrotropin-releasing hormone receptors. Physiol Rev 76:175–191, 1996.

Hinuma S, Habata Y, Fujii R, Kawamata Y, Hosoya M, Fukusumi S, Kitada C, Masuo Y, Asano T, Matsumoto H, Sekiguchi M, Kurokawa T, Nishimura O, Onda H, and Fujino M: A prolactin-releasing peptide in the brain. Nature 393:272–276, 1998.

Hsueh AJW, and Jones PBC: Extrapituitary actions of gonadotropin-releasing hormone. Endocr Rev 2:437–461, 1981.

Kaiser UB, Conn PM, and Chin WW: Studies of gonadotropin-releasing hormone (GnRH) action using GnRH receptor-expressing pituitary cell lines. Endocr Rev 18:46–70, 1997.

Kourides IA, Gurr JA, and Wolf O: The regulation and organization of thyroid-stimulating hormone genes. Recent Prog Horm Res 40:79–120, 1984.

Krieger DT, Liotta AS, and Brownstein MJ: ACTH, β-lipotropin and related peptides in brain, pituitary and blood. Recent Prog Horm Res 36:272–344, 1980.

Maruyama M, Matsumoto H, Fujiwara K, Kitada C, Hinuma S, Onda H, Fujino M, and In-
    oue K: Immunocytochemical localization of prolactin-releasing peptide in the rat brain.
    Endocrinology 140:2326–2333, 1999.

Müller EE, Locatelli V, and Cocchi D: Neuroendocrine control of growth hormone secretion.
    Physiol Rev 79:511–607, 1999.

Rawlings SR, and Hezareh M: Pituitary adenylate cyclase-activating polypeptide (PACAP)
    and PACAP/vasoactive intestinal polypeptide receptors: Actions on the anterior pituitary
    gland. Endocr Rev 17:4–29, 1996.

Reichlin S: Neuroendocrinology. In: *Williams Textbook of Endocrinology,* 8th ed., JD Wilson
    and DW Foster, eds., Saunders, Philadelphia, pp. 135–219, 1992.

Reisine T, and Bell GI: Molecular biology of somatostatin receptors. Endocr Rev 16:427–442,
    1995.

Riskind PN, and Martin JB: Functional anatomy of the hypothalamic-anterior pituitary com-
    plex. In: *Endocrinology,* 2nd ed., Vol. 1, LJ DeGroot, ed., Saunders, Philadelphia, pp. 97–
    107, 1989.

Rivest S, and Rivier C: The role of corticotropin-releasing factor and interleukin-1 in the reg-
    ulation of neurons controlling reproductive functions. Endocr Rev 16:177–199, 1995.

Sealfon SC, Weinstein H, and Millar RP: Molecular mehcanisms of ligand interaction with
    the gonadotropin-releasing hormone receptor. Endocr Rev 18:180–205, 1997.

Smith RG, Van der Ploeg LHT, Howard AD, Feighner SD, Cheng K,Hickey GJ, Wyvratt Jr,
    MJ, Fisher MH, Nargund RP, and Patchett AA: Peptidomimetric regulation of growth hor-
    mone secretion. Endocr Rev 18:621–645, 1997.

Venihaki M, and Majzoub JA: Animal models of CRH deficiency. Front Neuroendocrinol
    20:122–145, 1999.

7

The Posterior Pituitary and Water Metabolism

WILLIS K. SAMSON

STRUCTURE OF THE POSTERIOR PITUITARY GLAND

The neurohypophysis, also called the *posterior pituitary* or *neural lobe,* is the ventral extension of hypothalamic tissue derived from a developmental downgrowth of the neuroectoderm forming the floor of the third cerebroventricle. It weights approximately 0.10–0.15 g in humans and is well developed at birth, having been present since the fifth month of intrauterine life. In addition to containing glial elements called *pituicytes,* the posterior pituitary is composed of unmyelinated nerve fibers and axon terminals of neurons whose cell bodies reside primarily in the supraoptic and paraventricular hypothalamic nuclei (Fig. 7-1). These hypothalamo-neurohypophyseal fibers deliver the two primary posterior pituitary hormones, oxytocin (OT) and arginine vasopressin (AVP), to the neural lobe in association with specific proteins, the neurophysins, once thought to be carrier proteins but now known to be portions of the OT and AVP precursor molecules.

The neurons produce either OT or AVP, never both, and recent studies indicate that in addition to one of these two hormones, other neuropeptides, such as corticotropin-releasing hormone (CRH), and neurotransmitters are also produced in OT- or AVP-containing cells The phenomenon of co-localization of neuromodulatory agents has aroused a great deal of clinical interest in the role of neuropeptides such as OT and AVP in brain function. Both OT- and AVP-containing nerve fibers originating in the supraoptic and paraventricular nuclei also project to a variety of other brain structures that are thought to be the sites of their observed central nervous system actions, and to the vicinity of the hypophyseal portal vessels in the median eminence. Release from these fibers of both OT and AVP explains the high levels of these hormones in portal blood and provides the framework for the actions of OT and AVP as modulators of anterior pituitary function.

The arterial blood supply of the posterior pituitary is via the inferior (and to some degree the superior) hypophyseal arteries, which originate from the cavernous and postclinoid portions of the internal carotid artery. The venous drainage is comprised of efferent vessels joining the intercavernous sinuses and eventually the internal jugular vein.

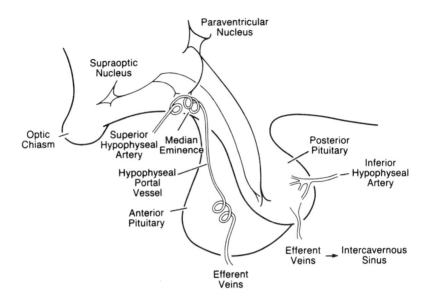

Fig. 7-1 Blood supply and innervation of the posterior pituitary by oxytocin- and vasopressin-containing neurons.

POSTERIOR PITUITARY HORMONES

Both OT and AVP (also called *antidiuretic hormone,* ADH) are nonapeptides containing internal disulfide bonds linking cystine residues at positions 1 and 6, giving them a ring structure that is necessary for some of the peptides biological activity (Fig. 7-2). Both are assembled on the ribosomes as parts of large precursor molecules that consist of the respective hormone and its associated carrier protein (a neurophysin, approximately 10,000 molecular weight). The AVP-associated neurophysin, nicotine-stimulated neurophysin, is a polypeptide with a C-terminal extension that contains the 39-amino acid, AVP-associated C-terminal glycoprotein. Estrogen-stimulated neurophysin, associated with OT, is a polypeptide that lacks the C-terminal glycoprotein extension. After ribosomal assembly the precursor molecules are transferred to the Golgi complex and packaged into neurosecretory granules that move along the axon at a flow rate of 8 mm/hour (faster than normal axoplasmic flow). The precursor and the associated neurophysins have not been demonstrated conclusively to possess biologic activity; however, during axoplasmic transport the neurophysin carrier is proteolytically cleaved from the associated neurohormone and both the neurophysin and neurohormones (OT or AVP) are released into the capillary spaces in the posterior pituitary. These hypothalamo-neurohypophyseal cells are neurons that can generate and propagate action potentials that upon arrival at the nerve terminals, cause depolarization and exocytosis of the secretory granule contents (stimulus–secretion coupling). Both OT and AVP circulate in the blood unbound to other proteins and are rapidly removed (mainly by the kidney, but also by the liver and brain) from the circulation. The older literature reflects a plasma half-life ($t_{1/2}$) for both hormones of about 5 minutes; however, studies

ARGININE VASOPRESSIN

$$\overbrace{}^{\text{S——S}}$$
Cys-Tyr-Phe-Gln-Asn-Cys-Pro-Arg-Gly-NH$_2$

m.w. 1084

OXYTOCIN

$$\overbrace{}^{\text{S——S}}$$
Cys-Tyr-Ile-Gln-Asn-Cys-Pro-Leu-Gly-NH$_2$

m.w. 1007

ATRIAL NATRIURETIC FACTOR (ANP 99-126)

Ser-Leu-Arg-Arg-Ser-Ser-Cys-Phe-Gly-Gly-Arg-Met-

$$\underbrace{}_{\text{S——S}}$$
Asp-Arg-Ile-Gly-Ala-Gln-Ser-Gly-Leu-Gly-Cys-Asn-Ser-Phe-Arg-Tyr-NH$_2$

m.w. 3081

Fig. 7-2 Structures of vasopressin, oxytocin, and atrial natriuretic factor.

employing sensitive radioimmunoassays for each peptide and calculations based on more physiological circumstances reveal a two-component disappearance curve with a much faster $t_{1/2}$ (less than 1 minute) and a second component of approximately 2–3 minutes.

VASOPRESSIN (AVP, ADH)

Primary Action: Antidiuresis

Vasopressin (AVP), which circulates in basal levels of around 1 pg/ml plasma (10^{-12} M), binds to a specific membrane receptor, the V_2 receptor, on the peritubular (serosal) surface of cells of the distal convoluted tubules and medullary collecting ducts inducing adenylyl cyclase activity. The cyclic AMP (cAMP) formed is responsible for activation of a protein kinase, which initiates a phosphorylation cascade resulting in the insertion of the protein, aquaporin, in the luminal membrane and thereby enhances permeability of the cell to water. This AVP-dependent increase in membrane permeability to water permits back diffusion of solute-free water remaining in the urine after proximal tubule handling down the osmotic gradient from hypotonic urine to the hypertonic interstitium of the renal medulla, resulting in an increase in urine osmolality (relative to glomerular filtrate or plasma). The net result is an increase in urine osmolality and a decrease in urine flow.

Control of Secretion

Plasma Osmolality

Water deprivation results in increased plasma osmolality, which is thought to be sensed by specialized brain cells, called *osmoreceptors,* located in two highly vascularized regions (where the blood–brain barrier is absent) of the central nervous system: the vascular organ of the lamina terminalis and the subfornical organ. The increased osmolality of plasma results in a loss of intracellular water from the osmoreceptors and a stimulation of AVP release. The osmoreceptor cells themselves do not release AVP; instead, as revealed in animal studies, they are thought to communicate with the AVP neurons using acetylcholine as their neurotransmitter. The sensitivity of the osmoreceptor to changes in plasma osmolality is increased by angiotensin II, which potentiates AVP release in response to osmotic stimuli. As can be seen in Figure 7-3, the AVP response to changes in plasma osmolality is extremely sensitive: indeed, increases as small as 1% result in enhanced AVP secretion.

Nonosmotic Factors

A fall in blood volume of greater than 8% (hemorrhage), quiet standing (orthostatic hypotension), and positive pressure breathing, all of which reduce cardiac output and therefore central blood volume, are potent stimuli for AVP release (Fig.7-3), whereas maneuvers that increase total blood volume (isotonic saline or blood infusion, cold water immersion) suppress AVP release. Low (left atrial) and high (carotid and aortic) pressure baroreceptors sense small alterations in blood volume and communicate with central nervous system structures via medullary afferents of the ninth and tenth cranial nerves. These pressure receptors normally exert a tonic inhibition on AVP release via medullary efferents to the hypothalamus; thus, decreases in blood volume *unload* the baroreceptors (decrease afferent flow), resulting in *less* inhibition (α-adrenergic) of AVP release and *increased* circulating AVP. Hypovolemia also results in renin release from the juxtaglomerular apparatus of the kidney (see Chapter 14) and the formation of angiotensin II, both of which sensitize the osmoreceptor cells of the hypothalamus leading to enhanced AVP release. Therefore, altering blood volume can "reset" the central osmotic threshold and possibly the sensitivity for AVP release (Fig. 7-3), such that the AVP response to any given increase in plasma osmolality is more accentuated as the level of volume depletion increases. A variety of other stimuli can affect AVP release. Increased $P_a CO_2$ or reduced $P_a O_2$, pain, stress, increased temperature, β-adrenergic agents, estrogens, progesterone, opiates, barbiturates, nicotine, and prostaglandins have been demonstrated to stimulate AVP release. A decrease in temperature, α-adrenergic agents, ethanol, and cardiac hormones can exert inhibitory actions on AVP release.

Secondary Actions

It has been demonstrated that AVP acts within the central nervous system to lower body temperature and to facilitate memory consolidation and retrieval. Indeed, studies in aged humans revealed the improvement of short-term memory after AVP administration. Vasopressin-containing fibers that project to the hypophyseal portal plexus in the median eminence deliver AVP to the portal blood and anterior pituitary where AVP acts via a subtype of vasopressin receptor, which differs from that in the kidney and vasculature, to potentiate the release of adrenocorticotropin in response to CRH. This action of AVP seems coordinated to potentiate the adrenocorticotropin (ACTH) response to stress.

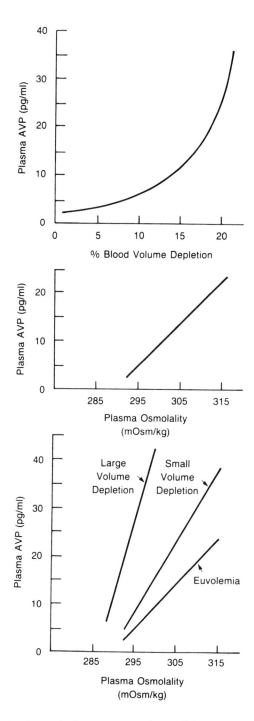

Fig. 7-3 Effects of volume depletion (*top*) and osmolality (*center*) on vasopressin release. Interaction of the two variables (*bottom*) is also illustrated. (Idealized for humans from rat data reported by Dunn FL, et al: J Clin Invest 52:3212–3219, 1973.)

In addition to its effects in the kidney, via V_2 receptors, AVP exerts potent vascular actions as well. Interaction of AVP with specific (V_1) receptors on vascular smooth muscle results in profound contraction, shunting of blood away from the periphery, and elevated central venous pressures. Total peripheral resistance increases in a linear fashion, with increases in circulating AVP. However, the rise in total peripheral resistance seen in response to AVP is buffered by baroreceptor-mediated falls in cardiac output and general sympathetic tone so that other than having a prolonged effect on regional distribution of blood flow, the overall increase in arterial pressure is minimal.

Disorders of AVP Secretion

Deficient Secretion

Usually caused by destruction or dysfunction of the hypothalamo-neurohypophyseal complex, diabetes insipidus is characterized by the inability to produce a concentrated urine, frequent urination (with low specific gravity and osmolality), and often excessive thirst. Treatment of this disorder involves use of a vasopressin analog, desmopressin, which fails at therapeutic doses to react with vascular (V_1) AVP receptors (therefore is a nonpressor) yet is recognized by renal tubular (V_2) receptors; it has the additional advantage of a prolonged duration due to a longer $(t_{1/2})$ in plasma, and enhanced antidiuretic potency.

Patients with diabetes insipidus cannot reduce urine flow during standard water deprivation testing because of their inability to concentrate their urine. Diabetes insipidus can result from central nervous system (CNS) lesions (failure to secrete AVP) or from a renal disorder (failure to respond to AVP). The differential diagnosis can be made by AVP administration. Patients with diabetes insipidus of central origin respond, whereas those with nephrogenic diabetes insipidus do not. The renal form of diabetes insipidus is primarily a local lesion characterized by unresponsiveness of the tubule to appropriate levels of vasopressin and is not associated with lesions of the hypothalamus or posterior pituitary gland.

Inappropriate Production

Release of AVP exceeding that predicted by plasma volume or tonicity can result from CNS disease or trauma, drug interactions, or ectopic production by tumors resulting in water retention and concentration of urine in excess of plasma. Paradoxically, sodium excretion into the urine increases despite the low serum sodium (probably due to elevated levels of atrial natriuretic factors caused by the expanded plasma volume; see below). Symptoms include altered mental status, headache, drowsiness, nausea, and often coma. Fluid restriction is appropriate treatment; however, acute administration of hypertonic saline is often considered to raise plasma osmolality. In the longer term, treatment with naloxone (to decrease central AVP release) or demeclocycline (to block AVP action on the kidney) is often employed. This so-called Syndrome of Inappropriate AntiDiuretic Hormone (SIADH) secretion is characterized by normal renal and adrenal function, yet by

1. Hyponatremia (serum sodium concentrations of 100–115 mEq/liter)
2. Continued renal sodium excretion

3. Absence of clinical evidence of volume depletion or edema
4. Inappropriately high urine osmolality

OXYTOCIN (OT)

Primary Action

Oxytocin stimulates milk ejection by contracting the myoepithelial cells surrounding the alveoli and ducts in the mammary gland. Additionally, it stimulates rhythmic myometrial contractions in the uterus, aiding in expulsion of the fetus. Although not necessary for its initiation, labor proceeds more slowly in the absence of OT. Therapeutically, oxytocin (also called *pitocin*) is employed postpartum to sustain contractions and to decrease bleeding.

Control of Release

Oxytocin is normally present in barely detectable levels (1–10 pg/ml plasma) but is present in readily detectable quantities during ovulation, parturition, and lactation, as well as in males and females during certain mild stresses. Vaginal stimulation during intercourse or delivery and stimulation of touch receptors in the nipples result in afferent neural input (via the spinothalamic tract and a variety of brain stem relays) to OT-producing cells in the paraventricular and supraoptic nuclei. The stimulatory neurotransmitter involved is thought to be acetylcholine or dopamine. Extremely severe pain, increased temperature, and loud noise can inhibit OT release (probably via an opioid mechanism), whereas hemorrhage and psychogenic stress (restraint, novel environment, mild apprehension and fear) stimulate oxytocin secretion. The OT release seen during the immediate preovulatory period is possibly due to rising estrogen levels present at that time (remember the OT-associated carrier is also known as the *estrogen-stimulated neurophysin*). Indeed, administration of exogenous estrogens can stimulate OT release.

Secondary Actions

In addition to possessing some renal and vascular actions that mimic AVP, probably due at least in part to an interaction with the vasopressin receptor, OT can potentiate CRH-induced adrenocorticotropin release, again by interacting with the AVP receptor. Central nervous system actions of OT include amnestic effects and a stimulation of maternal behavior. Recently, OT has been shown to act within the CNS to curb salt appetite. Increases in oxytocin levels in plasma often parallel those of prolactin (during mild stress, ovulation, lactation), and recent evidence indicates that OT can act directly at the lactotroph to stimulate prolactin release, suggesting a physiological role for OT as a prolactin-releasing factor.

Disorders of Oxytocin Secretion

Oxytocin excess has not been clearly demonstrated. A deficiency in OT secretion normally results in difficulty in nursing due to inadequate milk ejection.

CARDIOVASCULAR HORMONES AND THE INTEGRATED CONTROL OF FLUID AND ELECTROLYTE HOMEOSTASIS

It has been recognized for some time that hypothalamic peptides (AVP and OT) interact with hormones from the adrenal gland (glucocorticoids and mineralocorticoids) and angiotensin II to coordinate the homeostastic mechanisms regulating fluid and electrolyte homeostasis. Only recently has it become clear that several additional families of peptides, derived primarily from vascular tissues but produced also in adrenal gland, kidney and brain, play important roles and, indeed, contribute to the physiology and pathophysiology of sodium and water balance. These discoveries have led to the definition of a new discipline, *cardiovascular endocrinology,* which has as its central focus the interactions of hormonal and cardiorenal mechanisms protecting vascular status (tissue perfusion) and plasma osmolarity (electrolyte balance). Cardiovascular hormones can be functionally divided into procontractile/promitogenic factors and vasodilatory/antimitogenic factors, a categorization that identifies two important characteristics of their biologic actions.

Procontractile Cardiovascular Peptides

Leading the list in this category is angiotensin II (A II). Produced in circulation and in some tissues (i.e., brain and vascular cells) as a result of conversion of the precursor angiotensin I by angiotensin converting enzyme (ACE), this octapeptide has potent vasoconstrictive and promitogenic effects. As detailed in Chapter 14, angiotensin I is cleaved from the plasma protein angiotensinogen by renin released from the juxtaglomerular apparatus of the kidney in response to decreased renal perfusion pressure or decreased renal tubular sodium delivery to the macula densa. The hallmark actions of angiotensin II are many, most related to a physiologic compensation for loss of fluid and electrolytes (Table 7-1).

There are two major subclasses of angiotensin receptors, AT1 and AT2, with the first class further subdivided on the basis of gene cloning into the AT1A and the AT1B receptors. All are seven transmembrane domain receptors and members of the G–protein coupled receptor family. In kidney, adrenal cortex, and vascular smooth muscle cells, the action of A II is transduced via the AT1 receptor coupled to a pertussis-toxin–insensitive class of G-proteins (G_q of G11) and subsequent activation of phospholipase C (PLC). There and in other tissues such as the pituitary gland, A II also activates AT1 receptors coupled via G-proteins (G_s or G_i) to adenylyl cyclase. Coupling of the AT1 receptor to phospholipase A2 and phospholipase D has also been reported. The mitogenic actions of A II are expressed via activation of mitogen-activated protein kinases (MAP kinases) and tyrosine kinases. The function of the AT2 receptors is less clear; however, it is known that AT2 receptors is present in fetal tissues and adult brain, suggesting developmental and neurotropic effects. The AT2 receptor activation initiates G-protein–linked signaling as well as non G-protein–linked signaling via tyrosine phosphatase and MAP-kinase inactivation. This perhaps explains the observed functional antagonism of the AT1 and AT2 receptors, with AT1 receptor activation leading to a hyperplastic response and AT2 receptor activation leading to cell inactivation and death (i.e., apoptosis).

The second major procontractile vascular hormone is actually a family of pep-

Table 7-1 Physiologic Actions of Angiotensin II

Vascular

Vasoconstriction (increased total peripheral resistance by direct actions on the contractile elements and indirectly via enhancement of norepinephrine release from nerve terminals innervating the blood vessels, increased sympathetic discharge, and increased medullary epinephrine release)

Remodeling (enhanced migration, proliferation and hypertrophy of vascular smooth muscle cells, cardiomyocytes and fibroblasts; increased matrix formation; indirect stimulation of cardiomyocyte proliferation and hypertrophy by the increased cardiac afterload due to volume expansion secondary to sodium retention)

Renal/Adrenal

Antinatriuresis (direct proximal tubule effect to stimulate sodium reabsorption and indirect effect via stimulation of aldosterone release and subsequent sodium reabsorption in distal tubule)

Hemodynamic (renal vasoconstriction; increased renal sympathetic tone)

Brain:

Sympathostimulation and attenuation of the baroreceptor reflex

Dipsogenesis

Stimulation of salt appetite

Stimulation of AVP and OT secretion

Pituitary Gland

Synergism with CRH to stimulate ACTH secretion

tides know as the *endothelins* (ETs). Three unique and ancestrally related gene products, ET-1, ET-2, and ET-3, comprise this family. All are 21-amino acid peptides containing two intramolecular disulfide bonds necessary for biological activity. These peptides are produced in endothelial cells lining the blood vessels; fortunately, because of their potent vasoconstrictive effects, under normal conditions they are secreted abluminally—that is, away from the vessel lumen. Thus, in most cases these peptides act as local paracrine or autocrine factors. One of the peptides, ET-3, appears to be preferentially produced in brain where it exerts potent mitogenic actions on astrocytes. Two distinct endothelin receptors have been identified, both seven transmembrane spanning domain proteins. The ET-A receptor displays a rank order of binding affinity preferring ET-1 (ET-1 $\geq$ ET-2 $\gg$ ET-3). This is the primary ET receptor on vascular smooth muscle cells and cardiomyocytes. The ET-B receptor binds all three isoforms with equal affinity. The actions of the ETs are diverse in nature and mediated via multiple signaling mechanisms (Table 7-2).

Because of their powerful vasoconstrictive effects, the ETs were hypothesized to play a role in the pathogenesis of hypertension. However, mice lacking the ET-1 gene are not hypotensive; rather, they are paradoxically hypertensive, and thus a definitive role for the ETs in blood pressure regulation remains unestablished. Good evidence does exist for a role for endogenous ET in reperfusion injury. Blockade of the action of locally released ET with antibodies or antagonists significantly reduced tissue damage distal to transient coronary artery ligation and in a model of myocardial infarction. Thus, ET antagonists may have clinical utility in the prevention of reperfusion injury.

Some of the best evidence for a therapeutic value of the ET antagonists comes from the improvement of renal function in genetic models of hypertension and the prevention, by these antagonists, of ischemia-induced renal failure. Finally,

Table 7-2 Biologic Actions of the Endothelins

Tissue	Receptor subtype	Signaling mechanism	Actions
Lung	ET-A	Phospholipase D and A2	Prostanoid production
Vascular smooth muscle	ET-A	Phospholipase C Activation of K^+ channels Activation of adenylyl cyclase	Contraction, mitogenesis
Myocardium	ET-A	G-protein mediated closing of Cl^- and L-type Ca^{++} channels, with opening of K^+ channels leading to decreased electrical activity	Tissue damage in myocardial infarction
Endothelium	ET-B	Nitric oxide synthase (NOS) activation, PLC activation and Ca^{++} mobilization, CNP release Opens Na^+-H^+ antiporter Inhibits adenylyl cyclase	Transient vasodilation
Astrocytes	ET-B	PKC activation of MAP-kinase	Mitogenesis

cyclosporine-induced nephrotoxicity must at least be due in part to the local release of endogenous ET (and the subsequent constriction of the afferent arteriole) as the renal toxicity of immunosuppressant therapy was blocked by ET antagonist administration. The potential pathologic roles for the endothelins in disease states are listed in Table 7-3.

Table 7-3 Endothelins in Human Disease

Proven pathologic roles	Proposed pathologic roles
Myocardial damage from vascular insult	Acute vascular insult (vasospasm in brain)
Cyclosporine-induced nephrotoxicity	Patent ductus arteriosus
Postischemic renal failure	Pulmonary hypertension and fibrosis
Vasospasm secondary to subarachnoid hemorrhage	Gastric ulceration
Hirschsprung's disease	Heart failure manifestations
	Hepatorenal syndrome (cirrhosis)
	Unstable angina
	Raynaud's phenomenon
	Shock
	Glomerulonephritis
	Inflammatory bowel disease
	Dysmenorrhea
	Asthma
	Pre-eclampsia

While angiotensin II can be viewed as a physiologically relevant, circulating hormone that regulates cardiovascular and renal function by not only affecting volume status (and therefore pressure) but also sodium homeostasis, the effects of the ETs are more related to abnormal alterations in blood pressure and regional flow, as well as renal perfusion. Thus, only under pathologic conditions may the ETs be important regulators of fluid and electrolyte balance.

Vasodilatory Cardiovascular Peptides

Two families of peptides, the natriuretic peptides and peptides derived from the adrenomedullin gene product, express not only vasodilatory and antimitogenic actions opposed to those of A II and the ETs, but also exert potent actions related to the control of fluid and electrolyte homeostasis. Biologic activities shared between the two families of peptides are exerted at numerous tissue sites, all seemingly coordinated to regulate sodium intake and excretion, and at the same time volume status.

The Natriuretic Peptides

It has been recognized for some time that atrial distension resulted in profound *diuresis* (increased urine flow), and the proposed mechanisms for this effect included not only neuronal reflex activation of CNS structures (vagal afferents) but also the possible release of a volume regulatory substance from the heart. Infusion of extracts of mammalian cardiac atrial tissue were found to stimulate significant increases in urine volume and urinary sodium excretion (*natriuresis*). Additionally, these extracts were shown to relax precontracted vascular and gastrointestinal smooth muscle strips *in vitro* (a *spasmolytic* actions). The peptide responsible for the diuretic, natriuretic, and spasmolytic actions was identified to be 28 amino acids in length and to be produced primarily in atrial myocytes under normal physiologic conditions. Because of the original localization and the spectrum of biologic activity, this peptide was named *atrial natriuretic peptide* (ANP). Expression of ANP increases under volume overload conditions, as does the production of a second member of the family, the 32 amino acid *B-type natriuretic peptide* (BNP). The third member of the family, *C-type natriuretic peptide* (CNP, 22 amino acids), was later isolated and found to be produced in endothelial cells and brain, but not normally in cardiac myocytes. ANP is the major circulating member of the family, and normal plasma levels range from 50 to 150 pg/ml. Highest levels are present in the aorta (vena cava to aorta concentration gradient 76–177 pg/ml, identifying the heart as the major site of release) and the plasma half-life is about 1–3 minutes. In addition to being filtered into the urine, major degradation sites include kidney, liver, lung, and brain.

Stimuli for Release. Cardiac myocytes are located in a position to detect pressure changes accompanying increases in venous return or afterload. Indeed, stretch associated with increases in venous return is the major stimulus for ANP release, as interventions (head down tilt, passive leg elevation, cold water immersion, saline or blood loading) that result in increases in right atrial pressure and an increase in right atrial dimension result in concomitant increases in ANP release and diuresis. Therefore, the heart responds to an increase in venous return (Fig. 7-4) by releasing hormones that act at the kidney (and other sites, see below), resulting in a lowering of fluid volume (via diuresis) and a decrease in venous return. Recent evidence indicates that an increase in plasma osmolality also releases ANP, perhaps reflecting the natriuretic action as well. Increasing sodium intake in normal volunteers from 10 to 200 mmol sodium per day resulted in significant, twofold elevations in plasma ANP. Furthermore, these subjects released even more ANP in response to subsequent interventions that elevated venous return.

Natriuretic Peptide Receptors. Three subtypes of natriuretic peptide receptors have been cloned and sequenced. Two have extracellular binding domains linked via a

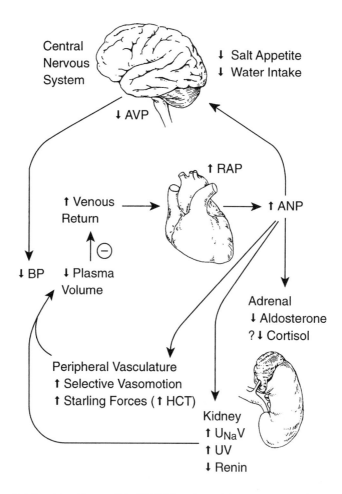

Fig. 7-4 Atrial natriuretic peptide (ANP) is released in response to increased venous return and the associated increase in right atrial pressure (RAP). ANP acts in the brain, adrenal, kidney, and peripheral vasculature to result in a drop in blood pressure (BP) and venous return, thus eliminating the signal for its release. AVP, vasopressin; HCT, hematocrit; $U_{Na}V$, urine sodium excretion; UV, urine volume.

Table 7-4 The Natriuretic Peptide Receptor Family

Receptor subtype	Ligand preference	Signalling mechanism
NPR$_A$ receptor (guanylyl cyclase A, GC-A)	ANP>BNP>>CNP	particular guanylyl cyclase
NPR$_B$ receptor (guanylyl cyclase B, GC-B)	CNP>ANP>BNP	particular guanylyl cyclase
NPR$_C$ receptor (clearance receptor)	ANP=BNP=CNP	inositol phosphase turnover, adenylyl cyclase

transmembrane spanning segment with an intracellular, particulate guanylyl cyclase. The third lacks the intracellular extension, and although it has been designated the *nonbiologic, clearance receptor* (originally thought to function only as a biologic sponge that removed the natriuretic peptides from the circulation), it is now apparent that this subtype transduces important antimitogenic signals of the natriuretic peptides and is linked to activation of inositol phosphate hydrolysis and inhibition of adenylyl cyclase. Table 7-4 summarizes the three receptor subtypes.

Renal Actions. The hallmark renal actions of ANP are natriuresis and diuresis. Infusion of ANP into healthy volunteers results in increases in urine volume, creatinine clearance, free water clearance, and the excretion rates of sodium and chloride. These effects are at least partially due to ANP's ability to increase glomerular filtration rate, a reflection of its action to stimulate postglomerular vasoconstriction. Additionally, ANP exerts a direct tubular action to inhibit sodium transport in the distal nephron and antagonizes the effect of AVP in the tubule and duct. A final renal action of ANP is exerted directly at the level of the juxtaglomerular apparatus to inhibit renin secretion, thus reducing angiotensin II formation.

Adrenal Actions. In addition to preventing angiotensin II formation by inhibiting renin release, ANP blocks the action of angiotensin II in the adrenal. Indeed, both basal and stimulated (angiotensin II and ACTH) aldosterone secretion are inhibited by cardiac hormones. Although the renal effect of ANP (natriuresis) is too rapid to be explained by alterations in aldosterone levels, in chronic volume expansion ANP may play a part in the suppression of aldosterone levels.

Vascular Actions. Intravenous infusion of ANP in humans results in decreased mean arterial blood pressure and a decreased cardiac output. This decrease in mean arterial pressure could be due solely to an *in vivo* vasodilatory effect of ANP that matches its *in vitro* spasmolytic action. Increases in forearm blood flow have been observed; however, in certain vascular regions, vasoconstrictive effects are seen (efferent renal artery). Alternatively, the drop in mean arterial pressure could be secondary to the observed decrease in cardiac output caused by decreased venous return. Strong evidence in favor of this exists. Detailed experiments have revealed that ANP reduces circulatory capacitance as a result of decreased blood volume (and vascular recoil) and active vasoconstriction, thereby decreasing venous return. In addition to urinary fluid loss, the observed increase in hematocrit during ANP infusion may be due to transcapillary fluid shifts initiated by increases in postcapillary resistance. No direct chronotropic or inotropic effects have been observed *in vitro* in isolated heart preparations.

The abundant production of CNP in vascular endothelial cells reflects a paracrine action of the peptide to control vascular tone in concert with several other vasorelaxant and vasoconstrictive factors produced locally. Circulating endothelin-3 or locally produced endothelin-1, members of a powerful family of vasoconstrictor peptides, stimulate the release from the endothelial cells of both CNP and nitric oxide (NO). These factors are released abluminally, away from the vascular lumen toward the surrounding smooth muscle, and induce vasodilation by unique but potentially convergent mechanisms. While CNP activates particulate guanylyl cyclase via the NPR_B receptor, NO diffuses into the vascular smooth muscle cell and activates soluble guanylyl cyclase, both resulting in elevated cytosolic cGMP. Thus, there exists at the endothelial interface with the vascular smooth muscle a balance of redundant vasodilatory substances including CNP and nitric oxide, and additional endothelial-derived factors such as prostacyclins and adrenomedullin (see below), with local vasconstrictors such as endothelin-1. An interplay of these agents, together with local neural influences, determines vascular tone, and therefore, blood pressure. The ability of CNP to potently dilate coronary vessels suggests a possible therapeutic use for CNP or selective NPR_B agonists in the treatment of myocardial ischemia.

Central Nervous System Actions. In addition to its renal, adrenal, and vascular actions, ANP exerts a profound influence on central nervous system–mediated events that relate to fluid and electrolyte homeostasis. Natriuretic peptide receptors have been localized to discrete brain regions, and the production of ANP and to a greater extent CNP in neuronal elements is well established. Natriuretic peptide-containing neurons terminate in regions known to be important in the neuroendocrine and neuronal control of renal and cardiovascular function. Indeed, ANP exerts a profound inhibitory action on AVP release (Fig. 7-4) and significantly impairs fluid consumption by inhibiting water intake and salt appetite. These central actions match well the peripheral effects of the hormone, such that in addition to exerting an opposite action (diuresis) in the kidney, ANP inhibits the release of AVP (the antidiuretic hormone). Also, the renal diuretic and natriuretic actions are suitably paired with ANP's central nervous system actions to inhibit water and salt intake.

Pathophysiology of the Natriuretic Peptide. Whereas derangements in ANP and BNP secretion have been observed (i.e., elevation during congestive heart failure, supraventricular tachycardia, chronic renal failure and primary hyperaldosteronism), these conditions of elevated plasma peptide levels usually reflect exaggerated drive for release of the hormone. In fact, it is in volume overload states such as congestive heart failure (CHF), that expression of BNP, particulary in ventricular myocytes, increases. The elevated circulating levels of BNP in CHF are considered by many to be diagnostic of the early stages of the disease. The extreme elevations in circulating ANP and BNP in the face of continued water reabsorption during CHF suggests not a derangement of hormone levels per se, but instead a combination of possibly altered natriuretic peptide receptor mechanisms (i.e., down-regulation), reduced renal perfusion, or simultaneous activation of the renin–angiotensin system. Just the same, exaggerated ANP release might be an important factor in the syndrome of inappropriate anti-diuretic hormone secretion (SIADH) (see above) and aldosterone escape (see Chapter 14).

Plasma levels of CNP are remarkably elevated in septic shock, but not CHF or hypertension. A variety of circulating cytokines and growth factors (including interleukin 1α and 1β, tumor necrosis factor-α (TNF-α), and transforming growth factor-β) as well as ANP and BNP can stimulate CNP release from endothelial cells. As a result, the endothelial cells can, via CNP secretion, both transduce the antimitogenic effects of circulating ANP and BNP and buffer the proliferative effects of circulating cytokines and growth factors.

How Physiologically Relevant Are These Effects? Transgenic overexpression models reveal that ANP must play some role in the maintenance of normal blood pressure as animals with the ANP transgene display lower mean arterial blood pressure than do nontransgenic littermates under basal conditions. However, under basal condition renal function is not altered. It is only when challenged, in this case by volume expansion, that the renal excretory function of the animals with excessive ANP production exceeds that of normal, nontransgenic littermates. Another way to address the issue of physiologic relevance is to create animals lacking ANP, so-called gene knockouts (i.e., null mutations). Homozygous mice lacking the ANP gene are more likely to develop hypertension when maintained on a high salt diet than normal, ANP gene-intact animals. These findings tell us that ANP is not necessary for normal embryologic and postnatal development (i.e., knockouts survive and thrive under unstressed conditions) but that endogenous ANP must protect against the development of hypertension.

The Adrenomedullins

Recently, a second family of vascular hormones has been identified with even more potent vasodilatory and diuretic actions than the natriuretic peptides. Discovered originally in extracts of a pheochromocytoma (tumor of the adrenal medulla) the first member of the family was named *adrenomedullin* (AM). This 52-amino acid peptide was later found to be produced in endothelial cells and in neurons and to exert many actions similar to those of ANP. Once the structure of the AM-gene product was identified it became clear that a second peptide was also encoded, this being 20 amino acids in length, residing in the N-terminus of the prohormone. That peptide, called *proadrenomedullin N-terminal 20 peptide* (PAMP), is also a potent vasodilatory agent, albeit via a differing mechanism than that of AM. Adrenomedullin circulates in plasma like other vasoactive peptides at very low levels (10–100 pg/ml) and has a plasma half-life of approximately 20 minutes.

Physiologic Actions. Both AM and PAMP appear to play important roles in the regulation of vascular tone, hormone secretion from the anterior pituitary gland, and adrenal function. Profound renal actions have been demonstrated as well. In general, these peptides, like the natriuretic peptides, seem to function to maintain appropriate vascular volume and therefore assure adequate tissue perfusion. This is accomplished by multiple tissue sites of action related to both fluid and electrolyte homeostasis.

Vascular Actions. Adrenomedullin is a potent hypotensive agent. This action is blocked by pretreatment with false substrates for the enzyme *nitric oxide synthase* (NOS); thus, the majority of the actions of AM in the vascular tree are mediated via nitric oxide. The effects of endogenous AM on vascular tone are probably not due to changes in circulating hormone levels, but instead to a paracrine action of the peptide, since it was necessary in human trials to elevate plasma levels of AM past those observed in pathologic states to cause hypotension. Does this mean that this vascular effect is solely pharmacologic in nature? Indeed, it does not. It is clear that proinflammatory cytokines such as interleukin-1 and TNF-α are potent stimulators of AM gene transcription and peptide release both from cultured vascular smooth muscle and endothelial cells *in vitro*, and from the blood vessels *in vivo*. Thus, the hypotensive crisis of septic shock has been directly correlated with AM release in this condition, and it is thought that the elevated AM levels of septic shock not only are responsible for the profound drops in mean arterial pressure, but, more importantly, for the maintenance of renal perfusion during this life-threatening event (AM increases renal blood flow). Hence, the release of AM in inflammatory states is in fact a positive compensatory event. The other peptide encoded by the AM gene product, PAMP, also exerts vasodilatory actions; however, these effects are not due to a direct action on the vascular smooth muscle or endothelial cells. Instead, PAMP, released in the adrenal medulla, actually decreases the amount of epinephrine released (i.e., local autocrine negative feedback, since both epinephrine and PAMP are released from the chromaffin cells) and additionally acts in the vasculature to inhibit norepinephrine release from sympathetic fibers innervating the vessels.

Renal Actions. Although in humans the threshold for vascular actions may be lower than that for renal actions, it is clear that AM, but not PAMP, is a renotropic agent. The diuretic and natriuretic effects of AM are due to inceases in renal blood flow and direct tubular actions. The tubular actions occur at lower doses than do the blood flow changes, suggesting that AM produced in the kidney, particularly in glomerulus, cortical, and medullary collecting ducts (but not medullary thick ascending limb), acts in a paracrine fashion to control sodium excretion and free water clearance. Osmotic permeability of the inner medullary collecting duct is increased by AM, and a complementary action of the peptide is expressed in brain where it inhibits AVP release and in adrenal gland where it inhibits aldosterone secretion.

Increases in renal blood flow stimulated by AM are due to a prostaglandin-mediated and inhibitory effect on renal vascular resistance and an inhibition of mesangial cell proliferation. Also, AM directly stimulates renin secretion, an effect that joins other actions in brain and heart to provide a measure of cardioprotection during septic shock.

Adrenal Actions. Both AM and PAMP are potent inhibitors of angiotensin II and potassium-induced release of aldosterone. These actions complement both the natriuretic actions of AM in the renal tubule and the actions of both peptides to inhibit ACTH secretion from the anterior pituitary gland. Thus, in several tissues the actions of these peptides seem coordinated to assure the appropriate excretion of sodium into the urine and therefore the normalization of plasma volume and electrolyte content.

Cardiac Actions. Plasma AM levels are elevated in human disease states characterized by volume or pressure overload, including pulmonary hypertension, heart failure, essential hypertension, renal failure, liver disease with ascites, and thyrotoxicosis. This suggested that, like ANP, AM may be produced in cardiac myocytes and, indeed, this is the case. Direct cardiac actions have also been described. Adrenomedullin blocks angiotensin II-induced protein synthesis in cultured cardiomyocytes and coronary smooth muscle cell migration, and thus may play an important role in the prevention of cardiac muscle growth and coronary vessel remodeling. Also, AM may prevent pathologic vascular remodeling in the general circulation as it inhibits vascular smooth muscle cell migration and proliferation. In endothelial cells, AM acts as a survival factor, suppressing apoptosis.

Just as in kidney, where the effect of AM on renal perfusion may protect against failure in septic shock, positive cardioprotective effects have been demonstrated. Adrenomedullin exerts direct effects in heart to increase heart rate, cardiac output, and force of contractility. These effects, together with the peptide's ability to act in brain to activate the sympathetic nervous system, provide a measure of protection against circulatory collapse in sepsis or heart failure. This portfolio of biologic actions makes AM an excellent candidate for the potential treatment of volume expanded and pressure overload states such as congestive heart failure (Table 7-5).

How Physiologically Relevant Are These Effects? Although the only pharmacologic action of AM yet to be demonstrated to have physiologic relevance is its ability to inhibit salt appetite and therefore regulate ingested sodium load, many clinical conditions exist in which plasma levels of AM are markedly elevated. Do these elevations reflect compensatory roles for AM gene products or merely tissue damage? Recent experiments strongly suggest a potential role for AM and PAMP in the body's response to pathologic conditions and the possible therapeutic benefit of selective AM or PAMP agonists.

Table 7-5 Actions of the Adrenomedullins (AM and/or PAMP)

Tissue	Effect
Vasculature	Hypotension (vasodilation)
	Decreased total peripheral resistance
	Increased renal blood flow
	Antimitogenesis
Heart	Positive chronotropism and inotropism
	Inhibition of myocyte hypertrophy and vascular hyperplasia
Lung	Pulmonary vasodilation
Adrenal gland	Inhibition of cholinergic stimulation of catecholamine release
	Inhibition of stimulated aldosterone secretion
Kidney	Diuresis
	Natriuresis
Pituitary gland	Inhibition of ACTH release
Brain	Inhibition of water drinking and salt appetite
	Stimulation of sympathetic nervous system activity
	Inhibition of AVP release

Plasma AM levels are elevated in a variety of human hypertensive conditions. In stroke prone, spontaneously hypertensive animal models, plasma AM levels are very low, perhaps reflecting the loss of the protective, vasodilatory effect of the peptide. In another genetic model of spontaneous hypertension, AM gene delivery significantly lowered blood pressure to levels observed in normal littermates. This suggests that the elevated AM plasma levels in hypertensive humans reflect a compensatory mechanism counteracting the elevation in pressure.

Patients in heart failure also display elevated plasma AM levels. When heart failure is induced in laboratory animals, AM gene transcription in heart increases in parallel with the observed cardiac hypertrophy. Additionally, infusion of AM into these animals at doses too low to cause hypotension initiates ameliorative responses in kidney (i.e., diuresis and natriuresis). It had long been hoped that ANP infusion would be a clinical tool for lowering plasma volume and therefore cardiac afterload in heart failure; however, the natriuretic peptide receptors in kidney appear to be down-regulated in response to continued elevation of plasma ANP and BNP levels in this condition, thereby limiting the efficacy of this approach. It is now possible that AM infusion will provide the therapeutic benefit originally hypothesized for ANP.

The antimitogenic actions of AM demonstrated *in vitro* may have a physiologic correlate. The peptide is produced in cardiomyocytes, endothelial cells, and mesangial cells and has been demonstrated to express its antimitogenic actions in these cell types. It was recently shown that antiserum against AM accentuated angiotensin II-induced protein and platelet-derived growth factor (PDGF)-stimulated DNA synthesis in cultured myocytes and endothelial and mesangial cells, respectively. Thus, endogenously produced AM may act in an autocrine fashion to prevent cell proliferation and uncontrolled growth.

The best evidence for a physiologic role for AM comes from studies of sepsis, in which plasma AM levels parallel the inflammatory and hypotensive course of the disease. It is now recognized that proinflammatory cytokines stimulate AM gene transcription and peptide secretion. Additionally, a positive correlation exists between circulating hormone levels and survival rate. It appears that the increased plasma AM levels, in addition to causing a vasodilation, spare the kidney by concomitantly elevating, even in the face of exaggerated drops in mean arterial pressure, renal plasma flow and therefore preventing renal failure.

INTEGRATED CONTROL OF WATER AND SODIUM HOMEOSTASIS

The integrated control of body fluid homeostasis requires a balance of renal, adrenal, vascular, cardiac, brain, and endocrine influences (Fig. 7-5). Most importantly, all of these converge on the kidney as the final site of regulation. It is not surprising, therefore, that multiple endocrine peptides with profound effects on fluid and electrolyte homeostasis have as a major site of action the kidney. Thus, angiotensin II (A II) itself is antinatriuretic, as is aldosterone. Both of these hormonal actions contribute to sodium, and as a result both water retention and the restoration of plasma volume and perfusion pressure. The counter-regulatory hormones ANP and AM act in the opposite fashion, stimulating urinary sodium and water excretion and thereby

Fig. 7-5 The endocrine regulation of fluid and electrolyte homeostasis. The volume-conservatory hormones angiotensin II (A II), aldosterone, vasopressin (AVP), and endothelin (ET) act to restore plasma volume and maintain tissue perfusion. The volume-reducing hormones atrial natriuretic peptide (ANP), adrenomedullin (AM), and proadrenomedullin N-terminal 20 peptide (PAMP) act directly or indirectly to lower plasma volume and to decrease tissue perfusion, with the exception of renal blood flow, which is stimulated by AM.

contributing to volume regulation by unloading the vascular tree. These two hormones also act to inhibit the antidiuretic actions of AVP, the major determinant of free water reabsorption from the urine, again assuring the reduction in plasma volume in electrolyte and/or volume overload states.

The level of integration of the actions of these potent volume regulatory hormones is even more complex than those renal actions would suggest. In fact, in numerous tissues these opposing hormones "push and pull" physiologic mechanisms by which fluid and electrolyte homeostasis is maintained (Fig. 7-5). The natriuretic and diuretic actions of AM and ANP expressed in kidney are complemented in brain by effects of the peptides to inhibit water drinking (thirst) and salt appetite. These actions in brain are antagonistic to those of A II, which oppositely stimulates both thirst and salt appetite. In the adrenal gland as well, the stimulatory effect of A II on aldosterone secretion is blocked by both ANP and AM, and by the other adrenomedullin gene product PAMP. In anterior pituitary gland the ability of A II to stimulate ACTH secretion is opposed by ANP, AM, and PAMP. The release of AVP from nerve terminals in the posterior pituitary gland is stimulated by A II and inhibited by ANP and AM.

The opposing actions of the volume conservatory versus the volume depleting hormones extend into the vasculature as well (Fig. 7-5). Whereas A II and ET are vasoconstrictors, ANP, AM, and PAMP exert vasodilatory effects, actions well suited to their roles in other tissues to regulate plasma volume and tissue perfusion pressures. The antimitogenic actions of ANP and AM also are opposed by the promitogenic effects of A II and ET, and thus a common thread is revealed. In most cases, the overall physiologic effects of the procontractile/promitogenic/volume-conservatory peptides are opposed by those of the vasorelaxant/antimitogenic/volume-reducing hormones, and only the integration of these multiple signals can explain the normal maintenance of fluid and electrolyte homeostasis. Clearly, any alteration in the production, release, or bioactivity (including response to) of any one of these hormones can result in imbalances in volume status and plasma osmolar state. In addition, states of over- or underproduction of these hormones lead to hypertensive states that threaten life if left untreated. Thus, the peptides themselves may be diagnostic of underlying cardiovascular disease and may prove useful as therapeutic agents in a variety of disease states.

SUGGESTED READING

Bayliss PH, and Thompson CJ: Osmoregulation of vasopressin secretion and thirst in health and disease. Clin Endocrinol 29:549–576, 1988.

Dawood MY, Khan-Dawood FD, Wahi RS, and Fuchs F: Oxytocin release and anterior pituitary and gonadal hormones in women during lactation. J Clin Endocrinol Metab 52:678–682, 1981.

Ganten D, and Pfaff D: *Neurobiology of Vasopressin,* Springer-Verlag, Berlin, 1985.

Gavras H: Pressor systems in hypertension and congestive heart failure: Role of vasopressin. Hypertension 16:587–593, 1990.

Ivell R, and Russell J: *Oxytocin*, Plenum Press, New York, 1995.

Levin ER, and Nadler JL: *Endocrinology of Cardiovascular Function*, Kluwer Academic Publishers, Boston, 1998.

Reichlin S: *The Neurohypophysis, Physiological and Clinical Aspects,* Plenum Press, New York, 1984.

Samson, WK. Adrenomedullin and the control of fluid and electrolyte homeostasis. Annu Rev Physioly 61:363–389, 1999.

Samson WK, and Levin ER: *Natriuretic Peptides in Health and Disease*, Humana Press, Totowa, NJ, 1997

Samson WK: Cardiovascular hormones. In: *Endocrinology: Basic and Clinical Principles,* PM Conn and S Melmed, eds., Humana Press, Totowa, NJ, pp. 361–376, 1997.

Schrier RW: *Vasopressin,* Raven Press, New York, 1985.

Sowers JR: *Endocrinology of the Vasculature,* Humana Press, Totowa, NJ, 1996.

8

Sexual Differentiation

KEITH L. PARKER

Sexual differentiation is a sequential process that begins at fertilization with the establishment of chromosomal sex, continues with the determination of gonadal sex, and culminates in the development of secondary sexual characteristics that comprise the male and female phenotypes. This basic paradigm (Fig. 8-1) was formulated by Alfred Jost to explain the results of castration experiments in fetal rabbits. If the gonads (ovaries or testes) were removed before sexual differentiation, female sexual differentiation inevitably ensued. The male pathway could be partly restored by testosterone implants, suggesting that hormones produced by the testes mediated male sexual development. Thus, the concept arose that the testes induced a male pattern of differentiation on an embryo that otherwise would follow the female pathway. Cytogenetic studies shortly thereafter showed that the critical genetic determinant of sex was the presence or absence of the Y chromosome. Thus, it was proposed that the Y chromosome directed the gonad to differentiate into a testis, which then produced hormone(s) that caused male sexual differentiation.

The chromosomal sex of the embryo generally corresponds to its phenotypic sex. Occasionally, however, the process of sexual differentiation goes awry, resulting in individuals with abnormal sexual differentiation. Clinically recognized disorders of sexual development occur at many levels, ranging from relatively common disorders in the terminal steps of male differentiation (e.g., testicular descent, growth of the penis) to more fundamental abnormalities that lead to varying degrees of ambiguity of phenotypic sex. Although most of these abnormalities impair reproduction, they usually are not life-threatening. Thus, humans and experimental animals with naturally occurring defects in sexual differentiation survive to reach the attention of physicians and scientists. This chapter reviews the sequence of events in normal sexual development and describes disorders of this process—many of which result from single-gene mutations—that have provided valuable insights into the mechanisms of sexual differentiation.

DEVELOPMENT OF CHROMOSOMAL SEX

Normally, human somatic cells have 22 pairs of autosomes and one pair of sex chromosomes. The critical genetic determinant of sex is the presence or absence of the

CHROMOSOMAL SEX
↓
GONADAL SEX
↓
PHENOTYPIC SEX

Fig. 8-1   The Jost paradigm for sexual differentiation.

Y chromosome; thus, the female genotype is 46,XX, while the male genotype is 46,XY. Meiosis in the germ cells reduces their chromosomal complement to the haploid state, so that oocytes are 23,X and spermatocytes are either 23,X or 23,Y. Fertilization restores the diploid state and—depending on the presence or absence of the Y chromosome—specifies the genetic sex as either 46,XX (female) or 46,XY (male).

The most striking function of the Y chromosome is in sex determination. Analyses of human subjects whose phenotypic sex did not correlate with genetic sex (i.e., the presence or absence of a Y chromosome) led to the isolation of a gene called *SRY* (sex-determining region, Y chromosome) that is both necessary and sufficient for male sex determination. The *SRY* gene encodes a putative transcriptional regulator proposed to trigger a cascade of events that result in development of the testes. The term "sex determination" is used to describe the initiation of the male pathway by *SRY*, and the subsequent events in the production and action of testicular hormones are referred to as *male sexual differentiation.*

Although it is one of the smallest human chromosomes, the Y chromosome contains more than 30 genes that contribute to functions such as spermatogenesis, skeletal growth, and tooth development. The Y chromosome also contains a putative locus near the centromere—designated *GBY* for *gonadoblastoma, Y chromosome*—that predisposes to the development of germ-cell tumors in subjects with disorders of gonadal sex.

The Y chromosome presumably arose from an ancestral homolog of the X chromosome and retains regions of homology at its ends—termed the *pseudoautosomal regions*—that permit it to pair with the X chromosome during meiosis. Between these pseudoautosomal regions lie discontinuous stretches of X-Y homology mixed with regions that are unique to the Y chromosome. The *SRY* gene, the critical mediator of male sex determination, is located on the short arm of the Y chromosome just inside the pseudoautosomal region. Because of its position directly adjacent to the pseudoautosomal region, in which X-Y recombination normally occurs, *SRY* occasionally is transferred from the Y to the X chromosome, leading to either 46,XX males or 46,XY females (see below under disorders of genetic sex).

DEVELOPMENT OF GONADAL SEX

An overview of the events in the development of the male and female phenotypes is shown in Figure 8-2.

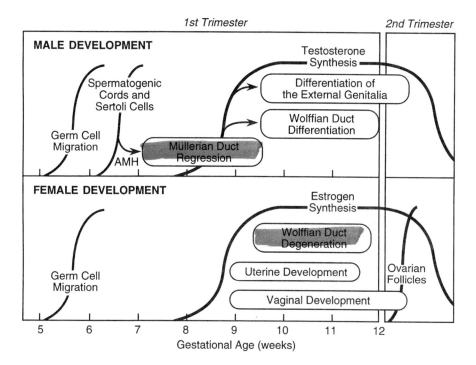

Fig. 8-2 Gonadal differentiation and the timing of the events of phenotypic sexual differentiation. AMH, anti-müllerian hormone.

Indifferent Phase

Both male and female gonads develop from the urogenital ridges—structures containing cell lineages that ultimately contribute to the kidneys, the gonads, and the adrenal cortex. The gonads initially are identical in both sexes and therefore are termed *indifferent gonads*. These indifferent gonads arise from different cell types that have functional counterparts in testes and ovaries: supporting cells (Sertoli or granulosa cells), stromal cells (Leydig or theca cells), and primordial germ cells (spermatogonia or oocytes). The supporting cells derive from the coelemic epithelium of the gonadal ridge (although cells derived from the mesonephros also may contribute in some species), stromal cells derive from the mesenchyme of the gonadal ridge, and primordial germ cells originate in the allantois and migrate into the gonadal ridge by the fifth week of gestation. The differentiation of these cell lineages to form the indifferent gonad requires the action of several transcription factors, which presumably regulate the expression of target genes needed for gonadogenesis.

Before ~7–8 weeks of gestation, during the indifferent phase, the sexual phenotype of the embryo cannot be recognized. At this time, all embryos acquire dual ductal systems that are the precursors to the male and female internal genitalia (Fig. 8-3, top). The first ducts to form are the wolffian (or mesonephric) ducts, which serve as excretory ducts for the mesonephric (embryonic) kidney and are attached

INTERNAL GENITALIA

EXTERNAL GENITALIA

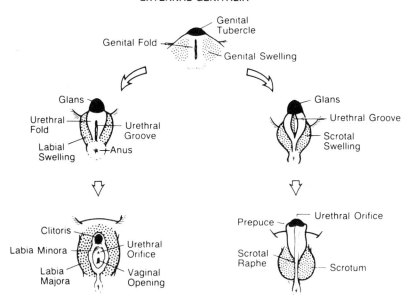

Fig. 8-3 Differentiation of the internal and external genitalia of the human fetus.

directly to the indifferent gonad. Caudally, as the wolffian ducts join the primitive urogenital sinus, an outgrowth of their dorsomedial wall—the ureteric bud—gives rise to the excretory ducts and collecting tubules of the metanephric (permanent) kidney. The internal male accessory organs of reproduction—the seminal vesicles, vas deferens, and epididymis—develop from these wolffian ducts.

The paramesonephric (müllerian) ducts begin to form at 6 weeks of gestation as an evagination of the coelomic epithelium into the mesonephros just lateral to the wolffian ducts. These müllerian ducts in females ultimately give rise to the internal reproductive tract (fallopian tubes, uterus, and upper vagina), whereas they regress in males. The external genitalia of both sexes, which arise from the genital tubercle, urethral folds and groove, and the labioscrotal swellings, again are indistinguishable before sexual differentiation. Thus, the male and female internal genitalia develop from different embryonic anlagen, whereas the external genitalia arise from a common anlage (Fig. 8-3, bottom).

Male Development

The initial event in the virilization of the male urogenital tract is regression of the müllerian ducts, which coincides with the organization of the testes into spermatogenic cords at approximately 8 weeks of gestation. Shortly thereafter, the male genital tract begins to develop from the wolffian ducts (Fig. 8-2). Those mesonephric tubules adjacent to the testis lose their primitive glomeruli and establish contact with the developing rete and spermatogenic tubules of the testis to form the efferent ductules. The portion of the wolffian duct immediately caudal to the efferent ductules becomes elongated and convoluted to form the epididymis, and the middle portion of the duct develops thick muscular walls to become the vas deferens (Fig. 8-3, top). At about the thirteenth week of gestation, the lower portions of the wolffian ducts near the urogenital sinus begin to form the seminal vesicles. The terminal portions of the ducts between the seminal vesicles and the urethra become the ejaculatory ducts and ampullae of the vas deferens.

The prostatic and membranous segments of the male urethra develop from the pelvic portion of the urogenital sinus. At approximately 10 weeks of gestation, the prostatic buds begin to form in the mesenchyme surrounding the pelvic urethra. This budding is most extensive in the area surrounding the entry of the wolffian ducts (the ejaculatory ducts) into the male urethra. Although initial differentiation of the prostate occurs early in embryogenesis, growth and development of the gland continue after birth.

Beginning in the ninth week of gestation and continuing through the twelfth week, the external genitalia of the male and female become sexually differentiated (Fig. 8-3, bottom). The genital swellings in the male enlarge and migrate posteriorly to form the scrotum, and the genital folds fuse over the urethral groove to form the penile urethra. The line of closure remains marked by the penile raphe. Incomplete fusion of the genital folds over the urethral groove results in a condition known as *hypospadias*. When the formation of the penile urethra is almost complete, the prepuce begins to develop, completely covering the glans penis by 15 weeks of gestation.

Although the formation of the male genital tract is largely accomplished between 7 and 13 weeks of gestation, two additional aspects of male development occur later in gestation—growth of the external genitalia and testicular descent.

At approximately 11 weeks of gestation, when formation of the male urethra is largely complete, the male and female phalluses are comparable in size. During the last two trimesters of pregnancy, the male external genitalia, prostate, and structures derived from the wolffian ducts grow progressively. As a consequence of this growth, the male external genitalia at birth are considerably larger than those of the female.

The complex events of testicular descent remain incompletely understood, although this descent is essential to reproductive function because spermatogenesis requires the lower temperature present in the scrotum. A failure of the process—termed *cryptorchidism*—occurs in at least one testis in approximately 3% of full-term male infants, making it one of the most common congenital abnormalities. Testicular descent involves two stages: the *transabdominal* phase, which occurs between 10 and 15 weeks of gestation, and the *inguinoscrotal* phase, which usually occurs between 26 and 35 weeks of gestation. During the transabdominal phase, the cranial suspensory ligaments regress, and outgrowth of a posterior fold of peritoneum called the *gubernaculum* causes the testes to migrate from the dorsal abdominal wall to the internal inguinal ring. During the third month of gestation, prompted at least partly by increased intra-abdominal pressure, the processus vaginalis develops as a herniation in the coelemic cavity along the course of the gubernaculum. In the inguinoscrotal phase, the portion of the gubernaculum that contacts the testes regresses, and they pass through the inguinal canal into the scrotum. This event normally occurs at about the seventh month of gestation, although it does not take place in some infants until the first year of life.

At least two hormones contribute to testicular descent. The increased incidence of cryptorchidism in human subjects with impaired testosterone biosynthesis or action implicates androgens in this process. In addition, studies in knockout mice demonstrate that the Leydig insulin-like hormone Insl3, a secreted member of the insulin-like hormone superfamily, is essential for development of the gubernaculum and subsequent testicular descent.

Female Development

In females, the internal reproductive tract forms from the müllerian ducts, and the wolffian ducts largely degenerate. The cephalic ends of the müllerian ducts—which are derived from coelemic epithelium—are the anlagen of the fallopian tubes, while the caudal portion fuses to form the uterus (Fig. 8-3, top). The uterine cervix is recognizable by 9 weeks of gestation, and the formation of the myometrium from mesenchyme surrounding the müllerian ducts is completed by 17 weeks of development.

Vaginal development begins at approximately 9 weeks of gestation with the formation of a solid mass of cells—the uterovaginal plate—between the caudal buds of the müllerian ducts and the dorsal wall of the urogenital sinus. The cells of the uterovaginal plate subsequently degenerate, thus increasing the distance between the uterus and the urogenital sinus. The upper one-third of the vagina derives from the müllerian ducts, and the remainder derives from the urogenital sinus.

After 10 weeks of gestation, the genital tubercle begins to bend caudally, the lateral portions of the genital swellings enlarge to form the labia majora, and the posterior portions fuse to form the posterior fourchette. The urethral folds flanking the urogenital orifice do not fuse but persist as the labia minora (Fig. 8-3, bottom). Thus, most of the urogenital sinus of the female remains exposed on the surface as a cleft into which the vagina and urethra open.

Breast Development

At 5 weeks of development, paired lines of epidermal thickening extend on the ventral surface of the embryo from the forelimb to the hindlimb. Between 6 and 8 weeks of development, these "mammary lines" largely disappear, except for a small portion on each side of the thoracic region that condenses and penetrates the underlying mesenchyme. This single pair of mammary buds undergoes little change until the fifth month of embryonic development, when secondary epithelial buds appear and the nipples begin to form. Although some species exhibit sexual dimorphism in embryonic breast development, such dimorphism has never been demonstrated in humans, and breast development is identical in males and females before the onset of puberty.

ENDOCRINE CONTROL OF PHENOTYPIC DIFFERENTIATION

The fetal castration experiments of Jost demonstrated definitively that the fetal testes are necessary for male phenotypic development. Two products of the fetal testis are essential for male development: the glycoprotein hormone *anti-müllerian hormone* (AMH; also called *müllerian-inhibiting substance,* or MIS)—which causes regression of the müllerian ducts—and testosterone—which virilizes the wolffian ducts, urogenital sinus, and genital tubercle. In contrast, female differentiation apparently does not require hormone production by the fetal ovaries, as female phenotypic development occurs in the absence of gonads.

Onset of Endocrine Function of Testes and Ovaries

Fetal ovaries and testes first become distinct histologically at approximately 7 weeks of gestation, when the testes form primitive spermatogenic tubules that contain fetal Sertoli cells and primordial germ cells. The fetal Sertoli cells produce AMH, which causes the first discernible event in male phenotypic differentiation: regression of the müllerian ducts. Shortly thereafter, at ~8–9 weeks of gestation, mesenchymal cells in the interstitium differentiate into Leydig cells and initiate testosterone synthesis (Fig. 8-2). Although the role of pituitary or placental gonadotropins in the earliest stages of androgen production is debated, virilization in the latter two-thirds of gestation—such as penile growth—probably requires gonadotropins (see Chapter 11). No effects on female sexual differentiation have been attributed to ovarian hormones, and the fetal ovaries do not actually form primordial follicles until the fifth month of development, but they nonetheless initiate estrogen biosynthesis at approximately 9 weeks of gestation (Fig. 8-2).

Role of Testicular Hormones in Male Development

Müllerian Duct Regression

Müllerian duct regression in male fetuses begins at 8–9 weeks of gestational age, and is mediated by AMH, a member of the transforming-growth factor β (TGF-β) family of signaling molecules that is secreted by fetal Sertoli cells. By interacting with its type 2 receptor on mesenchymal cells surrounding the müllerian ducts, this 140,000 glycoprotein activates an apoptotic pathway that ultimately causes müllerian duct regression. As discussed below, mutations in either the *AMH* gene or its receptor cause the persistent müllerian duct syndrome. In the female, it is essential that AMH is not expressed during fetal development of the urogenital tract, as the female internal genitalia otherwise would not develop. Perhaps to maintain this extremely tight regulation, the *AMH* gene is a target gene for a number of transcription factors involved in gonadal development, including steroidogenic factor-1 (SF-1), Wilms tumor–related 1 (WT1), and SOX9 (see below).

Virilization

Virilization of the male fetus results from the action of androgens on the wolffian ducts, urogenital sinus, and external genitalia. Although testosterone is the principal androgen secreted by the fetal and adult testes, many of the differentiating, growth-promoting, and functional actions of androgens are mediated by its 5α-reduced metabolite, dihydrotestosterone (Fig. 8-4).

Androgens act via a specific receptor found in androgen-responsive cells (Fig. 8-4). The androgen receptor is a member of the nuclear hormone receptor superfamily, a group of structurally related, zinc finger transcription factors that mediate the action of a large group of hydrophobic ligands, including steroid hormones, thyroid hormone, retinoids, vitamin D, bile acids, and oxysterols. Following secretion by the testes, testosterone enters target cells by passive diffusion. In certain target tissues, the type 2 isozyme of 5α-reductase converts testosterone to dihydrotestosterone. After binding testosterone or dihydrotestosterone, the androgen receptor reg-

Fig. 8-4 Mechanisms of androgen action in target tissues. T, testosterone; D, dihydrotestosterone.

ulates the expression of target genes by binding to recognition sequences in their promoter regions.

Genetic studies (see below) clearly demonstrate that a single androgen receptor mediates the action of both testosterone and dihydrotestosterone. Nonetheless, there is a dichotomy of androgen action in different androgen-responsive tissues. Testosterone itself regulates gonadotropin release and virilizes the wolffian ducts during male sexual differentiation, whereas conversion to dihydrotestosterone is required for virilization of the external genitalia during embryonic development and for the development at puberty of most male secondary sex characteristics. Definitive support for the differential roles of the two androgenic hormones comes from the study of patients with inherited deficiency of dihydrotestosterone due to the absence of 5α-reductase activity; such patients have normally differentiated structures derived from the wolffian ducts but exhibit failure of external virilization.

DISORDERS OF CHROMOSOMAL SEX

Two disorders of chromosomal sex resulting from nondisjunction of the sex chromosomes during meiosis—Klinefelter syndrome (47,XXY) and Turner syndrome (most commonly 45,X)—illustrate the roles of the sex chromosomes in controlling gonadal development.

Klinefelter Syndrome

Individuals with Klinefelter syndrome, which affects one in 500 newborn males, typically have a 47,XXY karyotype and a predominantly male phenotype. Before puberty, patients have small testes and decreased number of spermatogonia but otherwise have a normal male phenotype. After the time of normal puberty, patients often exhibit incomplete virilization and breast enlargement (gynecomastia). After puberty, consistent clinical features include male phenotype, bilaterally small testes (always <3 cm in length and generally <1.5 cm in length) and absence of sperm in the ejaculate (azospermia).

Endocrine findings include low to normal plasma testosterone and elevated circulating levels of estradiol; the relative imbalance of androgen to estrogen causes varying degrees of impaired virilization and enhanced feminization. Circulating gonadotropins—particularly follicle-stimulating hormone—are elevated owing to impaired feedback at the hypothalamic/pituitary levels.

Various karyotypes are associated with Klinefelter syndrome, almost all of which include two or more X chromosomes and a Y chromosome (e.g., 47,XXY [classic form]; 46,XY/47,XXY [mosaic form]). Other individuals with the Klinefelter phenotype have a single Y chromosome and more than two X chromosomes, demonstrating that a single Y chromosome is sufficient to induce testicular differentiation and male phenotypic development irrespective of the number of X chromosomes. The classic variant of Klinefelter syndrome results most frequently from nondisjunction of the sex chromosomes during the first or second meiotic division; thus, increased maternal age is an important risk factor.

Turner Syndrome

Classically, Turner syndrome is seen in phenotypic females who exhibit short stature, primary amenorrhea, lack of secondary sexual characteristics (sexual infantilism), multiple congenital abnormalities, and bilateral streak gonads (i.e., bands of fibrous tissue that lack histological features of either testicular or ovarian organization). These congenital defects include aortic coarctation, bicuspid aortic valve, horseshoe kidney, webbed neck, and various skeletal abnormalities. Originally ascribed to a 45,X genotype, we now recognize that Turner syndrome is associated with a range of karyotypes—all of which involve complete or partial absence of one sex chromosome or monosomy X. Moreover, Turner syndrome patients frequently carry two or more cell lines with distinct karyotypes (i.e., they are mosaic). A larger percentage of 46,XX cells in these mosaic patients correlates with a milder phenotype.

With the advent of more frequent karyotypic analysis, it now is apparent that spontaneous abortion also is a leading manifestation of Turner syndrome. Because an estimated 2% of all human conceptuses are 45,X—less than 1% of which survive to term—Turner syndrome collectively accounts for up to 10% of spontaneous abortions.

Although the only universal feature in live-born Turner patients is short stature, individuals with Turner syndrome frequently present with sexual infantilism, and a large majority have primary ovarian failure. Primordial germ cells migrate normally into the gonads—and the number of oogonia is relatively normal until the stage of primary follicle formation at approximately 20 weeks of gestation—but oocytes undergo markedly accelerated atresia after birth, leading to premature ovarian failure. The deficiency of ovarian steroid hormones results in primary amenorrhea and failure to develop female secondary sexual characteristics. Turner syndrome is the most common cause of primary amenorrhea.

DISORDERS OF GONADAL SEX

Disorders of gonadal sex occur when chromosomal sex is normal (i.e., either 46,XX or 46,XY), but differentiation of the gonads is abnormal. Phenotypic sex will vary depending on when the gonadal defect becomes manifest during embryogenesis.

Pure Gonadal Dysgenesis

Pure gonadal dysgenesis denotes a syndrome in which bilateral streak gonads are associated with an immature female phenotype. In contrast to patients with 45,X gonadal dysgenesis, these patients are of normal height, do not have associated somatic defects, and, most importantly, have a normal 46,XX or 46,XY karyotype. Because gonadal development is arrested before AMH and androgens are produced, the sexual phenotype is female. Little is known about the pathogenesis of 46,XX gonadal dysgenesis. A few of these subjects have homozygous mutations in the follicle-stimulating hormone (FSH) receptor, resulting in hypoplastic ovaries that retain some primary follicles. Within the same kindreds, 46,XY males homozygous for the identical mutation exhibit variably impaired spermatogenesis without azospermia.

SRY and 46,XY Complete Gonadal Dysgenesis

The demonstration of point mutations in *SRY* in some subjects with 46,XY complete gonadal dysgenesis provided definitive support for the essential role of *SRY* in testis determination and subsequent male sexual differentiation. More extensive studies have identified *SRY* mutations in approximately 10%–20% of these subjects; most cases of 46,XY gonadal dysgenesis therefore result from mutations in other genes (see below). Subjects with 46,XY pure gonadal dysgenesis—whether associated with *SRY* mutations or with mutations in other genes described below—have an increased incidence of gonadoblastoma, possibly associated with the GBY locus near the centromere of the Y chromosome.

Other Genes Implicated in Complete Gonadal Dysgenesis

Three autosomal genes and one gene on the X chromosome have been implicated in 46,XY complete gonadal dysgenesis (Table 8-1). Intriguingly, these genes all encode putative transcription factors that are proposed to regulate the expression of target genes essential for gonadal survival. The cascade of gene regulation within the developing gonads apparently is very sensitive, because changing either the relative amounts of these transcription factors or the time when their expression commences can impair normal gonadal development.

Wilms Tumor–Related 1 (WT1). The first autosomal gene to be linked specifically to 46,XY complete gonadal dysgenesis was the Wilms tumor–related gene *WT1*, which maps to chromosome 11p13; it was isolated through analyses of patients with familial Wilms tumor, an embryonic kidney tumor arising from abnormal proliferation of the metanephric blastema. Although Wilms tumors generally present sporadically, approximately 1% occur in patients with similarly affected first-degree relatives, suggesting that these families carry mutations in a tumor-suppressor gene.

The *WT1* mutations cause two distinct syndromes of gonadal dysgenesis— Denys–Drash syndrome and Frasier syndrome. Denys–Drash syndrome is an autosomal dominant disorder characterized by gonadal and urogenital abnormalities in conjunction with diffuse mesangial sclerosis. The gonadal abnormalities vary but are relatively severe, with streak gonads and female external and internal genitalia at one extreme and varying degrees of impaired virilization in less severely affected 46,XY males. Denys–Drash syndrome almost always results from point mutations

Table 8-1 Genes Associated with 46,XY Gonadal Dysgenesis

Gene	Chromosomal location	Associated disorder	Target genes
WT1	11p13	Denys–Drash syndrome Frasier syndrome	AMH
SF-1	9q33	Adrenal insufficiency	AMH, steroid hydroxylases, ACTH receptor, StAR
SOX9	17q21	Campomelic dysplasia	AMH
DAX-1	Xp21	Adrenal hypoplasia congenita	StAR (inhibits)

in the zinc finger region of WT1 that abrogate DNA binding; these mutated proteins are predicted to inhibit function of the protein encoded by the wild-type allele. The degree of inhibition of WT1 action generally correlates with the impairment of genitourinary development, with the most severe mutations leading to early gonadal dysgenesis and sex reversal of external and internal genitalia. Genetic modifiers also affect the severity of the phenotype, as demonstrated by studies of Denys–Drash families in which the fathers were phenotypically normal despite carrying the same *WT1* mutation as the affected offspring.

Patients with Frasier syndrome present with gonadal dysgenesis, impaired virilization, and focal glomerular sclerosis, but they do not develop Wilms tumors. The *WT1* mutations that cause Frasier syndrome cluster within intron 9 of the *WT1* gene, apparently interfering with the synthesis of specific splice variants of WT1 that are essential for gonadal development but are not required to suppress the development of Wilms tumors.

Steroidogenic Factor 1 (SF-1). Development of the indifferent gonads also requires steroidogenic factor 1 (SF-1). Initially, SF-1 was identified as a transcription factor that regulated the cell-specific expression of the cytochrome P450 steroid hydroxylases that catalyze most steroidogenic conversions. Like the androgen receptor, SF-1 belongs to the nuclear hormone receptor superfamily. Subsequent studies have shown that SF-1 regulates the expression of a diverse array of genes involved in steroidogenesis, including 3β-hydroxysteroid dehydrogenase, the ACTH receptor, the steroidogenic acute regulatory protein (StAR), and the high-density lipoprotein receptor SR-B1. Cell transfection and transgenic analyses suggest that SF-1 also regulates expression of the *AMH* and *Insl3* genes; thus, SF-1 very likely regulates the production of multiple hormones that are essential for male sexual differentiation: androgens and AMH. The SF-1 transcripts also are expressed in pituitary gonadotropes and the ventromedial nucleus of the hypothalamus (VMH), suggesting that it regulates endocrine function at all three levels of the hypothalamic–pituitary–gonadal axis.

Knockout mice lacking SF-1 exhibit adrenal and gonadal agenesis, with female internal and external urogenital tracts, confirming its essential roles in gonadal development and sexual differentiation. The human *SF-1* gene, located on chromosome 9q33, shares extensive homology with its mouse counterpart and is expressed in many of the same sites, suggesting that SF-1 also has important roles in human endocrine development. This model is supported by a human subject with adrenal insufficiency and 46,XY gonadal dysgenesis. This patient has a heterozygous mutation in one SF-1 allele that precludes DNA binding, while the other allele is apparently normal. These studies suggest strongly that SF-1 in humans also plays essential roles in embryonic development of the adrenal glands and gonads.

SOX9. Gonadal dysgenesis also is seen in most 46,XY patients with *campomelic dysplasia,* an autosomal dominant syndrome that includes skeletal, renal, and cardiac abnormalities. Campomelic dysplasia results from heterozygous mutations in *SOX9,* a close relative of *SRY* that maps to chromosome 17q21. SOX9 is expressed at high levels in testes—where it is proposed to regulate the transcription of key mediators of male differentiation such as AMH—and at lower levels in ovaries. Presumably, homozygous *SOX9* mutations are incompatible with fetal survival owing to its essential roles in chondrogenesis.

DAX-1 and Dosage-Sensitive Sex Reversal. 46,XY gonadal dysgenesis also is associated with duplication of the short arm of the X chromosome (Xp21), a phenomenon termed *dosage-sensitive sex reversal.* The critical region of Xp21 for dosage-sensitive sex reversal contains a gene, *DAX-1*, that is mutated in boys with adrenal hypoplasia congenita (AHC). In addition to adrenal insufficiency, AHC patients have a compound hypothalamic/pituitary defect that causes hypogonadotrophic hypogonadism at the time of normal puberty. The *DAX-1* gene encodes a atypical member of the nuclear receptor family that retains the conserved ligand binding domain but lacks the typical zinc finger DNA-binding motif. This finding suggests that DAX-1 may interact directly with other proteins involved in the cascade of gonadal development. Consistent with this model, DAX-1 and SF-1 are coexpressed in many sites, including the gonads, adrenal cortex, pituitary gonadotropes, and the VMH. Moreover, several studies indicate that DAX-1 inhibits the expression of SF-1–dependent target genes, providing a potential mechanism by which an excess of DAX-1 in patients with Xp21 duplication could cause 46,XY gonadal dysgenesis and sex reversal.

The Vanishing Testis Syndrome

A spectrum of phenotypes has been described in 46,XY males with absent or rudimentary testes in whom endocrine function of the testis was present at some time during sexual differentiation. The disorder varies in its manifestations from complete failure of virilization, through varying degrees of incomplete virilization of the external genitalia, to otherwise normal males with anorchia. The most severely affected individuals are 46,XY phenotypic females who lack testes and accessory male reproductive organs and are sexually infantile. The disorder in these individuals differs from the 46,XY form of pure gonadal dysgenesis in that no müllerian duct derivatives are present. Thus, testicular failure in these individuals must have occurred in the interval between the onset of AMH biosynthesis and the secretion of testosterone. In other patients, the clinical features suggest that testicular failure occurred later in gestation, while at the other extreme are phenotypic men with anorchia who lack müllerian derivatives and are completely virilized except for the absence of the epididymis.

DISORDERS OF PHENOTYPIC SEX

Disorders of phenotypic sex are classified as those disorders in which the phenotypic sex is ambiguous or is completely in disagreement with chromosomal and gonadal sex. Conceptually, as detailed below, such disorders generally result from a failure of synthesis or action of hormones that mediate male sexual differentiation (male pseudohermaphroditism) or the inappropriate synthesis of androgens (female pseudohermaphroditism).

Female Pseudohermaphroditism

This condition occurs in individuals who have ovaries and müllerian derivatives, but exhibit varying degrees of virilization of the external genitalia. This process requires exposure *in utero* to androgens, and the degree of virilization depends on the stage of sexual differentiation at the time of androgen exposure. Following the twelfth week of gestation, when the vagina has formed from the urogenital sinus, androgen exposure causes only clitoromegaly. Because AMH is not produced, the uterus and fallopian tubes are normal.

The most common cause of virilization in newborn females is a condition called congenital adrenal hyperplasia (CAH), which results most frequently from mutations in the 21-hydroxylase enzyme (see pathway of steroid biosynthesis in Fig. 8-5). Less commonly, CAH with female pseudohermaphroditism results from defects in 11β-hydroxylase or 3β-hydroxysteroid dehydrogenase. The common feature in these disorders is an enzymatic defect that impairs cortisol synthesis in the adrenal cortex and disrupts the normal feedback mechanism by which circulating cortisol inhibits corticotropin (ACTH) secretion by the pituitary. Elevated ACTH levels stimulate the flow of cholesterol precursor down the steroidogenic pathway in adrenocortical cells, with consequent buildup of steroids proximal to the enzymatic block (e.g., progesterone and 17-hydroxyprogesterone in 21-hydroxylase deficiency). The 17-hydroxyprogesterone is a precursor to the predominant adrenal androgen, *androstenedione,* which can be converted peripherally to testosterone. The resulting increase in circulating androgens *in utero* virilizes the female.

The genitalia of females with virilizing CAH exhibit a spectrum of masculinization from simple clitoral enlargement to complete labioscrotal fusion and a penile urethra. The internal female structures and ovaries are unaltered, and male

Fig. 8-5 Pathway for synthesis of glucocorticoid and androgenic hormones from cholesterol in adrenal and testis.

wolffian duct derivatives are not present. These facts indicate either that the onset of increased adrenal androgen occurs after the critical period for wolffian duct differentiation or that these ducts are not capable of responding to the adrenal androgens. The labial folds are rugated and resemble an empty scrotum. Thus, the external appearance of affected females is similar to that of males with bilateral cryptorchidism and hypospadias. Occasionally, when virilization is so severe that a complete penile urethra is formed, errors in sex assignment are made at birth.

Placental aromatase deficiency, a rare autosomal recessive disorder, provides striking evidence for the protective role of the placenta against excess androgen exposure in utero. During pregnancy, the placenta receives large amounts of androgen precursors from the fetal and maternal adrenal glands, which it converts into androgens such as androstenedione. Placental aromatase converts the C19 androstenedione into C18 estrogens, thus removing the potential source of excess androgen. In the absence of this protective barrier, androgen exposure in 46,XX subjects results in clitoromegaly, varying degrees of posterior fusion, scrotalization of the labioscrotal folds, and occasionally a single perineal orifice. At puberty, subjects with aromatase deficiency develop hypergonadotropic hypogonadism and polycystic ovaries with progressive virilization.

Male Pseudohermaphroditism

Defective virilization of the 46,XY embryo with testes (male pseudohermaphroditism) can result from defects in androgen synthesis in the testis, defects in androgen action in target cells, or defects in müllerian duct regression.

Disorders of Androgen Biosynthesis

Defects in Testosterone Synthesis. Figure 8-5 summarizes the pathway by which testosterone is synthesized from cholesterol in the testis. As discussed above, many of the same enzymes are involved in corticosteroid production in the adrenal cortex. Thus, defects in the early steps of the pathway—which are required for the biosynthesis of both corticosteroids and androgens—cause both adrenal insufficiency and male pseudohermaphroditism. Although mutations in the cholesterol side chain cleavage enzyme have not been described in humans, clinical disorders do result from mutations in 3β-hydroxysteroid dehydrogenase and 17α-hydroxylase. The regulated production of all classes of steroid hormones also requires a mitochondrial phosphoprotein—the steroidogenic acute regulatory protein (StAR)—that is essential for the delivery of cholesterol to the steroidogenic complex inside the mitochondria. Mutations in *StAR* cause the rare disorder *congenital lipoid adrenal hyperplasia.*

Defects in the glucocorticoid pathway distal to 17-hydroxyprogesterone result in both adrenal insufficiency and virilization of females by adrenal androgens (see section "Female Pseudohermaphroditism"). Finally, isolated male pseudohermaphroditism results from defects in the androgen synthetic pathway distal to the formation of 17-hydroxyprogesterone (e.g., the C17–20 lyase reaction of 17α-hydroxylase and the conversions catalyzed by the type 3 isozyme of 17β-hydroxysteroid dehydrogenase).

Impaired androgen production also is associated with Leydig cell hypoplasia or agenesis. This condition results from inactivating mutations in the gene encoding the receptor for luteinizing hormone (LH). In 46,XY subjects with the most severe form of this disorder, the external genitalia appear female; milder defects may cause microphallus and hypoplastic external genitalia. Some virilization of structures derived from the wolffian ducts can occur, suggesting some capacity at early stages of gestation for autonomous production of androgens. The absence of Leydig cell hypoplasia/aplasia in patients with deficient secretion of pituitary gonadotropins suggests that fetal testosterone production during the critical period of virilization of the external genitalia may be driven by human chorionic gonadotropin.

Unlike patients with gonadal dysgenesis, AMH production is normal and müllerian structures regress normally. Presumably, impaired development of Leydig cells due to the absence of LH receptor signaling prevents adequate production of testosterone, with consequent failure of virilization. Thus, 46,XX individuals with homozygous inactivating mutations of the LH receptor have normal development of secondary sexual characteristics at puberty, but have elevated LH levels and amenorrhea

Defects in Androgen Action

Testosterone synthesis is normal in more than 80% of male pseudohermaphrodites; thus, most disorders of male phenotypic development presumably result from impaired androgen action. In these disorders, testosterone synthesis and müllerian duct regression are normal, but male development is incomplete owing to impaired action of androgen in target cells. These subjects can have defects either in the conversion of testosterone to dihydrotestosterone by 5α-reductase or in the androgen receptor.

5α-Reductase Deficiency. Deficiency of 5α-reductase—which converts testosterone to the potent androgen dihydrotestosterone in peripheral tissues—is a rare cause of androgen resistance in humans. This disorder results from mutations in the gene encoding the type 2 isozyme of 5α-reductase, which maps to chromosome 2p23. Subjects with this disorder have a predominantly female phenotype. The urethral opening is commonly at the base of a small phallus, and a blind-ending vaginal pouch usually opens near the urethral orifice in the urogenital sinus. Female internal genitalia are not present, and the male internal genitalia (epididymis, vas deferens, and seminal vesicles) are well developed. The fact that the defect in embryonic virilization in these individuals is limited to the urogenital sinus and the external genitalia proved that testosterone can mediate virilization of the wolffian ducts but dihydrotestosterone is required for differentiation of the prostate and external genitalia.

Androgen Receptor Defects. The most severe form of androgen resistance—the complete androgen insensitivity syndrome, previously called *testicular feminization*—is caused by mutations that severely impair androgen receptor action. Subjects with this condition generally come to medical attention at the time of puberty when they are evaluated for primary amenorrhea. The karyotype is 46,XY, but the external genitalia are those of a normal female, except that the vagina is short and blind ending. The testes are of normal size and can be located in the abdomen, along the course of the inguinal canal, or in the labia majora. In contrast, neither müllerian- nor wolffian duct–derived structures are present internally. Although breast development is normal, axillary, pubic, and facial hair is absent or scanty. Biochemically, circulating testosterone levels are elevated, and 5α-reductase activity in peripheral tissues is normal.

Molecular analyses of the androgen receptor—which is encoded on the X chromosome—have defined the molecular basis for complete androgen insensitivity in most patients. These androgen receptor mutations run the full gamut, including deletions, expansion of a CAG triplet repeat, those that interfere with splicing, nonsense, missense, and frameshift mutations. Most of these subjects have point mutations in the hormone-binding domain of the androgen receptor that impair androgen binding. Less commonly, point mutations in the DNA-binding domain interfere with its activation of target genes despite normal hormone binding.

Less severe mutations in the androgen receptor—the partial androgen insensitivity syndrome—can cause relatively minor degrees of undervirilization and/or infertility. Although most patients with these conditions have normal androgen receptors, the partial androgen insensitivity syndrome includes hypospadias, cryptorchidism, and oligospermia. Patients with partial androgen insensitivity often develop gynecomastia at the time of puberty due to increased production of estradiol.

Syndrome of Persistent Mullerian Ducts

The persistence of the müllerian ducts (uterus and fallopian tubes) in a genotypic, and otherwise normal phenotypic male, is a rare condition. This syndrome generally is diagnosed at the time of surgery, often when it is noted that inguinal hernias contain müllerian derivatives (fallopian tubes and/or uterus). The testes are often cryptorchid, most likely secondary to interference of normal descent by the female structures rather than a direct requirement for AMH in testicular descent. The patients generally are fully virilized, although the intra-abdominal location of the testes often impairs spermatogenesis. Approximately half of the patients with persistent mullllerian ducts have mutations in the *AMH* gene on chromosome 19p13 that interfere with its biosynthesis or processing. The remainder have mutations in the type 2 AMH receptor—a serine threonine kinase that bears homology to receptors for other members of the TGF family—which presumably interfere with AMH binding or downstream signaling events.

CONCLUSION

Figure 8-6 summarizes our current understanding of the processes of sex determination and differentiation, indicating specific sites where dysfunction can lead to abnormal sexual development. Some genes, such as *SF-1* and *WT1*, are expressed very early in gonadogenesis and are essential for survival of the indifferent gonads; mutations of these genes cause early gonadal degeneration with impaired male sex differentiation. Thereafter, *SRY* in males induces the indifferent gonads to differentiate into testes and synthesize the two key effectors of male sexual development: AMH and androgens. SOX9 has been proposed to support SRY in the induction of

Fig. 8-6 Summary of the molecular events in mammalian sex determination and differentiation. As discussed in this chapter, the positions of genes believed to mediate key events in sex determination and differentiation are indicated. AMH, anti-müllerian hormone; AMH-R, AMH receptor; 5α-R, 5α-reductase; D, dihydrotestosterone; AR, androgen receptor.

testes development, whereas SF-1 has been proposed to act as a direct upstream regulator of genes involved in both arms of male sexual differentiation. AMH—secreted by fetal Sertoli cells—interacts with specific receptors to induce regression of the müllerian ducts. Testosterone—secreted by fetal Leydig cells—interacts with the androgen receptor to virilize the male internal genitalia, while virilization of the external genitalia and prostate further requires the conversion of testosterone to dihydrotestosterone by 5α-reductase. Anything that impairs the synthesis or function of these two testicular hormones causes aberrant or incomplete male sexual development.

Conversely, virilization of females can result from exposure *in utero* to androgens at critical periods of development, as seen most commonly in patients with congenital adrenal hyperplasia due to 21-hydroxylase deficiency. Thus, phenotypic sex differentiation is controlled by the presence (in males) or absence (in females) of specific hormonal signals during embryogenesis.

Although recent studies have identified in considerable detail the hormonal and genetic factors necessary for mammalian sexual differentiation, many fundamental issues in the embryogenesis of the urogenital tract remain poorly understood. Issues such as the nature and timing of chromosomal signals and cellular changes that cause gonadal differentiation and the mechanisms by which the same hormonal signal from androgens is translated into distinct physiological effects in different tissues must be clarified before we understand fully the developmental program that underlies phenotypic sexual differentiation.

SUGGESTED READING

Donohoue PA, Parker KL, and Migeon CJ: Congenital adrenal hyperplasia. In: *The Metabolic and Molecular Bases of Inherited Disease,* 8th ed., CR Scriver, AL Beaudet, WS Sly, and D Valle, eds., McGraw-Hill, New York, in press, 2000.

Grumbach, MM, and Conte FA: Disorders of sex differentiation. In: *Williams Textbook of Endocrinology,* 9th ed., JD Wilson, DW Foster, HM Kronenberg, and PR Larsen, eds., Saunders, Philadelphia, pp. 1303–1425, 1998.

Josso N, Picard JY, Imbeaud S, di Clemente N, and Rey R: Clinical aspects and molecular genetics of the persistent müllerian duct syndrome. Clin Endocrinol 47:137–144, 1997.

Jost A, Vigier B, Prepin J, and Perchellet J: Studies on sex differentiation in mammals. Recent Prog Horm Res 29:1–41, 1973.

Mendonca BB, Inacio M, Costa EM, Arnhold IJ, Silva FA, Nicolau W, Bloise W, Russel DW, and Wilson JD: Male pseudohermaphroditism due to steroid 5-alpha-reductase-2 deficiency: Diagnosis, psychological evaluation, and management. Medicine 75:64–76, 1996.

Parker KL, Schedl A, and Schimer BP: Gene interactions in gonadal development. Annu Rev Physiol 61:417–433, 1999.

Quigley CA, de Bellis A, Marschke KB, El-Awady MK, Wilson EM, and French FS: Androgen receptor defects: Historical, clinical, and molecular perspectives. Endocr Rev 16:271–321, 1995.

Swain A, and Lovell-Badge R: Mammalian sex determination: A molecular drama. Genes Dev 13:755–767, 1999.

Teixeira J, and Donahoe PK: Molecular biology of MIS and its receptors. J Androl 17: 336–341, 1996.

9

Female Reproductive Function

SERGIO R. OJEDA

The production of germ cells is essential for the continuation of a species. This function, in the female, is accomplished by the ovaries. In addition, the ovaries secrete steroidal and nonsteroidal hormones that not only regulate the secretion of anterior pituitary hormones but also act on various target organs including the ovaries themselves, the uterus, fallopian tubes, vagina, mammary gland, and bone.

STRUCTURAL ORGANIZATION OF THE OVARY

Morphologically, the ovary has three regions: an outer cortex that contains the oocytes and represents most of the mass of the ovary, the *inner medulla,* formed by stromal cells and cells with steroid-producing characteristics, and the *hilum*, which in addition to serving as the point of entry of the nerves and blood vessels, represents the attachment region of the gland to the mesovarium (Fig. 9-1).

The cortex, which is enveloped by the germinal epithelium, contains the functional units of the ovary—the follicles—that are present in different states of development or degeneration (atresia), each enclosing an oocyte. In addition to the oocyte, ovarian follicles have two other cellular components: granulosa cells, which surround the oocyte, and thecal cells, which are separated from the granulosa cells by a basal membrane and are arranged in concentric layers around this membrane. The follicles are embedded in the stroma, which is composed of supportive connective cells similar to that of other tissues, interstitial secretory cells, and neurovascular elements.

The medulla has a heterogeneous population of cells, some of which are morphologically similar to the Leydig cells in the testes. These cells predominate in the ovarian hilum; their neoplastic transformation results in an excessive production of androgens that induce virilization.

OVARIAN HORMONES

The ovary produces both steroidal and peptidergic hormones. Whereas the steroids are synthesized in both interstitial and follicular cells, peptidergic hormones are primarily produced in follicular cells and, after ovulation, by cells of the corpus luteum.

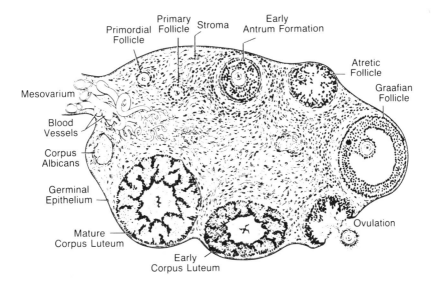

Fig. 9-1 Microscopic view of the human ovary. (Redrawn from Ham AW, and Li TS: *Histology,* 4th ed., Lippincott, Philadelphia, pp. 847–899, 1961, with permission.)

Biosynthesis, Transport, and Metabolism of Steroid Hormones

Biosynthesis

The initial precursor for steroid biosynthesis is cholesterol (Fig. 9-2), which derives from animal fats of the diet or from local synthesis. The cholesterol that arrives at the ovary via the bloodstream is mostly transported in association with low-density lipoproteins (LDL), which bind to specific receptors located in the plasma membrane of ovarian cells. Thereafter, the LDL–receptor complexes are internalized and hydrolyzed within lysosomes that release cholesterol for steroid biosynthesis. Excess cholesterol is esterified and stored in lipid droplets for later use. Under normal conditions cholesterol utilized in steroid biosynthesis comes from the plasma LDL-associated pool and intracellular lipid droplets. A less important source originates from *de novo* local synthesis.

For cholesterol to be used in steroid biosynthesis, it must be transported to the mitochondria. This process is achieved by a recently identified protein termed *steroidogenic acute regulatory protein* (StAR), which promotes the transfer of cholesterol from the outer to the inner mitochondrial membrane. Upon reaching this location, cholesterol becomes available to the cholesterol side-chain cleavage enzyme for conversion to pregnenolone (see below). The StAR is therefore essential for the acute regulation of steroid biosynthesis. The gene encoding StAR spans 8 kb in the human genome; its mRNA product comprises several transcripts ranging from 1.6 to 7.5 kb, and generates a 3.7-kDa precursor protein that is cleaved in the mitochondria to a 30-kDa mature protein. The cytosolic precursor form is thought to be the steroidogenic active protein acutely synthesized in response to hormonal, cAMP-mediated stimulation. Formation of the 30-kDa mature form in the mitochondria

Fig. 9-2 Biosynthesis of steroids in the ovary. 1: Cholesterol side-chain cleavage enzyme complex; 2: 3β-hydroxysteroid dehydrogenase; 3: 17α-hydroxylase; 4: 17,20-lyase; 5: aromatase; 6: 17β-hydroxysteroid dehydrogenase.

signals the termination of cholesterol transfer, so that new transfer requires additional synthesis of the precursor form.

The main steroids produced by the ovary are progesterone and estradiol (Fig. 9-2). Whereas androgens, particularly androstenedione and testosterone, are also secreted into the bloodstream, a significant portion is converted to estradiol through the action of an aromatase enzyme complex. In addition to these steroids, the ovary also secretes estrone, 17α-hydroxyprogesterone, 20α-hydroxyprogesterone, and 5α-reduced androgens such as 5α-dihydrotestosterone and 3α-androstanediol.

The first step in the synthesis of ovarian steroids is the conversion of cholesterol, which has 27 carbons, to the C-21 compound pregnenolone in a reaction catalyzed by an enzyme complex known as *cholesterol side-chain cleavage enzyme.* The reaction occurs in the mitochondria. Pregnenolone can then be converted into progesterone by the action of a 3β-hydroxysteroid dehydrogenase enzyme, or into 17α-hydroxypregnenolone by a 17α-hydroxylase. Both progesterone and 17α-hydroxypregnenolone can, in turn, be metabolized to 17α-hydroxyprogesterone (Fig. 9-2).

In contrast to cholesterol, progestogen compounds have only 21 carbons. Additional metabolism to androgens and estrogens results in further reduction in the number of carbons to 19 (androgens) and 18 (estrogens).

17α-Hydroxyprogesterone is the substrate for a 17,20-lyase enzyme that, by cleaving the C-20,21 side chain, yields androstenedione. This androgen is either directly metabolized to estrone or, preferentially, converted into testosterone in a reaction catalyzed by the enzyme 17β-hydroxysteroid dehydrogenase. Both androstenedione and testosterone are substrates for estrogen production. Whereas androstenedione is converted into estrone, testosterone metabolism results in estradiol formation. In both cases the reaction is catalyzed by an aromatase enzyme that generates the estrogens through a complex series of reactions involving hydroxylations, oxidations, removal of the C-19 carbon, and aromatization of the A ring of the androgen. All of the reactions involved in the metabolism of progesterone to estradiol, including the initial formation of progesterone from pregnenolone, occur in the endoplasmic reticulum.

With the exception of the 3β- and 17β-hydroxysteroid dehydrogenases, the enzymes involved in ovarian steroid biosynthesis belong to a group called *mixed function oxidases* that utilize different forms of cytochrome P450 and require molecular oxygen and nicotinamide adenine dinucleotide phosphate (NADPH) for their activity. They consist of the cytochrome P450, which binds to the substrate, and an electron transport system. In the case of the cholesterol side-chain cleavage enzyme, the electron transport system consists of an iron–sulfur protein and a flavoprotein, NADPH-adrenodoxin reductase. In the case of the 17α-hydroxylase, 17,20-lyase, and aromatase enzyme systems, the electron transport system is provided by a flavoprotein NADPH–cytochrome P450 reductase.

The synthesis of P450 steroid hydroxylases is regulated by the activation of an orphan nuclear receptor known as *steroidogenic factor-1* (SF-1). Alternative promoter usage and different 3' splicing patterns of the gene encoding SF-1 originates multiple transcripts that appear to serve different functions. In addition to being essential for P450 steroid hydroxylase expression, SF-1 is also involved in the regulation of other steroidogenic enzymes such as 3β-hydroxysteroid dehydrogenase and StAR. Unexpectedly, targeted disruption of the *SF-1* gene revealed that SF-1 is essential for ovarian and adrenal morphogenesis; in its absence both glands fail to develop. In addition, SF-1–deficient mice show a reduction in pituitary gonadotropin synthesis and loss of the ventromedial nucleus of the hypothalamus (for additional information see Chapter 8).

The bulk of androgen production occurs in interstitial cells and the cells of the follicular theca (see p. 208 and Fig. 9-3). Estradiol is mainly produced by granulosa cells of antral follicles. Progesterone, in contrast, is secreted by all steroidogenic cells of the ovary regardless of their localization.

For those students interested in the subject, a detailed description of steroid chemistry, pathways, and biosynthetic enzymes can be found in the review by Kellie, and in the book *The Physiology of Reproduction*, by Knobil and Neill, listed at the end of this chapter.

Transport and Metabolism of Steroid Hormones
Both 17β-estradiol and estrone are present in the bloodstream. Whereas estradiol is secreted directly by the ovary, estrone derives largely from peripheral conversion of

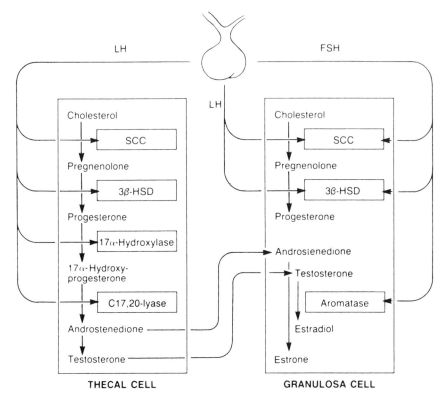

Fig. 9-3 The control of ovarian estrogen, progesterone, and androgen production by LH and FSH. The LH acts on both thecal and granulosa cells; FSH acts only on granulosa cells.

estradiol or androstenedione. Estrone is further metabolized to estriol, a reaction that occurs predominantly in the liver. Most circulating estrogens (>70%) are bound to proteins, preferentially albumin, for which they have a low affinity, or to a steroid-binding protein known as *sex hormone-binding globulin* (SHBG), for which they have a higher affinity. Estrogens have a lower affinity for SHBG than androgens; this results in a greater availability of estrogens to the tissues because only free steroids can be transported into their target cells (see Chapter 5).

Metabolism of estrogens via oxidation or conversion to glucuronide and sulfate conjugates occurs predominantly in the liver. The resulting metabolites are excreted in the bile and reabsorbed into the bloodstream via the enterohepatic circulation. Their final excretion route, however, is the urine.

Androgens in women are produced by both the ovaries and the adrenals. There are three main circulating androgens in women: dehydroepiandrosterone produced by the adrenal, androstenedione derived from both the ovary and the adrenal, and testosterone, which in addition to being produced by the ovary and adrenal is formed in peripheral tissues, mainly from androstenedione and to some extent from dehydroepiandrosterone and Δ^5-androstenediol. Indeed, testosterone is the primary physiologically active androgen in women. It may act on target tissues directly or after its conversion to 5α-dihydrotestosterone. As in men (see Chapter 10), 97%–99% of the total circulating testosterone in women is bound to SHBG. As with estrogens, androgens are excreted mostly in the urine.

Progesterone also circulates bound to a plasma protein, corticosteroid-binding protein (transcortin). Binding proteins with significantly higher affinity for progesterone than for corticosterone have been described in pregnant rabbits and guinea pigs, but their identity has not yet been established. Progesterone is converted in the liver to pregnanediol, which, following conjugation to glucuronic acid, is excreted in the urine.

Peptide Hormones of Ovarian Origin

One of the first peptide hormones to be recognized as a product of the ovary was *relaxin*. It is mainly produced by the corpus luteum during pregnancy but has also been found in decidual tissue and human seminal plasma. The secretion of relaxin from the corpus luteum is stimulated by human chorionic gonadotropin (hCG). Although several peptides showing relaxin-like activity have been reported, they do not appear to be the products of related genes, but rather the result of limited proteolysis of relaxin during the process of isolation. In humans, however, there is good evidence for the existence of two relaxin-related genes. Human relaxin consists of an α- and a β-peptide chain covalently linked by disulfide bonds. Interestingly, both the position of the bonds and the processing of the prohormone to yield mature relaxin are identical to those of insulin, suggesting that both proteins, as well as the insulin-like growth factors (IGFs; see Chapter 12), derive from the duplication of a common ancestral gene. The main effect of relaxin is to induce relaxation of the pelvic bones and ligaments, inhibit myometrial motility, and soften the cervix. In addition, relaxin has been shown to induce uterine growth. It is clear, therefore, that the hormone plays an important role in both maintaining uterine quiescence and favoring the growth and softening of the reproductive tract during pregnancy.

For many years it was suspected that the ovary produces a peptide hormone that exerts selective inhibitory control over the secretion of follicle-stimulating hormone (FSH). This protein, originally described in testicular extracts and termed *inhibin,* was isolated from follicular fluid and found to be a heterodimeric protein consisting of an α- and a β-polypeptide chain connected by disulfide bonds. Two forms of inhibin (A and B) exists, each with a molecular weight of 32,000. The α-subunits are identical and the β-subunits are different. Combination of the β-subunits of inhibin among themselves via disulfide bond linkage results in the formation of another family of proteins with completely different functions. The first of these functions to be recognized was the selective stimulation of FSH secretion from the adenohypophysis. Because of this activity, this inhibin-associated protein was termed *FSH-releasing protein* (FRP) or *activin*. There are three forms of activins resulting from the differential dimerization of β-subunits, which can form βA/βA, βA/βB, and βB/βB dimers, respectively.

It now appears that the functions of activin are much more diverse than originally anticipated. The messenger RNA (mRNA) encoding the βA subunit of activin is expressed in the brain, pituitary gland, germ cells of the testis, and erythropoietic tissue, suggesting a role for activin in cell differentiation. Such a role is supported by studies showing that the differentiation of erythrocytes is promoted by a factor encoded by the same mRNA that encodes the βA-subunit of activin. These nonreproductive functions, though initially surprising, are consistent with the finding that inhibins and activins are members of a large family of peptides that includes transforming growth factor-β (TGF-β), anti-müllerian hormone (AMH, see Chapter 8), and many other peptides involved in the control of growth and differentiation.

In addition to activins and inhibins, follicular cells produce another group of proteins with molecular weights ranging from 32 to 43 kDa, which inhibit FSH secretion. These proteins, termed *follistatins,* bind activins with high affinity and thus are able to neutralize their biological activity.

Still another peptidergic factor, termed *gonadotropin surge-attenuating factor* (GnSAF), has been postulated to be physiologically involved in the control of luteinizing hormone (LH) secretion during the menstrual cycle. This factor appears to be distinct from the inhibin family of peptides and produced by medium-sized antral follicles. It may function during the follicular phase of the cycle to prevent a premature LH surge.

Quite unexpectedly, the ovary has been found to produce peptides of the proopiomelanocorticotropin (POMC) family including β-endorphin, adrenocorticotropin (ACTH), and α-melanocyte-stimulating hormone (α-MSH). The ovary also produces vasopressin and oxytocin. These two peptides are synthesized in luteal cells. In the case of oxytocin there is clear evidence that the hormone is secreted into the general circulation. The physiological role that these peptides may play in the ovary is uncertain. However, they appear to exert paracrine effects.

Pituitary Control of Ovarian Hormone Formation

Steroids

The production of ovarian steroids is under the control of two main hormones secreted by the anterior hypophysis, luteinizing hormone (LH) and FSH. In rodents, prolactin and growth hormone (GH) have also been shown to act directly on the ovary. Experiments in rats demonstrated that, depending on its level, prolactin may either inhibit or support the stimulatory effect of LH on ovarian steroidogenesis, through modulation of the number of LH receptors. In contrast, GH has been found to facilitate FSH actions in rats by a mechanism involving local production insulinlike growth factor (IGF)-I.

Although the secretion of progesterone can be stimulated by both LH and FSH, the secretion of androgens is enhanced only by LH. The formation of estradiol, conversely, depends on both LH and FSH. The LH stimulates production of androgens that are utilized in estrogen production; FSH directly activates the aromatase enzyme complex that catalyzes the conversion of androgens to estrogens.

The LH receptors are found on steroidogenic cells of the stroma and thecal cells of the follicles, both of which produce progesterone and androgens. When the follicles become antral, the granulosa cells acquire LH receptors. As these cells have a limited 17,20-lyase activity, their exposure to LH results primarily in increased production of progesterone and little, if any, production of progesterone and little, if any, production of androgens. In contrast, FSH receptors are located exclusively on granulosa cells, which are the only ovarian cells with substantial aromatase activity.

These interactions have formed the basis for the formulation of a "two cell–two gonadotropin" hypothesis to explain the gonadotropic control of ovarian steroidogenesis. According to this hypothesis the follicular theca, under the influence of LH, produces androgens that upon diffusion to the granulosa cell compartment of the follicle are converted to estrogens via an FSH-supported aromatization reaction (Fig. 9-3).

Peptide Hormones

Production of inhibin is stimulated by FSH. The role of LH in the control of inhibin production is more complex. Inhibin production in preovulatory follicles decreases sharply soon after the preovulatory surge of gonadotropins (see below, "Dynamics of the Hypothalamic–Pituitary–Ovarian Relationship"). This decrease appears to be brought about by LH, which, however, simultaneously increases inhibin production in smaller follicles not destined to ovulate in that cycle. It also appears that formation of POMC peptides, vasopressin, and oxytocin is under gonadotropin control. While gonadotropins stimulate the formation of oxytocin and β-endorphin, they decrease the production of vasopressin.

Mechanism of Action of Gonadotropins

Both LH and FSH act on the ovary by first binding to high-affinity, low capacity–specific membrane receptors. Follicle-stimulating hormone (FSH) initiates its actions by binding to a seven-transmembrane domain G protein–coupled receptor. The receptor is a glycoprotein of a predicted molecular weight of 75 kDa encoded by a single gene that maps to chromosome 2 in the human genome. Although the LH receptor maps to the same chromosome, it is not located in the same region of the chromosome. The predicted human FSH receptor protein is encoded by an open reading frame of 2085 nucleotides, which generates a 678-amino acid mature protein. Expression of the receptor is highly specific, as it can only be found in Sertoli cells of the testis and granulosa cells of the ovary. Binding of FSH results in cAMP formation and calcium mobilization. It is not clear whether the calcium mobilization is a consequence of the increase in cAMP formation or a cAMP-independent phenomenon. It is known, however, that cAMP activates protein kinase A, which, in turn, induces the phosphorylation of several downstream proteins involved in regulating the expression of cAMP-responsive genes.

The LH receptor is also a seven-transmembrane, G-protein–coupled receptor. Its amino acid sequence shows significant homology to the FSH receptor, particularly in the transmembrane domain. The mature protein is a polypeptide of 674 amino acids with a predicted molecular mass of 75 kDa. Its short intracellular domain contains a number of potential sites for phosphorylation. Interestingly, although activation of the LH receptor causes a clear increase in cAMP levels, the intracellular domain of the receptor contains weak consensus sequences for cAMP-dependent protein kinase–mediated phosphorylation. The receptor is expressed in both differentiated granulosa and thecal cells, as well as in luteal cells of the ovary. However, immature granulosa cells from preantral and small antral follicles contain very low levels of the receptor, which is induced in granulosa cells of large preovulatory follicles.

Actions of Ovarian Steroids

Ovarian steroids exert intra- and extraovarian actions. The best-known intraovarian actions are those exerted on follicular development. Among the extraovarian actions are those exerted on the hypothalamic–pituitary unit (negative and positive feedback on gonadotropin secretion), on reproductive tissues such as fallopian tubes, uterus, vagina, and mammary gland, and on other tissues such as bone, kidney, and liver.

Intraovarian Actions

Estrogens. Estradiol (E_2) induces proliferation of the granulosa cells, increases E_2 receptors in these cells, and facilitates the action of FSH.

Androgens and Progestins. Testosterone and progesterone have been shown to affect ovarian steroidogenesis through binding to their respective receptors, which are present in granulosa cells. Progesterone inhibits FSH-induced estradiol production. Androgens, in contrast, enhance both the progesterone and estradiol secretion induced by FSH.

A very important intraovarian action of progesterone is in the ovulatory process. Mice lacking the progesterone receptor fail to ovulate despite their having preovulatory follicles. This failure appears to be related to the inability of the follicle to produce proteolytic enzymes necessary for rupture of the follicular wall.

Extraovarian Actions

The Uterus. The endometrium or uterine mucosa consists of a superficial layer of epithelial cells and a deeper stromal layer. The epithelial layer is interrupted by tubular invaginations or glands that penetrate into the stromal layer and that are lined by both epithelial cells and columnar secretory cells. The stroma is permeated by blood vessels (spiral arteries) and contains characteristically spindle-shaped cells.

During the first half of the menstrual cycle (i.e., before ovulation), estrogen stimulates proliferation of both the epithelial and stromal layers. The thickness of the endometrium increases 3- to 5-fold and the uterine glands become enlarged, but they maintain their straight shape.The spiral arteries also elongate. Because of such changes this has been called the *proliferative phase* of the endometrium.

The uterine cervix contains endocervical glands that elaborate a mucus, which, under the influence of estrogen, changes from a scanty, viscous substance to a much more abundant, watery material. The elasticity of the mucus, usually referred to as *spinnbarkeit,* is greatly increased, a change that can be easily determined by stretching a small drop of mucus between two fingers. When estrogen production is maximal, that is, close to the time of ovulation, the elasticity of the cervical mucus is such that the drop can be stretched maximally without rupture. If a drop of such mucus is spread on a slide, upon drying, the mucus forms a typical palm-leaf arborization or ferning pattern.

Under the influence of progesterone, which is produced in increasing amounts after ovulation, proliferation of the endometrium decreases and the uterine glands lose their straight configuration, becoming tortuous. Glycogen accumulates in large vacuoles at the basal portion of the cells. As the corpus luteum becomes firmly established, the glycogen vacuoles move toward the apical end of the cells and the secretory activity of the gland increases significantly. The stroma becomes edematous, and the elongating spiral arteries become coiled. These transformations establish the *secretory phase* of the endometrium. Coinciding with the loss of corpus luteum function and the resulting decline in plasma levels of estrogen and progesterone the endometrium undergoes focal necrosis, probably because of vasospasm of the spiral arteries. The areas of necrosis increase progressively and the mucosa exfoliates with loss of all superficial cells except those lining the base of the glands. Because necrosis also affects the endometrial blood vessels, blood loss occurs as menstrual bleeding.

Vasospasm of the endometrial blood vessels is believed to be mediated by prostaglandins, in particular prostaglandin $F_{2\alpha}$. It appears that the loss of luteal progesterone and estrogen destabilizes the lysosomal membranes of endometrial cells, which enhances phospholipid hydrolysis and subsequently prostaglandin formation. Reinitiation of follicular growth during menstruation is accompanied by an increased production of estrogen stimulating the endometrium to proliferate again.

In addition to its effects on the endometrium, progesterone decreases both the quantity and the elasticity of the cervical mucus and inhibits its ferning pattern.

The Vagina. The human vagina is lined by a stratified multilayered squamous epithelium that consists of superficial, intermediate, inner parabasal, and basal layers. In the presence of low levels of estrogen, such as before puberty or at menopause, the vaginal epithelium is thin and dry, and more susceptible to infections. Estrogens induce both proliferation and keratinization of the epithelium. As a result, mucosa thickness increases and there is increased exfoliation of superficial cells that can be readily identified under the microscope because of their acidophilia and pyknotic nuclei. Interestingly, the epithelium that lines the urethra is also sensitive to ovarian steroids. Thus, examination of urethral cells collected from a fresh urinary sediment can be used to assess alterations in circulating estrogen and progesterone levels in both prepubertal and mature women.

In general, progesterone has an effect on the vaginal epithelium that is opposite to that of estrogen. Under its influence the number of cornified cells decreases and the number of polymorphonuclear leukocytes increases.

The Mammary Gland. The human breast is composed of several lactiferous duct systems that are embedded in adipose and connective tissue. Each duct system contains thousands of sac-like milk-secreting alveoli, which are surrounded by myoepithelial cells and which drain into an increasingly larger milk-transporting system comprised of ductules, ducts, lactiferous sinuses, and a single ampulla that opens into the nipple at the center of the areola. At puberty, when estrogen secretion rises, growth of the ducts accelerates and the size of the areola increases. Furthermore, estrogen causes selective accumulation of adipose tissue around the lactiferous duct systems, and this contributes significantly to the overall growth of the breast.

While estrogen stimulates the development of the duct system, progesterone induces the formation of secretory alveoli, an effect more clearly observed during pregnancy. Progesterone also facilitates the proliferating effect of estrogen on the duct epithelium. However, in the absence of priming by estrogen, progesterone has little effect on the mammary gland.

Metabolic Effects. One of the best-known metabolic effects of estrogen is to increase the amount of plasma proteins produced by the liver that bind estradiol, testosterone, cortisol, progesterone, and thyroxine. Estrogens also increase the plasma proteins that bind iron and copper, and the levels of high-density lipoproteins (HDL) and very low-density lipoproteins (VLDL). The latter results in increased circulating levels of triglycerides, which are the lipids preferentially associated with these lipoproteins. In contrast to these effects, estrogen lowers the circulating levels of cholesterol and low-density lipoproteins (LDL). Estrogen also exerts appreciable effects on the electrolyte balance because of its stimulatory effects on the formation of angiotensinogen and aldosterone. Awareness of these metabolic effects has been heightened by the use of oral contraceptives that, as will be discussed later, are a combination of estrogen and progesterone.

Progesterone itself has little effect on plasma triglycerides. However, some synthetic progestins used in oral contraceptives have been shown to decrease triglyceride levels. More importantly, progesterone increases the levels of cholesterol and LDL and decreases the levels of HDL. Progesterone can also transiently increase sodium excretion in the urine, owing to its capacity to antagonize aldosterone action.

The best-known metabolic effect of progesterone is to increase basal body temperature. This is observed after ovulation and can serve as an index that ovulation has occurred.

Effects on Nonreproductive Tissues. We have already mentioned the effect of estrogen on the liver. Two additional target tissues are the bone and the kidney. Estrogen acts on bone both to accelerate linear growth and to induce closure of the epiphyseal plates. In addition, it prevents bone resorption. The importance of this effect becomes clearly evident at menopause. At this time, estrogen secretion decreases, resulting in osteoporosis and bone fragility in some women. It is now clear that at least part of this supportive effect of estrogen is exerted directly via binding of the steroid to specific receptors.

In the kidney, estradiol enhances the reabsorption of sodium from the renal tubules.

THE MENSTRUAL CYCLE

Reproductive function in the female is cyclic. A series of functional interrelationships among the hypothalamus, the anterior pituitary, and the ovaries leads to the monthly rupture of an ovarian follicle and extrusion of an ovum (i.e., "ovulation"), which is then transported to the fallopian tubes to be fertilized. Should fertilization fail to occur, menstruation ensues within 14 days and the hormonal and morphological events that led to ovulation are repeated. This coordinated series of events is known as the *menstrual cycle*. The normal menstrual cycle has an average duration of about 30 days, with a range that extends from 25 to 35 days. It can be divided into four phases: menstruation, which lasts about 4–5 days; a follicular phase of the ovary, which corresponds to the proliferative phase of the endometrium and lasts 10–16 days; an ovulatory phase, which lasts about 36 hours; and a luteal phase, which corresponds to the secretory phase of the endometrium. The latter is usually very constant, lasting about 14 days; thus, the length of the menstrual cycle is determined by the follicular phase, which can be highly variable. The greatest variability occurs during the few years that follow the first menstruation (menarche) and during the years preceding the loss of reproductive function (menopause).

An understanding of the menstrual cycle requires knowledge of the functional components responsible for its occurrence. These are (*1*) the gonadotropin-releasing system and its neural (hypothalamic) control, (*2*) the ovarian follicle, including its rupture at ovulation and its subsequent transformation into a corpus luteum, and (*3*) the ovarian negative and positive feedback control of gonadotropin secretion.

The Gonadotropin-Releasing System and Its Neural Control (Fig. 9-4)

As discussed in Chapter 6 the adenohypophysis has a population of cells—the gonadotrophs—that secretes both LH and FSH. Some cells secrete only LH, others FSH, and still others secrete both hormones.

Release of LH and FSH to the bloodstream is pulsatile. This is particularly noticeable in the case of LH, which has episodes of release every 70–100 minutes. Because the interpulse intervals are about an hour long, this rhythm has been called *circhoral*. The LH pulses are less frequent during the luteal phase of the menstrual cycle than during the follicular phase, presumably because of an inhibitory effect of progesterone that is secreted in large amounts by the corpus luteum.

In addition to this circhoral rhythm, LH secretion also exhibits a sleep-related rhythm. This mode of secretion is not clearly manifested in adult women, but it constitutes a fundamental feature at the onset of puberty. At this time, an increased amount of LH is released during sleep, the first overt neuroendocrine manifestation of the initiation of puberty (see p. 226).

Both types of release (circhoral and diurnal) are a function of luteinizing hormone-releasing hormone (LHRH), the hypothalamic peptide responsible for the control of gonadotropin secretion. Experiments performed in rats, sheep, and monkeys have demonstrated that LHRH is released into the portal circulation, and hence reaches the adenohypophysis, in a pulsatile fashion.

In nonhuman primates, surgical isolation of the medial basal hypothalamus fails to disturb the circhoral release of LH, indicating that the rhythm originates within this area of the brain. Lesion of the arcuate nucleus, which is located in the foremost ventral portion of the medial basal hypothalamus, abolishes basal release of both LH and FSH, indicating that the most essential neural center controlling gonadotropin secretion resides within the arcuate nucleus of the hypothalamus. It is also clear, however, that the function of this "pulse generator" is subject to modifying influences emanating from both extra- and intrahypothalamic loci. An increase in electrical activity in the arcuate nucleus area precedes, with astounding regularity, the discharge of LH into the bloodstream.

The involvement of several neurotransmitter systems in the control of LHRH secretion has also been demonstrated. Among them, the most important appear to be those neuronal networks that utilize excitatory amino acids and γ-aminobutyric acid (GABA) as neurotransmitters. While excitatory amino acids (most predominantly glutamate) stimulate LHRH secretion, GABAergic neurons exert a powerful

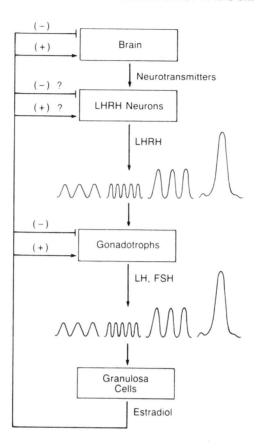

Fig. 9-4   The control of LH and LHRH secretion by ovarian estradiol. Both LH and LHRH are released in pulses. Estrogen (and combinations of estrogen plus progesterone) can alter the frequency and/or amplitude of the pulses by acting at both the hypothalamus and anterior pituitary. Within the brain, estradiol may inhibit (−) or stimulate (+) the activity of neurotransmitters that affect LHRH secretion. It is not clear whether estradiol can act directly on LHRH neurons (?). Estradiol can also induce a large, preovulatory surge of LH and LHRH secretion.

inhibitory influence. Other stimulatory neurotransmitters include the catecholamine norepinephrine (NE), and the peptide neuropeptide Y (NPY). Neurotransmitters, such as the amines *dopamine* (DA) and *serotonin,* can either stimulate or inhibit LHRH secretion, depending on the prevalent steroid milieu present.

In addition to GABA, opioid peptides are also able to inhibit LHRH release. β-Endorphin, synthesized in neurons of the medial basal hypothalamus, is a prominent example of this class of inhibitory inputs to LHRH neurons. If naloxone, a blocker of opioid receptors, is administered during the luteal phase of the menstrual cycle the frequency of LH discharges increases to levels similar to those seen during the early follicular phase. Because progesterone increases β-endorphin production in the hypothalamus it has been suggested that the inhibitory effect exerted by progesterone during the luteal phase on LH pulse frequency is mediated by β-endorphin.

Despite the complexity of the transsynaptic control of LHRH secretion, it is becoming increasingly evident that most of the above-mentioned neuronal networks play roles secondary to that of the glutamate–GABA regulatory systems. Recent experiments in rodents and nonhuman primates have implicated glial cells as an additional component of the regulatory complex controlling LHRH secretion. Glial cells of the astrocytic lineage were shown to affect LHRH release via production of trophic molecules, which, acting in a paracrine–autocrine fashion, stimulate the glial secretion of neuroactive substances able to stimulate LHRH release. TGF-α was identified as one of these glial regulatory molecules.

Follicular Development, Ovulation, and Atresia (Fig. 9-5)

Follicular Development

The primordial germ cells originate in the endoderm of the yolk sac, allantois, and hindgut of the embryo. By 5–6 weeks of gestation they migrate to the genital ridge and begin to multiply rapidly, so that by 24 weeks of gestation the total number of oogonia is about 7 million. They concentrate mostly within the cortical portion of the primitive gonad. As multiplication of the oogonia proceeds, some of them reach the prophase stage of meiosis and are called *primary oocytes*. Many others degenerate and die so that at birth only 2 million primary oocytes remain, a number that is further reduced before puberty to about 400,000. The first meiotic division is not completed until the moment of ovulation; at this time the oocyte has grown from a size of 10–25 μm to 150 μm in diameter. The factors determining their long suspension in meiotic prophase are unknown.

A single layer of flattened epithelial cells surrounds a primary oocyte, and a *primordial follicle* is formed. These cells, which will later generate the granulosa

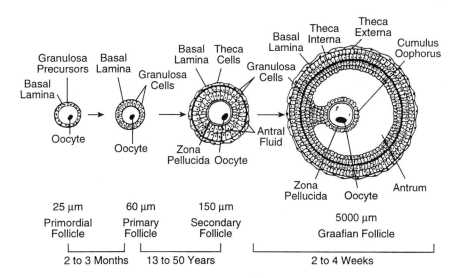

Fig. 9-5 Schematic representation of the development of an ovarian follicle (not to scale). (Redrawn and modified from Berne RM, and Levy MN: *Physiology*, Mosby, St. Louis, pp. 1069–1115, 1983, with permission.)

cells, provide nutrients to the oocyte via protoplasmatic processes that reach the oocyte plasma membrane. The primordial follicle becomes separated from surrounding spindle-shaped mesenchymal cells by a basement membrane called the *basal lamina*. When the flattened epithelial cells become cuboidal the follicle becomes a *primary follicle*. The oocyte secretes a mucoid substance rich in glycoproteins that forms a band that separates the oocyte from the granulosa cells. This band is called the *zona pellucida*.

The granulosa cells located next to the zona pellucida continue to extend protoplasmastic processes to the oocyte, presumably to maintain a nutrient flow and chemical signals to the growing oocyte. As these changes occur, the stromal cells adjacent to the basal lamina become differentiated in concentric layers around the primary follicle, constituting the *follicular theca*. The portion of the theca contiguous to the basal lamina is called the *theca interna*; the outer portion is called the *theca externa*.

Development of primary follicles is a very slow process lasting several years. At puberty, and throughout the reproductive years, cohorts of primary follicles enter into a new phase of development that is completed in approximately 3 weeks. During this phase, granulosa cells proliferate more rapidly, and some of the cells of the theca interna become cuboidal and filled with lipid droplets, indicative of enhanced steroidogenesis. In addition, the theca interna is invaded by the capillaries that terminate at the basal lamina. In some follicles the continuity of the granulosa cell layers is disrupted by the appearance of spaces filled with fluid. Gradually, these spaces become confluent, forming a single central cavity called the *antrum*. The follicles with these characteristics receive the name of *antral follicles*. As they grow further their antrum is greatly expanded. These follicles are known as *graafian follicles*. At this stage, the oocyte reaches its maximum size (150 μm).

The antrum is filled with a fluid that contains steroids, pituitary hormones, and local growth factors at concentrations several times greater than in plasma. As the granulosa cells continue to proliferate and the antrum enlarges, the oocyte is displaced from the center of the follicle and becomes surrounded by a hillock of granulosa cells called the *cumulus oophorus*. By the end of this stage, the antral follicle has reached a diameter of 5 mm. Because the granulosa cells and the oocyte are surrounded by the basal lamina throughout follicular development, they remain avascular; hormones, neurotransmitters, and blood-borne nutrients must reach them by diffusion.

During the second half of the follicular phase, one follicle becomes dominant and undergoes further growth so as to finally expel its oocyte at ovulation. The factors responsible for the selection of a single follicle (from a cohort of 6 to 10 follicles that become antral) in every cycle are poorly understood.

Ovulation

As discussed below, at the end of the follicular phase a large increase in plasma levels of gonadotropins takes place. This greatly increases the production of antral fluid in the dominant follicle; the follicle enlarges markedly, reaching a diameter of 10–20 mm in 48 hours. The granulosa become less cohesive and the cumulus oophorus loosens. Studies in the rabbit have shown that the first morphological changes in the thecal compartment of the ovulatory follicle occur by 4 hours after the initial gonadotropin stimulation. The theca interna begin to develop edema, and the fibroblastic cells of this region begin to dissociate. Thereafter, no major morphological changes occur until the last hour before rupture; at this time the fibroblasts and collagenous matrix of the apical portion of the follicular wall undergo dissociation. Simultaneously, there is extravasation of blood cells into the extracellular space of the follicular wall, which deteriorates at a specific site on its surface, called the *stigma*. Formation of the stigma begins with a local decrease of blood flow, followed by a gradual thinning and depolymerization of the connective tissue in the area, and reorganization of the vasculature around the edge of the stigma. Sixteen to 24 hours after the gonadotropin surge, the follicular wall at the stigma becomes exceedingly thin and finally appears to dissolve, allowing the extrusion of the oocyte surrounded by the cumulus oophorus.

It is now clear that ovulation requires the functional integrity of three different effector proteins: the progesterone receptor (PR); the cyclooxygenase enzyme, which catalyzes the formation of prostaglandins from arachidonic acid; and cyclin D2, a cell cycle activator. Null mutations of any of the genes encoding these proteins results in ovulatory failure, clearly establishing the absolute requirement for each of these molecules in the ovulatory process. All three genes are expressed in granulosa cells and are induced by the preovulatory LH surge. Of the three, only the cyclooxygenase gene is also expressed in thecal cells. The mechanisms by which the LH surge activates the expression of these three genes have not been elucidated. A transcription factor known as C/EBPβ (for CCAAT/enhancer binding protein) is strongly induced by LH in granulosa cells. Mice lacking this factor fail to ovulate, indicating that C/EBPβ is an essential early downstream signal used by LH to induce ovulation. However, C/EBPβ does not act by activating PR or cyclooxygenase expression. On the one hand, it does not bind to the PR promoter; on the other hand, mice lacking C/EBPβ exhibit persistently elevated levels of cyclooxygenase, instead of a decrease.

Despite the identification of these four key molecules (PR, cyclooxygenase, cyclin D2, and C/EBPβ), the signaling mechanisms they employ to set in motion the ovulatory rupture remain largely unknown. It is likely, however, that they involve the activation of specific proteolytic and collagenase activities able to disrupt the continuity of the follicular wall. Until recently, it was believed that plasminogen activators (PA), which are strongly induced by the preovulatory LH surge, were responsible for ovulatory rupture. Because mice carrying a deletion of the genes encoding either of the two PA candidates (tissue-type and urokinase-type PA) are fertile, it is now apparent that there are other proteases playing a more critical role in ovulation. *Matrix metalloproteases,* a class of proteases involved in tissue remodeling, are currently considered as potential candidates for such a role. Matrix metalloproteases include collagenases involved in the degradation of different types of collagens, such as MMP13, which degrades collagen type I, and MMP2 and MMP9, which degrade basement membrane collagens type IV and V. Although conclusive evidence for the involvement of MMP13 has not yet been provided, it appears that MMP2 and MMP9 may not be required for ovulation. MMP2 activity is decreased by LH; MMP9 null mutant mice are fertile.

Two additional groups of candidate substances are serine proteases of the kallikrein family and certain cytokines. The former are produced in the ovary and—

as in other systems—mediate vascular effects associated with inflammatory processes. The latter (such as interleukin-1 and -8) are produced by the preovulatory follicle in response to LH and attract leukocytes and macrophages to the follicle, where they induce the production of various proteases. Clearly, much more needs to be done to clarify the cellular and molecular mechanisms underlying the ovulatory process.

The first meiotic division is completed at the time of ovulation. The first polar body is eliminated, and the secondary oocyte is captured by the fimbria of the oviduct, which is closely applied to the surface of the ovary. The oocyte is then transported to the ampulla of the oviduct via ciliary movements. The second meiotic division occurs at the time of fertilization, yielding the ovum with a haploid number of chromosomes and a second polar body that is discarded.

Atresia

Because the human female has approximately 30 years of reproductive life, only 300–400 follicles reach maturity within a lifetime. The rest undergo a degenerative process called *atresia*. Atresia occurs via a regulated form of cell death known as *apoptosis,* a physiological process that occurs in all tissues throughout development. During apoptotic death very distinct morphological and molecular changes take place that allow one to follow the demise of the cell as it occurs. Within the nucleus there is an initial condensation of chromatin, followed by disruption of the nuclear membrane and fragmentation of the nucleus into pieces that form a dense structure known as *pyknotic nucleus.* During apoptosis the DNA is cleaved between nucleosomal units by calcium/magnesium–dependent endonucleases; if the DNA of cells undergoing apoptosis is isolated and analyzed on a gel, it will show a characteristic "ladder" pattern with fragments of sizes made of multiples of about 200 base pairs. The cytoplasm of an apoptotic cell also undergoes a series of characteristic changes: aggregation and disintegration of organelles; the plasma membrane shrinks; finally, there is cell fragmentation followed by phagocytosis by neighboring macrophages.

Atresia occurs in both germ cells and follicles. Apoptosis of germ cells is initiated during fetal life, during both migration and after arrival at the ovary, while they proliferate. In rodents, germ cells (termed *oogonia* after they reach the ovary) enter meiosis shortly before birth, but remain arrested at the diplotene stage of prophase until near ovulation (see above). Within a few hours after birth, some germ cells (now called *oocytes*) become surrounded by epithelial pregranulosa cells to form the primordial follicles. Many oocytes fail to be enclosed and undergo atresia. Only a small fraction (less than 10%) of the germ cells become finally encapsulated into a follicular structure. Thus, atresia of germ cells is massive before formation of the follicles.

Follicular atresia occurs at all stages of antral follicular development. The follicles to die are those that fail to be supported by survival factors. The FSH is the most critical of these factors; if a follicle receives sufficient FSH support during development it will escape atresia and reach the preovulatory stage. In addition, LH and growth hormone (GH) are also antiapoptotic, but less potent than FSH. The signaling pathway utilized by gonadotropins (FSH and LH) to prevent apoptosis involves the activation of cAMP formation. Gonadotropins can also exert survival effects indirectly by stimulating the production of insulin-like growth factor I (IGF-

I), interleukin-1 (IL-1), estrogen, and both *epidermal growth factor* (EGF) and *basic fibroblast growth factor* (bFGF), all of which are produced by the ovary. Atresia occurs mainly in granulosa cells. In marked contrast, thecal cells lose their differentiated condition, and instead of dying, return to the pool of interstitial cells not associated with follicles. The atretic follicle, in contrast, is invaded by fibroblasts and becomes an avascular, nonfunctional scar.

Factors that induce follicular atresia (atretogenic factors) include the cytokine *tumor necrosis factor-alpha* (TNFα), and a still unidentified ligand that activates a death domain-containing receptor known as *Fas.* It is now clear that TNFα acts via a signaling pathway that involves the production of ceramide, a lipid second messenger. Additional atretogenic factors are a cytokine produced in granulosa cells (IL-6) and androgens.

The signaling pathways utilized by survival and atretogenic factors involve the activation of an array of genes encoding antiapoptotic and proapoptotic protein molecules, respectively. The former group includes genes encoding proteins related to the apoptotic-suppressing protein Bcl-2. Intraovarian expression of Bcl-2 via a transgenic approach results in the development of many more follicles to the preovulatory stage and formation of germ cell tumors, indicating that prolonged survival of granulosa cells leads to tumorigenesis. Recent studies have identified the main ovarian antiapoptotic Bcl-2 protein (Mcl-1, myloid cell lymphoma gene-1) and a Bcl-2–related proapoptotic protein (termed *Bok,* Bcl-2 related ovarian killer) as principal components of the molecular process governing follicular atresia.

The Corpus Luteum

Following ovulation the collapsed follicle becomes reorganized to form the corpus luteum consisting of "luteinized" granulosa cells, and thecal cells, fibroblasts, and capillaries that invade the new structure. Luteinization of the granulosa cells involves the appearance of lipid droplets in the cytoplasm, development by the mitochondria of a dense matrix with tubular cristae, and hypertrophy of the endoplasmic reticulum. The outer portion of the corpus luteum is made up of thecal cells that are also luteinized. The basal lamina of the follicle, however, regresses. Should fertilization fail to occur, the corpus luteum remains functional for 13–14 days and then undergoes *luteolysis.* The luteal cells become necrotic, progesterone secretion ceases, and the corpus luteum is invaded by macrophages and then by fibroblasts. Endocrine function is rapidly lost, and the corpus luteum is replaced by a scar-like tissue called the *corpus albicans.*

Ovarian Feedback Control of Gonadotropin Secretion

The ovary regulates the secretion of gonadotropins through two basic mechanisms: an inhibitory or negative feedback effect, and a stimulatory or positive feedback loop (Fig. 9-4). The former is exerted mainly by estrogen, although other steroids such as progesterone and androgens and the gonadal protein inhibin also play a role. Positive feedback is exerted by estradiol, although progesterone can amplify the E_2 effect. In addition to these hormones, it is likely that the FSH-releasing protein activin has a physiological role to play in maintaining FSH secretion.

Negative Feedback

Ablation of the ovaries produces a prompt increase in plasma levels of LH and FSH. Conversely, administration of estradiol reverts the levels toward normal values. Estradiol acts on both the hypothalamus and the anterior pituitary to inhibit gonadotropin secretion. At the hypothalamus it suppresses LHSH secretion; at the pituitary it inhibits the release of LH induced by LHRH. The course of action of estrogen is fairly rapid. Within minutes of its intravenous injection, LH levels begin to decline. However, FSH levels are not brought to normal values by administering estradiol to ovariectomized women, as, in addition to estradiol, the secretion of FSH is also under the inhibitory control of inhibin. Inhibin controls the secretion of FSH via a direct inhibitory action on the pituitary gonadotrophs.

The mechanism by which estradiol inhibits LHRH secretion in the hypothalamus appears to involve activation of inhibitory neurotransmitter systems coupled to the LHRH neuronal network. The GABA neurons have been implicated as a major inhibitory neuronal group mediating the negative feedback effect of estradiol on LHRH secretion. At the pituitary level, estradiol decreases gonadotropin synthesis by suppressing gene expression of the LH β-subunit, and to a lesser extent, that of the FSH β-subunit (for an understanding of gonadotropin structure, see Chapter 6).

Positive Feedback

As with the negative feedback loop, positive feedback is for the most part estrogen dependent. Progesterone, however, can markedly potentiate the stimulatory effect of estradiol on gonadotropin release when given several hours after estradiol. In contrast to the negative feedback that occurs within minutes, the positive effect of estradiol has a latency of several hours. Typically, administering estradiol results in a rapid decline in plasma LH levels that last for at least 24 hours (negative feedback); this is followed by an abrupt, marked increase in the secretion of both LH and FSH (positive feedback). During the normal menstrual cycle this discharge of gonadotropins is a consequence of increases in plasma estrogen levels produced by the growing follicles (see below); the gonadotropin surge at the end of the follicular phase is essential for ovulation.

The anatomical site(s) where estradiol exerts its stimulatory effect have been a matter of controversy. In the Rhesus monkey, estradiol can elicit gonadotropin release even if the pituitary gland is disconnected from the hypothalamus provided that LHRH is administered in a pulsatile manner. An invariable pulsatile LHRH regimen administered to these animals is capable of sustaining the complete sequence of endocrine events characteristic of a normal menstrual cycle, suggesting that the hypothalamus—through the release of LHRH—plays a permissive rather than a commanding role in the genesis of the preovulatory surge of gonadotropins. In conflict with this view, however, are the more recent demonstrations by other investigators that administration of both estradiol or estradiol plus progesterone to monkeys increases the release of LHRH from the hypothalamus.

It thus appears that estradiol can act at both the hypothalamus and the anterior pituitary to affect gonadotropin secretion. At both loci the steroid is able to exert first inhibitory effects, and, then, a stimulatory action. Whereas the stimulatory effect of estradiol on LHRH release appears to be mediated by the activation of stimulatory neurotransmitter systems functionally coupled to LHRH neurons (glutamatergic, noradrenergic, and NPY neurons), at the pituitary level, estradiol may act by both increasing the releasable pool of gonadotropins and by stimulating the expression of the β-subunit genes. This stimulation only occurs in the presence of LHRH.

An involvement of activin in stimulating the preovulatory discharge of FSH has not been demonstrated but is suggested by the increased expression of activin βA subunit mRNA in graafian follicles close to the time of ovulation. Activin βA subunit mRNA has also been found in pituitary gonadotrophs where it may regulate FSH production through paracrine–autocrine actions.

Dynamics of the Hypothalamic–Pituitary–Ovarian Relationship

Hormonal changes occurring during the menstrual cycle are depicted in Figure 9-6. During menstruation and the early follicular phase, plasma FSH levels are 1.5- to 2-fold higher than at the end of the preceding luteal phase. The LH values are low. Thereafter, plasma FSH falls and LH increases moderately, so that by the end of the follicular phase the LH/FSH ratio has increased to a value of about 2. This increase in mean plasma LH appears to be mainly due to an increased frequency of episodic LH discharges, probably due to the rising estradiol levels.

Estrogen levels (estradiol and estrone) increase very little during the first half of the follicular phase, while progesterone, 17α-hydroxyprogesterone, and the aromatizable androgens, androstenedione and testosterone, remain essentially unchanged. During the second half of the follicular phase, and as follicles grow, plasma estrogen levels begin to rise, a change that becomes more pronounced toward the ovulatory phase, at which time estrogen levels rise up to nine-fold over basal values. Estradiol is produced directly by the ovaries, but most of the circulating estrone originates from peripheral conversion of estradiol and androstenedione. Progesterone and 17α-hydroxyprogesterone levels remain unchanged until the ovulatory phase; they are mostly derived from the ovary. Indeed, the concentration of progesterone in the follicular fluid increases markedly during the second half of the follicular phase, but not sufficiently to alter the systemic levels. Plasma androstenedione and testosterone also remain at relatively constant levels throughout the follicular phase. Normally, circulating androgens derive from both the ovary and the adrenal gland. The relative contribution of these glands, however, varies both during the day and during the cycle.

The initiation of the ovulatory phase is characterized by elevated estrogen levels that trigger an abrupt discharge of gonadotropins. This preovulatory gonadotropin surge is more pronounced in the case of LH than FSH, and lasts about 24 hours. As gonadotropins begin to rise, there is a concomitant increase in 17α-hydroxyprogesterone and a smaller rise in testosterone and androstenedione. Progesterone, in contrast, increases transiently during the LH surge, but not to the same extent as 17α-hydroxyprogesterone. Although LH and FSH are still elevated, there is a precipitous fall in circulating estrogen levels. Plasma levels of progesterone and androgens also decline, but this occurs after gonadotropin levels have returned to basal values.

Ovulation occurs 16–20 hours after the peak of the gonadotropin surge. At this time gonadotropins, estrogen, progesterone, and androgen levels have fallen. In contrast, 17α-hydroxyprogesterone values remain elevated.

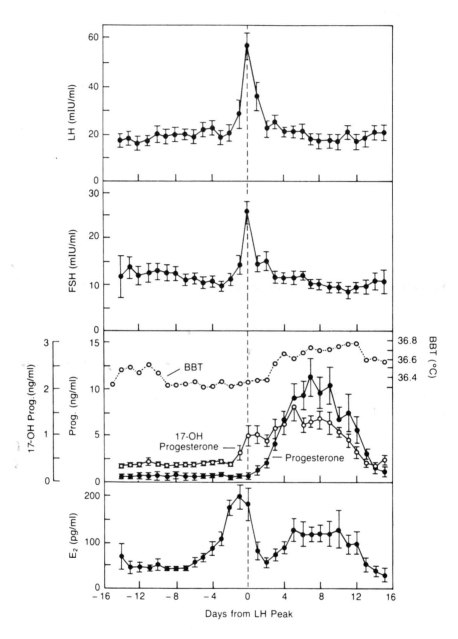

Fig. 9-6 Changes in plasma levels of LH, FSH, progesterone, estradiol, and 17-hydroxy-progesterone during the human menstrual cycle. The day of the LH peak is considered as day 0. Changes in basal body temperature (BBT) induced by progesterone are also represented. (Redrawn from Thorneycroft IH, et al: Am J Obstet Gynecol 111:947–951, 1971, and from Ross GT, et al: Recent Prog Horm Res 26:1–62, 1970, with permission.)

Both LH and FSH remain at low levels during the luteal phase. At the beginning of this phase the frequency of episodic LH discharges decreases, but they have a greater amplitude. Later on there is a progressive decrease in both amplitude and frequency of the LH pulses. A sustained elevation of progesterone and 17α-hydroxyprogesterone secreted by the corpus luteum becomes a predominant feature of this phase. Estrogens and androstenedione of luteal origin are also increased throughout the length of the luteal phase. After about 8–10 days, progesterone values begin to decrease, falling rapidly thereafter so that by day 14 after ovulation they have reached very low levels and menstruation ensues.

There is little doubt that the selective elevation in FSH levels observed during the early follicular phase plays a decisive role in initiating the growth of primary follicles. Although the formation of primoridal and primary follicles is independent of the pituitary, development of pituitary follicles to the antral stage cannot proceed in the absence of FSH. A first wave of follicular development is initiated by the midcycle preovulatory surge of FSH. Upon reaching the antral stage, however, these follicles undergo atresia in the midst of the luteal phase. A second crop of follicles that is recruited by the elevation of FSH levels at the beginning of the follicular phase progresses beyond the antral stage, but only one of them, the "dominant" follicle, reaches the ovulatory condition.

As the follicular phase progresses, aromatase activity increases under FSH control. As more estradiol is produced, the steroid further facilitates the proliferation of granulosa cells, enhances synthesis of its own receptor, and synergizes with FSH to amplify the stimulatory effect of the hormone on granulosa cell differentiation. More specifically, it facilitates the ability of FSH to stimulate estrogen secretion and to induce the formation of both FSH and LH receptors. A gradual increase in plasma LH levels promotes the differentiation of thecal cells and induces the synthesis of the 17,20-lyase enzyme, thereby increasing available androgens for estrogen biosynthesis.

At the end of the follicular phase, estrogen secretion is further increased as the dominant follicle reaches the preovulatory stage. Plasma FSH levels are depressed, perhaps as a consequence of the increase in estrogen and inhibin secretion (stimulated by FSH itself). Pituitary responsiveness to LHRH increases as a consequence of estrogen action, and within 48 hours the preovulatory surge of gonadotropins occurs.

It was previously mentioned that during the second half of the follicular phase a follicle is selected to reach the ovulatory stage. The factors involved in this selection are unknown; however, recent findings demonstrating the presence of noradrenergic and peptidergic nerves in the ovary of several species, including the human, raise the possibility that selection of a dominant follicle may have a neural component.

Once this selection has been made, the rest of the growing follicles undergo atresia. An important characteristic of follicles undergoing atresia is their increased androgen content and reduced estrogen and progesterone levels in comparison with healthy graafian follicles. This is associated with a decreased concentration of FSH and increased levels of prolactin in the follicular fluid. It seems evident, therefore, that the fate of follicles is *individually* determined by the action of local factors. The nature of these factors has been only partially elucidated. It appears to involve the activation of antiapoptotic genes, possibly encoding Bcl-2–related proteins, by survival factors such as FSH.

After ovulation, loss of the oocyte from the ruptured follicle appears to initiate luteinization of the granulosa cells. However, the LH discharge itself contributes significantly to the process. The mechanism involved in maintaining the function of the corpus luteum for 14 days and in precipitating its regression at the end of this period is incompletely understood. It is clear, however, that in humans LH is luteotropic–that is, it maintains the functional and morphological integrity of the corpus luteum. Prolactin has been found to be luteotropic in rodents, but its role in humans is unclear. The capacity of LH to maintain corpus luteum function declines as the luteal phase progresses. This phenomenon may be related to the influence of luteolytic factors that acquire predominance as the corpus luteum becomes older. Among these factors estrogen, oxytocin, and prostaglandin $F_{2\alpha}$ deserve mention. The luteolytic effect of both estrogen and oxytocin appears to be mediated at least in part by local formation of prostaglandin $F_{2\alpha}$.

DEVELOPMENT AND MAINTENANCE OF REPRODUCTIVE FUNCTION

Acquisition of reproductive competence is a long and extraordinarily complex process that takes an average of 12–14 years in the human female. Understanding of this process necessitates knowledge of both the initiation and progression of the neuroendocrine changes within the hypothalamic–pituitary–ovarian axis that lead to adult reproductive function.

Fetal, Neonatal, and Infantile Phases

The Hypothalamic–Pituitary Unit

The fetal pituitary gland synthesizes both FSH and LH as early as the fifth week of gestation, and circulating levels of these two hormones are detected by the end of the third month (the earliest fetus studied). Pituitary content of both LH and FSH rises from this gestational age, reaching maximum levels at 25–29 weeks, and then declines as pregnancy progresses. Newborn infants have two to five times less pituitary gonadotropin content than fetuses at 25–29 weeks.

Serum gonadotropins, and in particular FSH, begin to increase around the third month of gestation, reaching very high values (in the castrate range) by 150 days, that is, before the peak in pituitary gonadotropins. From then to birth, serum levels fall.

This pattern of gonadotropin release is thought to be related to the maturation of the negative feedback mechanism exerted by gonadal steroids. In the absence of this inhibitory feedback, FSH and LH secretion is relatively unrestrained. Later in fetal development the inhibitory feedback mechanism matures and becomes operative, leading to suppression of the synthesis and release of FSH and LH.

After birth, serum FSH (and to a lesser extent LH) levels increase again and remain elevated for at least the first 2 postnatal years. This increase seems to result from the loss of placental steroids, which greatly contributes to the inhibition of fetal gonadotropin release during the second half of pregnancy. It is unclear, however, why FSH levels remain elevated for such a long period after birth when the infantile ovary is capable of producing estrogens, which can keep gonadotropin secretion restrained. In fact, in ovariectomized neonatal nonhuman primates or agonadal patients, plasma gonadotropin levels are markedly increased (Fig. 9-7).

Two to 4 years after birth, gonadotropin secretion begins to decline and remains low throughout childhood (Fig. 9-7). This reduced output of gonadotropins is most likely due to events that occur within the central nervous system. A loss of excitatory inputs coupled with an increase of inhibitory influences on LHRH neurons may be an important factor determining the decline in gonadotropin secretion that characterizes the juvenile period.

By the eighth to tenth year of life, gonadotropin secretion begins to increase. The FSH levels rise before LH levels do and attain adult values while LH levels are still increasing. In fact, mean plasma LH may not increase noticeably until secondary sexual development is quite advanced. As before, the mechanism responsible for the pubertal reactivation of gonadotropin release is of central nervous system origin and independent of the ovary (see pp. 229–231).

The Ovaries

The prepubertal ovary shows morphological signs of activity such as follicular maturation to the stage of graafian follicle and subsequent atresia. The cellular residue of atretic follicles contributes substantially to the mass of the human ovary, which increases rectilinearly from birth to puberty.

Ovarian steroidogenic capability is present from birth. Estradiol is the major ovarian secretory product, although estrone, androstenedione, testosterone, and other steroids are also produced. Umbilical artery levels of estradiol, reflecting fetal production of the steroid, are more than 100 times higher than in adult females despite

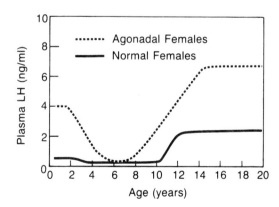

Fig. 9-7 Changes in circulating gonadotropin levels during postnatal development in normal and agonadal human females. Notice that gonadotropin levels in the agonadal subjects decrease during childhood and increase at puberty similar to normal subjects, indicating that these changes occur independently from the ovary. (Redrawn from Grumbach MM: The neuroendocrinology of puberty. In: *Neuroendocrinology*, DT Krieger and JC Hughes, eds., Sinauer, Sunderland, MA, pp. 249–258, 1980, with permission.)

considerable metabolism of estrogen by the fetus. Estrogen levels decline rapidly in the first postnatal week and remain at less than 10 pg/ml until the onset of puberty.

Puberty

Hormonal Changes

The first endocrinological manifestation of the onset of puberty is amplification of a sleep-related pattern of LH release. During childhood, LH is secreted in a pulsatile manner, but the magnitude of the pulses is small. In addition, greater LH levels are seen during sleep than during waking hours. At the end of childhood, before mean gonadotropin levels begin to increase, the difference in LH secretion becomes more pronounced and the magnitude of the LH pulses is enhanced (Fig. 9-8). These

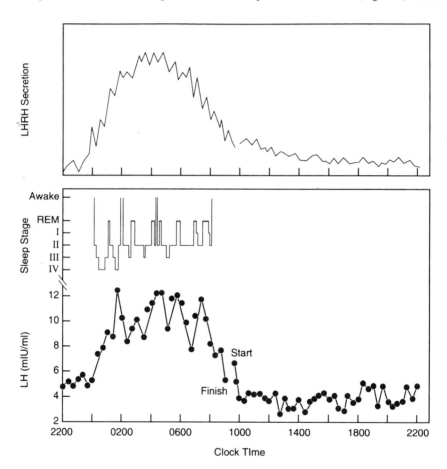

Fig. 9-8 Diurnal changes in pulsatile release of LH at puberty. The upper panel depicts the hypothetical changes in LHRH secretion assumed to occur during puberty at night. This increase in LHRH secretion does not require the presence of the gonads and is thought to be responsible for the nocturnal increase in LH secretion depicted in the lower panel. (Redrawn from the Boyar RM, et al: N Engl J Med 287:582–586, 1972.)

changes not only reflect the initial activation of the central mechanism governing LH secretion, but are also believed to be the initial event leading to the attainment of puberty.

As puberty progresses and plasma gonadotropin levels increase, there is a wide range of serum LH and FSH values, probably reflecting superimposed menstrual cyclicity. Episodic increases in LH levels (ovulatory spikes) have occasionally been recorded in girls within several months of the first menstruation. A short rise in progesterone levels following these LH peaks has also been found in these girls, suggesting corpus luteum formation and ovulation The luteal phase appears to be shortened. Accordingly, the infertility of the young adolescent girl may be related either to anovulatory cycles or to inadequate corpus luteum function.

The rising levels of plasma gonadotropins stimulate the ovary to produce increasing amounts of estradiol. Estradiol is responsible for the development of secondary sexual characteristics, that is, growth and development of the breasts and reproductive organs, fat redistribution (hips, breasts), and bone maturation. Using an ultrasensitive assay for estradiol, evidence has been provided that in childhood, plasma estradiol levels, though very low, are higher in girls than in boys. This difference may contribute to the earlier onset of puberty in girls. As puberty approaches, plasma estradiol levels fluctuate widely, probably reflecting successive waves of follicular development that fail to reach the ovulatory stage. The uterine endometrium is affected by these changes and undergoes cycles of proliferation and regression, until a point is reached when substantial growth occurs so that withdrawal of estrogen results in the first menstruation. This is called *menarche*. Plasma testosterone levels also increase at puberty although not as markedly as in males. In contrast, plasma progesterone remains at low levels, even if secondary sexual characteristics have appeared. A rise in progesterone after menarche is, in general, indicative that ovulation has occurred.

Menarche occurs at an average of 12 years of age. However, the first ovulation does not take place until 6–9 months after menarche because the positive feedback mechanism of estrogen is not developed. A single estrogen injection to premenarchial subjects fails to induce LH release. However, experiments with Rhesus monkeys have shown that if "priming" doses of estradiol are given, the surge mechanism can be activated shortly after menarche.

Somatic Changes

Somatic changes during puberty include a rapid general increase in the growth rate of skeleton, muscles, and viscera, known as the *adolescent growth spurt,* a sex-specific increase in hip width, and changes in body composition caused by an increase in muscle and in fat tissue, the latter being more pronounced in girls than in boys. The large increase in fat (120%) between growth spurt initiation and menarche in both early and late maturing girls may have a secondary significance. The mean fat for both early and late maturers at menarche is about 11 kg, which is equivalent to 99,000 calories. The number of calories estimated to sustain a pregnancy is 80,000. Thus, although speculative, it is possible that one of the main functions of the adolescent growth spurt in females might be the storage of energy to sustain pregnancy and lactation. Figure 9-9 shows schematically the sequence of events at

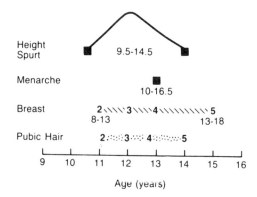

Fig. 9-9 Schematic sequence of somatic events during female puberty. The age range at which each event occurs is indicated at the beginning and end of each event. The numbers 2–5 correspond to the different stages of puberty as defined by Tanner. (Redrawn from Tanner JM: Sequence and tempo in the somatic changes in puberty. IN: *The Control of the Onset of Puberty*, MM Grumbach, GD Grave, and FE Mayer, eds., Wiley, New York, pp. 448–470, 1974, with permission.)

puberty in females. The development of the breasts is known as *thelarche*, and the growth of axillary and pubic hair is known as *pubarche*.

The age at which these morphological changes occur varies from individual to individual. A classification that is widely used by clinicians to assess the normalcy of the pubertal progression bases its five stages on the degree of breast development, age at peak velocity of linear growth, and growth and distribution of the pubic hair.

In addition to estrogens and androgens, GH may play a role in inducing pubertal growth. Plasma growth hormone levels are low but pulsatile in peripubertal subjects. Immediately upon falling asleep, there is an increase in GH release; usually several episodes of GH secretion can be detected during the sleep period. The magnitude of these episode reaches a maximum in advanced puberty.

Metabolic Signals

Earlier studies demonstrated that the mean weight of girls at the beginning of the adolescent growth spurt (around 30 kg), at the time of peak velocity of weight gain (around 39 kg), and at menarche (around 47 kg) are very similar in early- and late-maturing girls. This led to the notion that the attainment of a critical weight causes a change in metabolic rate per unit mass (or per unit of surface area), which, in turn, may affect the hypothalamic ovarian feedback by decreasing the sensitivity of the hypothalamus to gonadal steroids so that gonadotropin release increases, triggering the pubertal process.

The hypothesis of a critical weight was later modified to state that a particular ratio of fat to lean mass is normally necessary for puberty and the maintenance of female reproductive ability. Experiments conducted to test this hypothesis did not confirm it, but suggested that there may be metabolic signals used by peripheral tissues to influence the time of puberty. Two of these signals have been identified, namely IGF-I and leptin, the former produced mainly in the liver, the later by white adipose tissue. Although both peptides can act centrally to stimulate LHRH release and to accelerate the initiation of puberty, neither appears to initiate the pubertal process in the absence of other hormonal changes, an activity that seems essential for a substance to be considered a metabolic trigger of puberty.

In addition, experiments with nonhuman primates have demonstrated that LH pulsatile release is dramatically decreased by underfeeding and activated by administration of calorie-rich food, suggesting that caloric intake may be a mechanism by which the diet could affect the timing and/or progression of puberty. It seems clear that undernutrition delays the onset of puberty and disrupts menstrual cyclicity.

Of interest in this regard are the observations that in the past century, girls in the United States reached a weight of 46 kg at about 14 years, which was the age of menarche. In 1970, this body weight was reached at the age of 12.9 years, at which age menarche also occurred. Belgian girls who in the past century reached a weight of 46 kg at about age 16.5 years also attained menarche at that age.

Mechanisms Involved in the Regulation of the Onset of Puberty (Fig. 9-10)

Change in the Setpoint of Negative Feedback Mechanism. As previously discussed, the negative feedback of gonadal steroids is poorly developed during fetal life but becomes fully operative during childhood. Several years ago, from experiments in rats, the concept was advanced that a decrease in hypothalamic sensitivity to circulating sex steroids ("resetting of the gonadostat") results in the increased gonadotropin secretion seen at puberty.

Nevertheless, more recent experiments in rats, Rhesus monkeys, and humans demonstrated that the change in hypothalamic setpoint to steroid negative feedback is a late phenomenon in puberty. Thus, the "resetting" mechanism can no longer be considered as the cause of puberty, but rather a consequence of it.

Activation of the Hypothalamic "Pulse Generator." As discussed above, pulsatile release of LH becomes more prominent at the end of childhood. If juvenile monkeys are treated with LHRH, delivered in a pulsatile manner for several weeks, they show repetitive, normal ovulatory cycles. These cycles cease upon removal of the LHRH treatment. Direct measurement of LHRH released from the mediam eminence of the hypothalamus in nonhuman primates demonstrated that LHRH secretion does indeed increase as puberty approaches. These and other observations have led to the concept that the onset of puberty is determined by the enhancement of endogenous pulsatile LHRH release (Fig. 9-10). Such an activation would then drive the pituitary to secrete larger amounts of LH, particularly during sleep, and puberty would be initiated.

The pubertal activation of LHRH release may be brought about by the coordinated interplay of transsynaptic inputs and glial influences on LHRH neurons. According to this concept, LHRH release would increase as a consequence of an activation of stimulatory transsynaptic inputs (glutamate, but also NE and NPY), a decrease in GABA inhibition, and a growth factor–dependent increase in glial production of neuroactive substances, such as prostaglandins.

Another factor that operates at the time of puberty is an enhanced pituitary re-

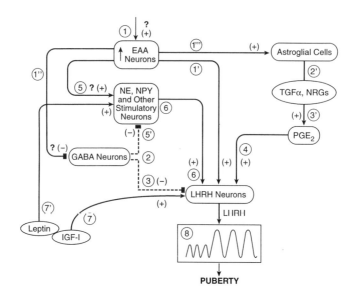

Fig. 9-10 The central events underlying the initiation of puberty. An increase in episodic LHRH secretion is postulated to be caused by the activation of an integrative mechanism involving both neuron-to-neuron and glia-to-neuron communication processes. The neuron-to-neuron (transsynaptic) component involves the simultaneous activation of excitatory transsynaptic inputs and a reduction in inhibitory inputs to LHRH neurons. The main excitatory transsynaptic input affecting LHRH release is postulated to be provided by neurons that use excitatory amino acids (EAA) as neurotransmitters. Noradrenergic (NE) and neuropeptide Y (NPY)-containing neurons provide a complementary facilitatory input to the LHRH neuronal network. The chief inhibitory neuronal input restraining LHRH release is provided by GABAergic neurons (GABA). The glia-to-neuron component of the process involves both the production of the epidermal growth factor related peptides, TGFα and neuregulins (NRGs), by astroglial cells, and the stimulatory effect of these peptides on the glial production of neuroactive substances, such as prostaglandin E_2, which then act on LHRH neurons to stimulate LHRH secretion. It is postulated that an increase in EAA release (1) occurs early in the sequence of events. Excitatory amino acids can act directly on LHRH neurons (1') to stimulate LHRH release. The change in EAA transmission is followed very closely by a decrease in GABA release (2) and the activation of the glial production of TGFα/NRGs (2'). The decrease in GABA release may be brought about by the increase in EAA transmission (1"). Initial evidence suggests that the glial activation of growth factor production is also caused, at least in part, by EAA (1'''), acting via a specific set of receptors located on hypothalamic astrocytes. While the decrease in GABA transmission begins to relieve LHRH neurons from GABAergic inhibitory control (3), the increased production of EGF-related glial peptides stimulates the formation of prostaglandin E_2 (3'), which acts directly on LHRH neurons to induce LHRH release (4), amplifying the stimulatory effect of EAA on the secretion of the neuropeptide (1') and magnifying the loss of GABAergic inhibitory control (3). Upon the initiation of these changes, a further increase in EAA stimulation (5) and further decrease in GABAergic inhibitory tone (5') lead to activation of NE and NPY neuronal systems (6). Both NE and NPY would then contribute to the progression of the pubertal process by stimulating LHRH secretion (6). The metabolic signals, leptin and IGF-I, further the process along by stimulating LHRH secretion either directly (7), or via functionally connected neuronal networks (7'). The resulting increase in pulsatile LHRH secretion (8) then results in the initiation of puberty. $-$ = inhibition; (+) = stimulation. (Reprinted from Ojeda SR and Bilger M: Neuroendocrine regulation of puberty. In: *Neuroendocrinology in Physiology and Medicine*, PM Conn and M Freeman, eds., Humana Press, Totowa, NJ, pp 199–224, 1999, with permission.)

sponsiveness to LHRH. The release of LH following the administration of LHRH is minimal in prepubertal children but increases markedly at puberty and is even greater in adult males. There is a sex difference in the rise of serum FSH: prepubertal and pubertal females release more FSH than do males at all stages of sexual maturation.

This increased gonadotropin release to LHRH is probably due to the elevated circulating levels of gonadal and adrenal steroids present at that time. As the response can be elicited before the development of secondary sex characteristics in both girls and boys, this change in pituitary responsiveness probably plays an important role in the progress of the pubertal process.

The Adrenal Gland and Puberty

Circulating levels of aromatizable androgens such as dehydroepiandrosterone and its sulfate, and androstenedione, are mostly of adrenal origin. Their concentrations in the bloodstream begin to increase at about 7–8 years of age, reaching maximum values by ages 13–15. This phenomenon is called *adrenarche.* It begins before the rise in gonadotropin secretion. Adrenal androgens are responsible to a significant extent for the growth of pubic and axillary hair; however, they do not appear to play a decisive role in determining the initiation of puberty. Premature adrenarche is not associated with advancement of gonadarche (i.e., the activation of the hypothalamic–pituitary–ovarian axis). Conversely, gonadarche occurs in the absence of adrenarche in children with chronic primary adrenal insufficiency, and in children with true idiopathic precocious puberty. It is evident, therefore, that adrenarche and gonadarche are separately controlled, albeit temporally associated phenomena.

Reproductive Cyclicity (Fig. 9-11)

This reproductive phase has already been discussed. Basically it entails the orderly repetition of the menstrual cycle, a sequence that may be interrupted by pregnancy. It begins with the first ovulation at puberty and extends on the average to about 50 years of age.

Menopause

Menopause can be defined as the time at which the final menstrual bleeding occurs. Like "puberty," however, the term is used in a much broader sense, and describes a period of the female climacteric during which reproductive cyclicity gradually disappears. The menstrual cycles become irregular, and the intervals between menses become shorter because of a reduction in the duration of the follicular phase.

Menopause is regarded as the result of the loss of ovarian function. There is an exhaustion of ovarian follicles, mainly due to the repeated cycles of atresia that occur twice in every menstrual cycle. Histologically, the stroma hypertrophies and primordial follicles disappear. Ovarian weight declines as menopause progresses, and plasma gonadotropin levels increase when estradiol production falls as follicles fail to mature (Fig. 9-11). The loss of estrogen is accompanied by atrophic changes of the breasts, uterus, and vagina, vasomotor instability (hot flashes), and in many instances, osteoporosis.

Fig. 9-11 Changes in the pattern of serum levels of gonadotropins during postnatal life in the human female. During neonatal and prepubertal phases, FSH levels are greater than LH, and pulsatile LH secretion is minimal (A). As puberty approaches, LH secretion increases during sleep (B). When puberty is completed, LH secretion is greater than FSH secretion (C) and cyclic gonadotropin release occurs (D). At menopause, cyclic gonadotropin release ceases (E) and plasma levels of both gonadotropins increase. (Redrawn from Yen SSC: In: *Neuroendocrinology*, DT Krieger and JC Hughes, eds., Sinauer, Sunderland, MA, p. 259–272, 1980, with permission.)

The occurrence of hot flashes is temporally related to pulses of LH secretion. Because such pulses appear to be the consequence of an increase in noradrenergic impulses arriving at hypothalamic LHRH neurons, the inference has been made that hot flashes are caused by a change in hypothalamic noradrenergic activity.

THE MAMMARY GLAND

Lactation is an evolutionarily conserved mammalian physiological function. The offspring of placental mammals are entirely dependent in early postnatal life on nutrients provided by the mother through the secretion of milk. The mammary gland replaces the nourishing function of the placenta after birth.

Development and Hormonal Control

During early fetal development, epithelial cells cluster in areas that will later give rise to the areola of the breast and proliferate to form cord-like structures that penetrate the underlying mesenchyme. These epithelial cords give origin to the duct system of the mammary gland that converges into a single ampulla that opens to the nipple. During the last part of gestation, the distal portion of the fetal ducts develops into alveolar structures that at birth are able to secrete. This secretion, known as *witch's milk,* can be observed in most infants by the first week of postnatal life and lasts for 4–6 weeks. Once the effect of placental steroids subsides, the secretory alveoli regress so that in children only scattered ducts without alveoli are observed embedded in stromal tissue.

As previously indicated, when estrogen secretion increases at puberty, breast development is markedly stimulated. When the ovulatory cycles begin and the corpus luteum secretes progesterone, the estrogen-dependent branching and lengthening of the ducts are enhanced, and alveoli development is accelerated.

During pregnancy the mammary gland undergoes further growth under the concerted influence of estrogen, progesterone, glucocorticoids, prolactin, and human placental lactogen (hPL). The duct system develops markedly, the alveoli form clusters called *lobules,* and their epithelial cells acquire vacuoles indicative of intense secretory activity. Actual secretion of milk (lactation) does not occur, however, until after birth, due to an inhibitory effect of placental estrogen and progesterone. Following delivery of the placenta, estrogen and progesterone levels drop precipitously and secretion of milk begins.

A pituitary hormone that plays a critical role in the process of breast development during pregnancy is prolactin. In combination with estrogen, prolactin causes primarily ductal but also lobuloalveolar growth. In the presence of progesterone its effect on alveolar growth is greatly enhanced. Prolactin not only induces cell proliferation but also controls the synthesis of key components of milk such as casein and α-lactoalbumin. Prolactin (PRL) initiates its biological actions by binding to a membrane-anchored receptor. The PRL receptor shows structural similarity to the GH receptor; it belongs to the class 1 cytokine receptor superfamily that also includes the receptors for leukemia inhibiting factor, granulocyte-colony stimulating factor, leptin, and erythropoietin, among others. The PRL receptor has a single transmembrane domain encoded by an mRNA transcript that can be alternatively spliced to produce multiple isoforms, referred to as *long, intermediate* and *short*, according to their size. Binding of PRL to its receptor results in phosphorylation of the receptor itself and several other cellular proteins. It is now known that upon PRL binding, the receptor interacts with JAK2, a member of a recently discovered family of protein tyrosine kinases known as *JAK kinases,* which transmit cytokine-initiated signals into the cell. Activation of JAK2 occurs within 1 minute of PRL stimulation and leads to receptor tyrosine phosphorylation. The phosphorylated tyrosines recruit a cytoplasmic protein known as Stat 5, which become part of the PRL receptor–JAK2 kinase complex and is phosphorylated by the kinase. The phosphorylated Stat protein is then released, dimerizes with other Stat molecules, and the dimer is translocated into the nucleus where it binds to the DNA to activate the transcription of PRL-responsive genes. Mice in which the PRL was deleted by gene targeting fail to become pregnant, have reduced ovulation, stunted follicular development, and are unable to sustain preimplantation development. Heterozygotic animals are unable to lactate after the first, but not after subsequent, pregnancies, possibly because of the activation of compensatory mechanisms. One of the hormones that may replace PRL under these conditions is GH.

Growth hormone (GH) produced by the anterior pituitary shares many of the actions of PRL, and, in fact, is as effective as prolactin in inducing duct development. Nevertheless, its presence is not essential for breast development or lactation to occur. The human placenta produces hPL, which has actions similar to growth hormone.

Insulin and glucocorticoids are also required for most phases of breast development. Their function, however, is of a permissive rather than a regulatory nature.

Lactation

Lactation can be divided into four stages: *milk synthesis,* which is initiated during the last part of pregnancy by prolactin and hPL action; *lactogenesis,* which comprises the synthesis of milk by the alveolar cells and its secretion into the alveolar lumen—it is initiated by the loss of placental steroids after birth; *galactopoiesis,* or maintenance of established lactation, which is mainly controlled by prolactin, whose release increases because of suckling by the infant; and *milk ejection,* which is controlled by the neurohypophyseal hormone oxytocin and comprises the passage of milk from the alveolar lumen to the duct system, its collection in the ampulla and larger ducts, and its delivery to the infant (see below).

Oxytocin and prolactin play fundamental roles in the maintenance and dynamics of lactation. The act of nursing itself is a powerful stimulus for oxytocin release. Sensory impulses arising from the nipple travel via the spinal cord through a multisynaptic pathway to the hypothalamic neurons that produce oxytocin and evoke its release. Oxytocin then reaches the mammary gland via the bloodstream and induces the contraction of the myoepithelial cells that surround the alveoli and the ducts. Contraction of these cells mobilizes milk from the alveoli and duct system to the nipple, producing the sensation of "milk let-down" in the mother. Oxytocin release is also induced by audiovisual stimuli such as the sight of the baby or hearing its cry, or even just by the anticipation of nursing.

Prolactin secretion is stimulated by the act of suckling (Fig. 9-12), but not by audiovisual or psychological stimuli. Throughout the lactational period plasma prolactin levels vary as follows: basal values are quite high during the first few weeks postpartum and each nursing episode further elevates the levels. After about 2 months of lactation, basal prolactin levels return to normal values (10–20 ng/ml), but nursing is still able to elicit a rise in prolactin levels. Such a response persists for many

Fig. 9-12 Changes in plasma prolactin levels during anticipation of nursing and nursing itself in women. The women played with their infants for 30 minutes before suckling began. Milk let-down, which results from an action of oxytocin on the breast, occurred before suckling. (Redrawn from Noel GL, et al: Prolactin release during nursing and breast stimulation in postpartum and nonpostpartum subjects. J Clin Endocrinol Metab 38:413–423, 1974, with permission.)

months following birth. It is clear that episodes of prolactin secretion are important for the maintenance of lactation as prolactin-inhibiting drugs such as ergot alkaloids (see below) result in cessation of lactation.

The mechanism by which nursing increases prolactin release appears to involve both secretion of prolactin-releasing substances from the hypothalamus into the portal vasculature (e.g., vasoactive intestinal polypeptide [VIP], oxytocin) and suppression of dopamine release from the tuberoinfundibular dopaminergic neuronal system. Because dopamine itself is a prolactin-inhibiting factor, suppression of its release enhances the secretion of prolactin.

A common abnormality of breast function is galactorrhea—the persistent discharge of milk in the absence of parturition or beyond 6 months' postpartum in a nonnursing mother. In most of these cases, plasma prolactin levels are elevated, and imaging of the pituitary occasionally reveals the presence of microadenomas. Most of these patients suffer from reproductive malfunction ranging from ovulatory failure to amenorrhea—that is, failure to menstruate.

The discovery that ergot alkaloids such as bromocriptine are potent suppressors of prolactin release provided a useful tool in the treatment of hyperprolactinemia. Bromocriptine treatment not only suppresses prolactin secretion, but often results in significant regression of the pituitary prolactin-secreting tumor. Ergot alkaloids suppress prolactin release because they are dopamine agonists.

Major Milk Components

The major milk proteins are casein, α-lactalbumin, and β-lactoglobulin. The protein content in the human colostrum (the first milk secreted at parturition) is 2.7 g/dl as compared to 1.2 g/dl in mature milk. The major carbohydrate is lactose (5.3 g/dl in the colostrum, 6.8 g/dl in mature milk). Milk is also rich in fat (2.9 vs. 3.8 g/dl) and contains many other substances including minerals (calcium, magnesium, phosphorus, iron), electrolytes (chloride, potassium, sodium), all vitamins with the exception of vitamin B_{12}, iron-binding proteins (transferrin), immunoglobulins (IgMs, IgEs, and particularly IgAs), and growth factors such as epidermal growth factor and IGF-I.

CLINICAL ASSESSMENT OF REPRODUCTIVE FUNCTION

A thorough history and physical examination are essential in the assessment of female reproductive function. Valuable information includes the age of first menstruation, the presence of secondary sexual characteristics such as breast development, and the presence of regular, cyclic menses. The latter implies that ovulation is occurring, that the secretion of gonadotropins and ovarian steroids is adequate, and that the outflow reproductive tract is intact. Should the symptoms be ambiguous, both plasma gonadotropin and steroid concentrations can be determined by radioimmunoassay.

As stated in Chapter 10 an accurate assessment of plasma gonadotropin values generally can be obtained by drawing multiple blood samples every 20 minutes for 2 hours and pooling them to obtain a mean value. This is usually not necessary in women. There are cases (e.g., precocious puberty and delayed puberty), however, in which each blood samples must be analyzed individually, and the sequential sampling needs to be extended for several hours.

Plasma estradiol levels can also be measured by sensitive immunoassays, but because of the normal variations in circulating levels of the steroid during the menstrual cycle it is preferable to use other less direct, but more informative tests. For example, adequate estrogen production can be inferred by the presence of a moist vagina and a copious, clear cervical mucus that shows a high degree of elasticity upon stretching and an arborization (ferning) pattern upon spreading on a glass slide. A test commonly used to assess the estrogen status is the progesterone withdrawal test. Administration of progesterone followed by menstrual bleeding upon termination of the treatment is indicative of adequate estrogen priming to allow the withdrawal bleeding.

The occurrence of ovulation can be assessed by measuring plasma progesterone by radioimmunoassay. A functional test that can be employed to assess progesterone status is the increase in basal body temperature associated with normal luteal function. If such an increase occurs and is maintained for 2 weeks, progesterone secretion and corpus luteum function can be considered to be adequate.

One very important diagnosis is that of pregnancy. Again, the history and physical examination are critical for a correct diagnosis. In this case, however, the laboratory measurement of the placental product human chorionic gonadotropin (hCG) is recommended because of its reliability and sensitivity.

DERANGED REPRODUCTIVE FUNCTION

There are many forms of reproductive dysfunction, but only the most common will be considered.

Sexual Precocity and Delayed Puberty

Early advent of sexual maturity can be isosexual, that is, feminization in girls and virilization in boys, or heterosexual, that is, feminization in boys and virilization in girls.

Isosexual Precocity

Isosexual precocity can be manifested in three forms: true precocious puberty, precocious pseudopuberty, and incomplete isosexual precocity.

True precocious puberty is characterized by an early but normal sequence of pubertal development, including the initiation of menstrual cycles in girls. In 90% of cases the factors determining the early advent of sexual maturation are unknown; the syndrome is called *constitutional* or *idiopathic precocious puberty*. Prompt treatment is essential and usually relies on the use of LHRH agonists. These analogs act by down-regulating pituitary LHRH receptors and desensitizing the gland to LHRH.

Precocious pseudopuberty is defined as a dysfunction in which girls feminize but fail to ovulate. In general, precocious pseudopuberty is caused by an enhanced secretion of estradiol, which in most cases originates from granulosa-theca cell tumors of the ovary. These tumors can be detected by rectoabdominal examination, sonography, or laparoscopy.

Incomplete isosexual precocity is defined as the premature development of a single clinical pubertal event. This event may be breast enlargement before the age of 7, known as *premature thelarche,* or appearance of axillary and pubic hair, known as *premature pubarche.* The former is thought to be caused by a transient increase in estrogen levels, or to a heightened breast sensitivity to normal plasma levels of estrogen. Premature pubarche is caused by a premature increase in androgens of adrenal origin. Neither syndrome requires treatment because in both cases these changes are transient and often regress, the patient entering puberty at the normal age.

Heterosexual Precocity

Heterosexual precocity of girls—that is, virilization—is usually caused by congenital adrenal hyperplasia (see Chapter 8) or androgen-secreting tumors of the ovary or adrenal.

Delayed Puberty

Delayed puberty is much less common in girls than in boys. The onset of puberty may be regarded as delayed if breast development has not begun by age 13. The progression of puberty is regarded as delayed if menses have not occurred 5 years after the onset of breast development. Delayed puberty may be due to disorders of the ovary or the hypothalamic–pituitary unit. In the former case, gonadotropin levels are elevated because of the absence or insufficiency of steroid secretion. The syndrome is called *hypergonadotropic hypogonadism;* the most common form in girls is gonadal dysgenesis, known as the *Turner syndrome* (see Chapter 8). The term *hypogonadotropic hypogonadism* is applied to disorders of the hypothalamic—pituitary unit that result in decreased secretion of gonadotropins. It must be differentiated from a constitutional delay in the onset of puberty that is characterized by a pattern of slow maturation but an otherwise normal attainment of puberty at a late age. Patients with hypogonadotropic hypogonadism do not reach puberty owing to their inability to produce gonadotropins. Because failure of gonadotropin secretion is usually the only pituitary hormone deficiency observed in these patients, the syndrome is termed *isolated gonadotropin deficiency*; it is the result of defective synthesis or release of hypothalamic LHRH, or the absence of LHRH neurons in the hypothalamus (see also Chapter 10).

Abnormal Uterine Bleeding

Abnormal uterine bleeding is a disorder of the menstrual cycle that may be associated with either ovulatory or anovulatory cycles. In the first case, abnormal bleeding may occur in the face of regular cycles, but it deviates from a normal menstruation because it is too abundant and prolonged (hypermenorrhea) or too light and interrupted (hypomenorrhea). Hypermenorrhea may be caused by polyps, submucus myomas, or adenomyosis of the uterus. Hypomenorrhea may result from obstruction of the uterinecervical lumen. Bleeding may also occur between normal menstruations and is usually due to cervical and/or endometrial lesions.

Uterine bleeding associated with anovulatory cycles is painless bleeding, unpredictable with respect to onset, amount, and duration. The syndrome is called *dysfunctional uterine bleeding* and is caused by alterations of ovarian function rather than to abnormalities of the uterus. As previously discussed, the sequential changes in estradiol and progesterone secretion during the menstrual cycle determine both the cyclic pattern of endometrial activity and the onset of menses upon their withdrawal.

Dysfunctional uterine bleeding may result from three different mechanisms: (*1*) estrogen withdrawal bleeding that results from interruption of ovarian estrogen production in the absence of progesterone. For example, if estrogen is given to a postmenopausal woman and the treatment is then interrupted, bleeding will occur. (*2*) Estrogen breakthrough bleeding occurs when the corpus luteum fails to form (or function) so that progesterone levels are low and the uterus is chronically exposed to continuous estrogen. It is the most common type of dysfunctional uterine bleeding. (*3*) Progesterone breakthrough bleeding occurs when the progesterone/estrogen ratio to which the endometrium is exposed is abnormally high, as in women on continuous progesterone-only contraceptives (see below).

Amenorrhea

Amenorrhea is the failure to menstruate. It may be classified as primary amenorrhea (i.e., a woman who has never menstruated) and secondary amenorrhea (i.e., a woman who had menses, but they ceased). Operationally, amenorrhea has been defined as the failure of menarche by age 16, irrespective of the presence of secondary sexual characteristics, or the absence of menstruation for 6 months in a woman with previous periodic menses.

Amenorrhea may result from *anatomical defects* (e.g., pseudohermaphroditism, congenital defects of the vagina, imperforate hymen), *ovarian failure* (the most frequent being gonadal dysgenesis in which the ovary does not develop normally), or *chronic anovulation* with or without estrogen present. More than 80% of all amenorrhea is the result of chronic anovulation. This disorder is characterized by the failure to ovulate spontaneously with the possibility of ovulating upon therapy. In the most common type of chronic anovulation estrogen is present. Women with this condition have withdrawal bleeding after progesterone administration, indicating the prior presence of estrogen. However, most of the estrogen produced is estrone formed by peripheral aromatization of androstenedione. In most cases the ovaries are sclerotic and show a thick capsule, multiple follicular cysts, and hyperplastic thecal and stromal tissue. The disorder is known as *polycystic ovarian disease* and is usually characterized by increased plasma levels of androgens, hirsutism, obesity, and amenorrhea. Its etiology is complex, but it does not appear to be caused by a primary defect in gonadotropin secretion as plasma LH and FSH are variable in patients suffering from the disease. Recent findings suggest that alterations in the ovarian microenvironment (e.g., growth factor dysfunction) may play a more important role.

Hirsutism

Hirsutism, or excessive growth of hair, is the result of an abnormally high production of androgens. The androgens may be produced by neoplastic tissue; in this case, the onset of hair growth is rapid. They may also have an adrenal origin in the absence of a tumor; in most such case the excessive androgen production results from heritable defects in adrenal steroidogenesis (congenital adrenal hyperplasia), which can occur as "late onset" forms. An excess of circulating androgens may also result from intake of some drugs or steroids with androgenic capacity.

A more common cause of hirsutism, however, is ovarian hyperandrogenism, and, in particular, polycystic ovarian disease. Its pubertal onset is associated with chronic anovulation.

The treatment of hirsutism depends on the source of excessive androgen production. If it is a tumor, the tumor should be removed. If the source is the ovary, suppression of ovarian function is attempted by administering oral contraceptives; adrenal hyperfunction is reduced by suppressing ACTH secretion with dexamethasone.

FERTILITY CONTROL

Few things are more important in today's world than birth control. There are several methods of contraception, including (*1*) natural rhythm, (*2*) withdrawal, (*3*) barriers such as condoms, foams, and diaphragms, (*4*) intrauterine devices known as IUDs, (*5*) sterilization, (*6*) abortion, and (*7*) oral and subdermal steroid contraceptives.

The most effective preventive method is that of oral and subdermal contraceptives. The least effective are the rhythm and withdrawal methods. Barrier methods are much more effective than the "natural" methods, but not as efficient as IUDs, which have a success rate of more than 95%.

Use of an IUD, however, carries significantly greater health risks than barrier methods. It is believed that IUDs prevent pregnancy by inducing a chronic inflammation of the endometrium, which then becomes unable to allow implantation of the blastocyst. The most serious side effect of the IUD is pelvic infection.

Oral contraceptives are the most widely used method of fertility control. When properly used their success rate is more than 99%, they are easy to administer, and in general the incidence of side effects is low. Oral contraceptives prevent pregnancy by inhibiting ovulation through suppression of gonadotropin secretion.

There are three types of oral contraceptive pills: a combination of estrogen–progestin, phasic estrogen–progestin, and progestin-only pills. The combination pill consists of a synthetic estrogen (mestranol or ethinyl estradiol) and a synthetic progestin (such as norethindrone or norgestrel). They are taken continuously for 21 days followed by 7 days of rest. During these 7 days the person may discontinue taking the pill altogether, or—as some manufacturers recommend—take a placebo pill for 7 days. Phasic pills consist of different concentrations of estrogen plus progesterone, which varies throughout a 21-day treatment schedule followed by 7 days of placebo. Progesterone-only pills are taken continuously on a daily basis.

The ideal combination pill has the least amount of steroids necessary to prevent pregnancy, but a sufficient amount to avoid breakthrough bleeding. Oral contraceptives are not free of side effects. Users of progesterone-only pills have a high incidence of breakthrough bleeding. Combination pills may in some patients increase the risk of deep-vein thrombosis, pulmonary embolism, thromboembolic stroke, and hemorrhagic stroke. Because of the stimulatory effect of estrogen on liver protein synthesis, including the renin substrate angiotensinogen, use of contraceptive pills results in a small rise in blood pressure. In some women, however, hypertension may develop after several years of use. As previously indicated, estrogen increases both HDL and VLDL levels and decreases cholesterol and LDL concentrations. Progestins increase cholesterol and LDL levels and decrease HDL. However, their combination in pills usually has minimal effects in the low doses used today. In some women glucose tolerance changes, manifested by elevated plasma insulin and glucose levels after a glucose load. Because of all these possible side effects oral contraceptives are contraindicated in women with diabetes mellitus, abnormal liver function tests, hypercholesterolemia, hypertension, or heavy smoking habits. Oral contraceptives do not appear to increase the incidence of uterine, cervix, breast, or ovarian cancer.

Although oral contraceptives are contraindicated in a small fraction of the population, they are the most reliable and effective method of birth control available to women throughout the world.

An alternative system of steroid administration is the subdermal implantation of the progestin levonorgestrel (Norplant). Implantation of six silicone capsules in the inside part of the lower arm provides continuous contraception for 5 years. The mechanism of action of the progestin is by inhibition of ovulation. It may be used by women who cannot receive estrogens or by women who do not want surgery and/or cannot use any other form of contraception. The main problem with this system is the surgery it requires; it also causes irregular menstrual bleeding and headaches in some patients.

An alternative form of contraception that provides a safe and efficient means of abortion is the administration of the antiprogestin mifepristone (known as RU486). When RU486 administration is followed 48 hours later by prostaglandin F2α given orally, intravaginally, or by injection, abortion occurs in almost 100% of the cases. Mifepristone in combination with prostaglandin F2α can be used to induce abortion in case of fetal death or for the voluntary termination of pregnancy during the first trimester of pregnancy.

SUGGESTED READING

Bole-Feysot C, Goffin V, Edery M, and Binart N: Prolactin (PRL) and its receptor: Actions, signal transduction pathways and phenotypes observed in PRL receptor knockout mice. Endocr Rev 19:225–268, 1998.

Boyar RM, Finkelstein J, Roffwarg H, Kapen S, Weitzman E, and Hellman L: Synchronization of augmented luteinizing hormone secretion with sleep during puberty. N Engl J Med 287:582–586, 1972.

Buffet NC, Djakoure C, Maitre SC, and Bouchard P: Regulation of the human menstrual cycle. Front Neuroendocrinol 19:151–186, 1998.

Carr BR, and Griffin JE: Fertility control and its complications. In: *Williams Textbook of Endocrinology,* 9th ed., JD Wilson, DW Foster, HM Kronenberg, and PR Larsen, eds., Saunders, Philadelphia, pp. 901–926, 1998.

Courie AT, Forsyth IA, and Hart IC: *Hormonal Control of Lactation,* Springer-Verlag, Berlin, 1980.

DiZegera GS, and Hodgen GD: Folliculogenesis in the primate ovarian cycle. Endocr Rev 2:27–49, 1981.

Filicori M, Santoro N, Merriam GR, and Crowley WF Jr: Characterization of the physiological pattern of episodic gonadotropin secretion throughout the human menstrual cycle. J Clin Endocrinol Metab 62:1136–1144, 1986.

Fink G: Neuroendocrine regulation of pituitary function. In: *Neuroendocrinology in Physiology and Medicine,* PM Conn and ME Freeman, eds., Humana Press Totowa, NJ, pp. 107–133, 1999.

Graham JD, and Clarke CL: Physiological action of progesterone in target tissues. Endocr Rev 18:502–519, 1997.

Grumbach MM, and Styne DM: Puberty: Ontogeny, neuroendocrinology, physiology, and disorders. In: *Williams Textbook of Endocrinology,* 9th ed., JD Wilson, DW Foster, HM Kronenberg, and PR Larsen eds., Saunders, Philadelphia, pp. 1509–1625, 1998.

Hirshfield AN: Development of follicles in the mammalian ovary. Int Rev Cytol 124:43–101, 1991.

Hsueh AJW, Adashi EY, Jones PBC, and Welsh TH Jr: Hormonal regulation of the differentiation of cultured ovarian granulosa cells. Endocr Rev 5:76–127, 1984.

Kaipia A, and Hsueh AJW: Regulation of ovarian follicle atresia. Annu Rev Physiol 59:349–363, 1997.

Kellie AE: Structure and nomenclature. In: *Biochemistry of Steroid Hormones,* HLJ Makin, ed., Blackwell Scientific, Oxford, UK, pp. 1–19, 1984.

Knobil E, and Neill JD: *The Physiology of Reproduction,* Vols. 1 and 2, Raven Press, New York, 1994.

Parker KL, and Schimmer BP: Steroidogenic factor 1: A key determinant of endocrine development and function. Endocr Rev 18:361–377, 1997.

Peters H: The human ovary in childhood and early maturity. Eur J Obstet Gynecol Reprod Biol 9:137–144, 1979.

Richards JS, Russell DL, Robker RL, Dajee M, and Alliston TN: Molecular mechanisms of ovulation and luteinization. Mol Cell Endocrinol 145:47–54, 1998.

Schwartz NB: Neuroendocrine regulation of reproductive cyclicity. In: *Neuroendocrinology in Physiology and Medicine,* PM Conn and ME Freeman, eds., Humana Press, Totowa, NJ, pp. 135–145, 1999.

Segaloff DL, and Ascoli M: The lutropin/choriogonadotropin receptors . . . 4 years later. Endocr Rev 14:324–347, 1993.

Stocco DM, and Clark BJ: Regulation of the acute production of steroids in steroidogenic cells. Endocr Rev 17:221–244, 1996.

Tucker HA: Neuroendocrine regulation of lactation and milk ejection. In: *Neuroendocrinology in Physiology and Medicine,* PM Conn and ME Freeman, eds., Humana Press, Totowa, NJ, pp. 163–180, 1999.

10

Male Reproductive Function

JAMES E. GRIFFIN

Like the ovaries, the testes are the source of both germ cells and hormones important for reproductive function. The production of both sperm and steroid hormones is under complex feedback control by the hypothalamic—pituitary system.

STRUCTURAL ORGANIZATION OF THE TESTIS AND MALE REPRODUCTIVE TRACT

The testis consists of a network of tubules for the production and transport of sperm to the excretory ducts and a system of interstitial or Leydig cells that contain the enzymes necessary for the synthesis of androgens. The spermatogenic or seminiferous tubules are lined by a columnar epithelium composed of germ cells and Sertoli cells and surrounded by peritubular tissue made up of collagen, elastic fibers, and myofibrillar cells (Fig. 10-1). Tight junctions between Sertoli cells at a site between the spermatogonia and the primary spermatocyte form a diffusion barrier that divides the testis into two functional compartments, the basal and adluminal. The basal compartment consists of the Leydig cells surrounding the tubule, the peritubular tissue, and the outer layer of the tubule containing the spermatogonia. The adluminal compartment consists of the inner two-thirds of the tubules including primary spermatocytes and more advanced stages of spermatogenesis. The base of the Sertoli cell is adjacent to the basement membrane of the spermatogenic tubule (Fig. 10-1) with the inner portion of the cell engulfing the developing germ cells so that spermatogenesis actually takes place within a network of Sertoli cell cytoplasm. The mechanism by which spermatogonia pass through the tight junctions between Sertoli cells to begin spermatogenesis is not known. The close proximity of the Leydig cell to the Sertoli cell with its imbedded germ cells is thought to be critical for normal male reproductive function.

The seminiferous tubules empty into a network of ducts termed the rete testis. Sperm are then transported into a single duct, the epididymis. Anatomically, the epididymis can be divided into the caput, the corpus, and the cauda regions. The caput epididymidis consists of 8 to 12 ductuli efferentes, which have a larger lumen tapering to a narrower diameter at the junction of the ductus epididymidis. The diameter then remains constant through the corpus, or body, of the epididymis. In the cauda epididymis the diameter of the duct enlarges substantially and the lumen ac-

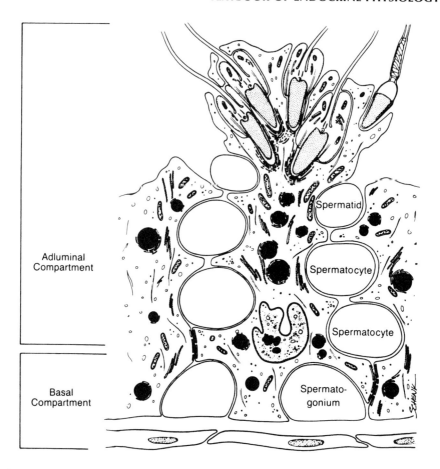

Fig. 10-1   Diagram of a Sertoli cell showing the relation between Sertoli cell cytoplasm and developing spermatocytes. (From Griffin JE, and Wilson JD: In: *Williams Textbook of Endocrinology,* 8th ed., JD Wilson and DW Foster, eds., Saunders, Philadelphia, p. 802, 1992.)

quires an irregular shape. The entire epididymal length is 5 to 6 cm. The epithelium exhibits regional differences of ciliated and nonciliated cells with evidence for a blood–epididymis barrier.

The vas deferens is a tubular structure about 30 to 35 cm in length beginning at the cauda epididymis and terminating in the ejaculatory duct near the prostate. In cross section there is a middle circular muscle layer surrounded by inner and outer longitudinal muscle layers. The pseudostratified epithelium lining the lumen of the vas deferens is composed of basal cells and three types of tall thin columnar cells, all three of which have cilia.

The normal adult prostate weighs about 20 g. The gland is composed of alveoli that are lined with tall columnar secretory epithelial cells. The acini of these alveoli drain into the floor and lateral surfaces of the posterior urethra. The alveoli and the ducts draining them are embedded with a stroma of fibromuscular tissue. The seminal vesicles are paired pouches 4–5 cm long that join the ampulla of the distal vas deferens to form the ejaculatory ducts. The seminal vesicles are composed of tubular alevoli containing viscous secretions. The ejaculatory ducts pass through the prostate and terminate within the prostatic urethra.

ANDROGEN PHYSIOLOGY

Testosterone Formation

The pathway of testosterone synthesis from cholesterol and the conversion of testosterone to active androgen and estrogen metabolites is depicted in Figure 10-2. Cholesterol, the precursor steroid, can be either synthesized *de novo* or derived from the plasma pool by receptor-mediated endocytosis of low-density lipoprotein particles. In contrast to the ovary which uses lipoprotein-derived cholesterol as its major source of substrate for steroid hormone formation (see Chapter 9), the testis appears to derive about half of the cholesterol required for testosterone formation from *de novo* synthesis. The rate-limiting process in testosterone synthesis is the delivery of cholesterol to the inner mitochondrial membrane by *Ste*roidogenic *A*cute *R*egulatory protein (StAR) (see Chapter 9). This protein and the enzymes involved in testosterone formation are stimulated by luteinizing hormone (LH). Five enzymatic steps are involved in the conversion of cholesterol to testosterone: 20,22-desmolase, 3β-hydroxysteroid dehydrogenase 2(3β-HSD2), 17α-hydroxylase, 17,20-lyase, and 17β-hydroxysteroid dehydrogenase 3 (17β-HSD3). The initial reaction in the process is the side-chain cleavage of cholesterol by the 20,22-desmolase complex of enzymes in mitochondria to form pregnenolone (cytochrome P450$_{scc}$). The remaining four enzymes in the pathway of testosterone synthesis are located in the microsomes. The 3β-hydroxysteroid dehydrogenase/isomerase (3β-HSD) enzyme complex oxidizes the A ring of the steroid to the Δ^4-3-keto configuration. Evidence indicates that the 17α-hydroxylase and 17,20-lyase activities are accomplished by a single cytochrome P450$_{17\alpha}$. Whereas the first four enzymatic activities in the pathway of testosterone synthesis are also common to the adrenals, the 17β-hydroxysteroid dehydrogenase activity is present primarily in the testes.

Although testosterone is the major secretory product of the testis, some of the precursors in the pathway as well as small amounts of dihydrotestosterone and estradiol are also directly secreted by the testis. The major sites of formation of dihydrotestosterone and estradiol are androgen target tissues and adipose tissue, respectively (see below). Concentrations of testosterone in testicular lymph and testicular venous blood are similar; however, because of its greater flow, the major route of testosterone secretion is via the spermatic vein. About 25 μg of testosterone is present in the normal testes, so that the total hormone content must turn over several hundred times each day to provide the 5–10 mg of testosterone secreted daily.

Testosterone Transport and Tissue Delivery

Testosterone circulates in the plasma largely bound to plasma proteins, primarily albumin and sex hormone-binding globulin (SHBG, also called testosterone-binding globulin [TeBG]). Plasma SHBG and its testicular counterpart, androgen-binding

Fig. 10-2 Pathway of testosterone formation in the testis and the conversion of testosterone to active metabolites in peripheral tissues. (Redrawn from Griffin JE, and Wilson JD: Disorders of the testes. In: *Harrison's Principles of Internal Medicine,* 13th ed., KJ Isselbacher, E Braunwald, JD Wilson, JB Martin, AS Fauci, and DL Kasper eds., McGraw-Hill, New York, pp. 2006–2017, 1994.)

protein (ABP), have identical primary structure and are encoded by the same gene on chromosome 17. SHBG is a β-globulin homodimer with a size of 95,000 Da containing 30% carbohydrate. SHBG has sequence homology to the coagulation factor protein S, laminin, and the growth arrest–specific gene 6 (GAS6). The unliganded SHBG can apparently interact with a cell surface receptor.

In normal men only about 2% of testosterone is unbound in *in vitro* tests of peripheral blood whereas 44% is bound to SHBG and 54% is bound to albumin and other proteins. Albumin has about 1000-fold lower affinity for testosterone than does SHBG, but albumin has an approximately 1000-fold greater binding capacity than does SHBG so that the capacity × affinity product is similar. The proportion of testosterone (or estradiol) bound to the SHBG fraction in serum is directly proportional to the SHBG concentration. As discussed in Chapter 5, we now know that debinding of steroid hormones occurs in the microcirculation *in vivo* and that tissue availability of steroid hormones is greater than the "free" fraction measured *in vitro*. The amount of hormone available for entry into cells depends on the given organ as a function of capillary transit time, dissociation rate from the given binding protein, and endothelial membrane permeability. In studies of *in vivo* tissue delivery, nearly all of the albumin-bound testosterone is available for brain uptake while the SHBG-bound testosterone is not significantly transported into the brain. (Brain is used as a representative nonhepatic organ.) Although capillary transit time in liver is longer than in brain, it is still short in relation to the half-time of dissociation from SHBG so that testosterone available for transport into hepatocytes is similar to that in brain or about 40%–50% of the total plasma testosterone in normal men (i.e., the free plus the albumin-bound fraction). In contrast, because estradiol dissociates more rapidly from SHBG, both albumin-bound and SHBG-bound estradiol are available for transport into liver cells.

This difference between testosterone and estradiol delivery to certain tissues from SHBG increases the significance of changes in SHBG levels. SHBG levels in men are one-third to one-half those in women, and they decrease from the prepubertal level to the lower level in normal adult men as a result of sexual maturation and the associated testosterone secretion. Decreased SHBG levels occur in hypothyroidism, and thyroid hormone excess increases SHBG levels, possibly because of increased estrogen formation. (The increased estrogen levels of normal pregnancy increase the SHBG levels by 5- to 10-fold.) In men with an intact hypothalamic–pituitary–testicular axis, increases or decreases in SHBG levels do not affect tissue delivery of testosterone in the steady state because of temporary compensatory changes in testosterone formation. However, as the level of plasma estradiol is not directly regulated in men (see below), changes in SHBG levels may have a more profound effect on estradiol tissue delivery. Because SHBG binds to estradiol less avidly than testosterone or dihydrotestosterone, increases in SHBG amplify the amount of estradiol cleared by the liver relative to the amount of testosterone. For example, increases in SHBG cause decreased hepatic clearance of testosterone but have no effect on the hepatic clearance of estradiol. Thus, even in normal men, changes in SHBG levels can produce alterations in the ratios of androgens to estrogens that persist even when androgen levels themselves are not permanently altered.

Metabolism of Androgens

Testosterone and its metabolites are excreted primarily in the urine. About half of the daily turnover is recovered in the form of urinary 17-ketosteroids (androsterone and etiocholanolone) and the other half in polar metabolites (diols, triols, and conjugates). These excretory metabolites are thought to be largely inactive. A small fraction of testosterone metabolism is initially to two types of active metabolites, which in turn mediate many androgen actions. These metabolites are formed in peripheral tissues, and in this regard testosterone serves as a prohormone (Fig. 10-2). The first category of active metabolites is 5α-reduced steroids, primarily dihydrotestosterone, that mediate many androgen actions in target tissues. The second category of active testosterone metabolites is estrogens formed by the aromatization of androgens in a number of peripheral tissues. Estrogens in some instances act in concert with androgen to affect physiological processes, but they may also exert independent effects or oppose the actions of androgens. Each of these reactions to form active metabolites (5α-reduction and aromatization) is physiologically irreversible; furthermore, 5α-reduced androgens cannot be converted to estrogens. Thus, physiological actions of testosterone are the result of the combined effects of testosterone itself plus those of estrogen and the active androgen metabolites. In some instances these metabolites are active only in the tissues in which they are formed, whereas in other cases the 5α-reduced and estrogen metabolites reenter the circulation to act in other tissues.

5α-Reductase accepts a number of Δ^4-3-ketosteroids as substrate and requires reduced nicotinamide-adenine dinucleotide phosphate (NADPH) as co-factor. There are two steroid 5α-reductase isozymes. Enzyme 1 is encoded by a gene on chromosome 5, and enzyme 2 is encoded by a gene on chromosome 2. 5α-Reductase has a distinct tissue localization with the most activity found in the accessory organs of reproduction, liver, and skin. In skin the highest activity is in the genital skin, but hair follicles from all anatomical sites contain the enzyme. 5α-Reductase 2 has a lower Km for testosterone and is primarily localized in androgen target tissues. In normal men about 6%–8% of the total testosterone produced is metabolized to dihydrotestosterone by 5α-reductase. Testosterone can also be converted to 5β-reduced metabolites in the liver; however, these 5β-reduced metabolites do not have androgenic activity. A key observation in the history of androgen physiology was the discovery in 1968 that 5α-dihydrotestosterone was the main intracellular androgen and the predominant androgen concentrated in the nucleus of the rat prostate. These findings, together with the observation that dihydrotestosterone is about twice as potent as testosterone in most bioassay systems, indicated that dihydrotestosterone is a major cellular mediator of androgen action. The importance of dihydrotestosterone in normal androgen physiology has been confirmed by studies of human mutations in which the steroid 5α-reductase 2 enzyme responsible for dihydrotestosterone formation is defective (see Chapter 8).

The aromatization of androgens to estrogens in testes and in extraglandular tissues of men is accomplished by the same enzyme complex present in placenta and ovary. Estrogen formation involves sequential hydroxylation, oxidation, and removal of the C-19 carbon and aromatization of the A ring of the steroid. Three moles of NADPH and 3 moles of oxygen are required to convert each mole of androstenedione or testosterone to estrone or estradiol, respectively. The oxidations are of the mixed function type (see Chapter 9) involving a specific cytochrome P450. The enzymes involved appear to be bound in a microsomal complex that include NADPH—cytochrome P450 reductase as well as cytochrome. Of the 45 μg of estradiol produced per day on average in normal young men, only about 10%–15% comes from direct secretion by the testes while the remaining 85%–90% is derived from peripheral aromatization of secreted androstenedione (via estrone) and testosterone. Estrogen formation in the testes is enhanced by increased levels of LH or human chorionic gonadotropin (hCG). The rate of overall aromatase in nongonadal tissue does not appear to be influenced by gonadotropins but rises with advancing age.

Androgen Action

The current concepts of androgen action in target cells are diagrammed in Figure 10-3. Among the major functions of androgen are regulation of gonadotropin secretion by the hypothalamic–pituitary system, stimulation of spermatogenesis, formation of the male phenotype during sexual differentiation, and promotion of sexual maturation at puberty. Inside the cell, testosterone can be converted to dihydrotestosterone by either steroid 5α-reductase 1 or 2; steroid 5α-reductase 2 is the predominant isozyme in most androgen target tissues. Either testosterone or dihydrotestosterone then binds to the androgen receptor protein. The androgen receptor is coded by a gene on the long arm of the X-chromosome and has a size of about 110,000 Da. It is similar to other members of the steroid–thyroid–retinoid family of receptors with distinct hormone-binding, DNA-binding, and functional domains (see Chapter 3).

The androgen receptor is predominantly in the nucleus in the unbound state. The binding of androgen to the hormone-binding domain of the receptor to form the hormone–receptor complexes is a prerequisite to the transformation reaction in which the hormone–receptor complexes acquire increased affinity for nuclear components. The DNA-binding domains of the receptors then bind to androgen response

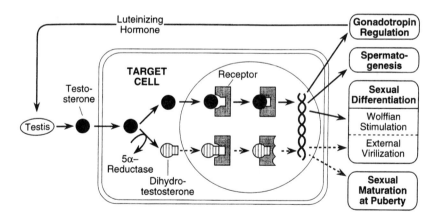

Fig. 10-3 Normal androgen physiology. Testosterone, secreted by the testis, binds to the androgen receptor in a target cell, either directly or after conversion to dihydrotestosterone. Dihydrotestosterone binds more tightly than testosterone, and the complex of dihydrotestosterone and the androgen receptor can bind more efficiently to the chromatin. The major actions of androgens, shown on the right, are mediate by testosterone (solid lines), or by dihydrotestosterone (broken lines). (Redrawn from Griffin JE: Androgen resistance—the clinical and molecular spectrum. N Engl J Med 326:612, 1992.)

elements (AREs) in the promoter region of target genes activating transcription. Estradiol, as discussed above, may be either secreted directly by the testis or formed in peripheral tissues. The mechanisms by which estrogens augment or block androgen action are not fully understood.

Based on studies in humans and animals, it appears that the testosterone–receptor complex is responsible for gonadotropin regulation, stimulation of spermatogenesis, and the virilization of the wolffian ducts during sexual differentiation, whereas the dihydrotestosterone–receptor complex is responsible for external virilization during embryogenesis and for most male secondary sexual characteristics of the adult (see below). Androgen receptor concentrations are highest in the accessory organs of male reproduction that depend on androgens for their growth. Other tissues such as skeletal muscle, liver, and heart rate have smaller amounts of the receptor. In the testis, androgen receptors are present both in isolated Sertoli cells and in interstitial cells. Whether the presence of androgen receptors identifies a tissue as androgen responsive is not clear, although androgen receptors are present in greater numbers in tissues known to respond to androgen. Single gene mutations in humans and animals (see Chapter 8) indicate that a single androgen receptor binds both testosterone and dihydrotestosterone and that the receptor protein is coded by a locus on the X chromosome. Dihydrotestosterone formation appears to be required for normal androgen action even though there is only a single receptor. In the case of the human androgen receptor, a partial explanation for this requirement of dihydrotestosterone may be the severalfold greater affinity of the receptor for dihydrotestosterone than for testosterone. Dihydrotestosterone may also facilitate transformation of the receptor for transactivation more efficiently (Fig. 10-3). Thus, a difference in the interaction of the two hormones with the androgen receptor may serve as an amplifying mechanism for androgen action in certain target tissues.

SPERMATOGENESIS, SEMINAL FLUID FORMATION, AND CAPACITATION

Stages of Spermatogenesis

After migration of the germ cells to the gonadal ridges during embryogenesis (see Chapter 8), the total number of germ cells is approximately 3×10^5 per gonad. This number increases to about 6×10^6 spermatogonia per testis by the time of puberty. With sexual maturation, sperm production of about 2×10^8 sperm per day develops. As depicted in Figure 10-4, each spermatogonium undergoing differentiation gives rise to 16 primary spermatocytes, each of which enters meiosis and gives rise to four spermatids and ultimately four spermatozoa. Thus, 64 spermatocytes can develop from each spermatogonium. It appears that contiguous groups of spermatogonia begin the differentiation process simultaneously, resulting in certain typical cellular associations in seminiferous tubules.

The conversion of the round spermatid to the mature spermatozoa (spermiogenesis) requires the reorganization of nucleus and cytoplasm and development of a flagellum. The nucleus comes to occupy an eccentric position near what will become the head of the spermatozoon and is covered by an acrosomal cap. The cilial

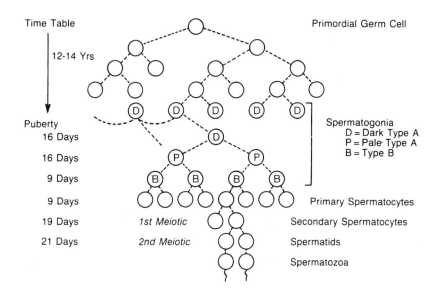

Fig. 10-4   Cell divisions during spermatogenesis. (From Griffin JE, and Wilson JD: In: *Williams Textbook of Endocrinology*, 8th ed., JD Wilson and DW Foster, eds., Saunders, Philadelphia, p. 810, 1992.)

structure that serves as the core of the sperm tail consists of nine outer fibers and two inner fibers. The mitochondria form a helix around this cilia in the middle piece of the spermatozoon, and most of the cytoplasm is lost. The differentiation of the spermatocyte to a motile sperm takes about 70 days, and the transport of the sperm through the epididymis to the ejaculatory ducts takes about 14 days. Sperm maturation occurs during passage through the epididymis, as evidenced by the development of capacity for sustained motility. The mechanism of sperm motility is believed to involve sliding action of microtubules (fibers) contained in the axial structure of the tail. The microtubules are attached to each other by dynein arms that contain the protein dynein, an ATPase. The energy for the process is derived from hydrolysis of ATP generated in the mitochondrial sheath.

Regulaton of Spermatogenesis

Normal spermatogenesis requires follicle-stimulating hormone (FSH), testosterone, and normal Sertoli cell function. FSH binds to the surface of Sertoli cells, stimulating adenylyl cyclase and thus activating protein kinase. One of the products of the Sertoli cell stimulated by FSH is ABP, which serves as a binding protein for testosterone in the seminiferous tubule lumen, maintaining the high androgen levels all the way to the epididymis. Testosterone interacts with androgen receptors in Sertoli cells to activate specific genes necessary for the differentiation process. Testosterone may also act indirectly by stimulating peritubular cells to produce peritubular factors that modulate Sertoli cell function (P-Mod-S). These factors are yet to be purified proteins. Following removal of the pituitary gland in the adult, no spermatocytes are formed. Spermatogenesis can be restored by treatment with the combination of hCG plus human menopausal gonadotropin (hMG), which contains FSH, and once restored, spermatogenesis can be maintained by hCG alone. This might seem to imply that FSH is required only for initiation of spermatogenesis but not its maintenance. But in studies of normal men in whom FSH is selectively suppressed by the sequential administration of exogenous testosterone followed by hCG, FSH administration is required for quantitatively normal spermatogenesis. Thus, it is likely that both FSH and luteinizing hormone (LH) play a continuing role in human spermatogenesis.

Based on animal studies, it appears that at least four other factors in addition to FSH and testosterone play an essential role in modulating spermatogenesis: vitamin-A, *c-fos*, and stem cell factor. Rats fed on a vitamin A–deficient diet develop defective spermatogenesis with germ cell arrest. The nuclear protooncogene *c-fos* was found to be necessary for spermatogenesis by studies of mice homozygous for germline mutations at the locus. Stem cell factor is the ligand for *c-kit*. Stem cell factor is made in Sertoli cells, and the *c-kit* receptor is present in germ cells. Mutations in either stem cell factor or *c-kit* genes result in abnormal spermatogenesis. The cAMP-response element modulator (CREM) is a protein that accumulates in large amounts during spermiogenesis, and mice carrying homozygous deletions of the CREM gene have a block in spermatogenesis.

A number of other factors have been studied *in vitro* and postulated to have paracrine/autocrine roles in modulating spermatogenesis. These include transferrin, insulin-like growth factor (IGF)-I, fibroblast growth factor (FGF), nerve growth factor (NGF), interleukin (IL)-1, opioids, transforming growth factors (TGF), growth hormone-releasing hormone (GHRH), inhibin/activin (see below), and others.

Seminal Fluid Formation

During the approximately 12 days of transit through the epididymis, sperm undergo maturation with development of the capacity for sustained motility, modification of the structural state of the nuclear chromatin and tail organelles, and loss of the remnant of spermatid cytoplasm. The epididymis also serves as reservoir for sperm. After transport of the sperm and secretory products of the testis and epididymis through the vas deferens, the fluid reaching the ejaculatory ducts is enriched by the secretions from the seminal vesicles. The seminal vesicles are the source of seminal fluid fructose and prostaglandins and contribute about 60% of the total volume of the seminal fluid. Approximately 20% of the total seminal fluid volume is derived from prostatic secretions added to the semen when the ejaculatory ducts terminate in the prostatic urethra. The prostatic fluid is the source of seminal fluid spermine, citric acid, zinc, and acid phosphatase.

Capacitation

Fertilization normally takes place within the fallopian tube. Spermatozoa usually require a period in the female reproductive tract before they can fertilize. This functional change, termed *capacitation,* is thought to have at least two components: (*1*) increased rate of flagellar beat and acceleration of sperm movement, and (*2*) an acrosome reaction in sperm that allows the underlying plasma membrane of the sperm to fuse with the ovum. The time required for optimal capacitation of normal sperm may vary from 2 to more than 6 hours. Whether capacitation is an absolute requirement in the human or serves only to enhance fertilizing capabilities has not been established.

The elements of the capacitation reaction that promote motility may include a change in the intracellular concentration or metabolism of calcium or cAMP. The acrosome reaction appears to be more complex but also involves calcium. Neither the fallopian tube nor the egg itself appears to be essential for this process. The acrosome reaction involves fragmentation and loss of the acrosome with release of a variety of hydrolytic enzymes and proteases allowing the sperm to penetrate and fuse with the ovum. Understanding of the mechanism of sperm penetration is largely based on studies of fertilization of human eggs *in vitro*. Ovulated eggs are surrounded by layers of cumulus cells embedded in a matrix of hyaluronic acid. The mechanism by which spermatozoa tunnel through the cumulus is not known. Possibly, hyaluronidase is released by the degenerating acrosome, and the mechanical agitation of the flagellum may disperse cumulus cells (see Chapter 11).

THE HYPOTHALAMIC–PITUITARY–TESTICULAR AXIS

LHRH and Gonadotropins and Their Actions

As discussed in detail in Chapter 6, peptidergic neurons in the hypothalamus secrete luteinizing hormone-releasing hormone (LHRH, also called gonadotropin-releasing hormone [GnRH]). The LHRH is transported to the pituitary by a portal vascular system and interacts with cell surface receptors on pituitary gonadotrophs to stimulate the release of LH and FSH (Fig. 10-5). LHRH is a decapeptide that is widely distributed in the central nervous system and may also be present in other tissues. However, a physiological role for LHRH in sites other than the pituitary has not been established. The amount of LH and FSH released in response to LHRH depends on age and hormonal status. In a primate model the sensitivity of the gonadotrophs to LHRH is high during the first few months of life and then declines and remains low until the onset of puberty when it increases and attains an adult level of response. The secretion of FSH in response to LHRH is relatively greater than that of LH before puberty.

Both LH and FSH are secreted by the same basophilic cells in the pituitary. Like thyrotropin (TSH) and hCG, LH and FSH are glycoproteins consisting of two polypeptide chains designated α and β. The α-subunit of each of the four hormones is identical, and distinct immunological and functional characteristics are determined by unique β-subunits. The turnover of FSH is slower than that of LH. The receptors for FSH and LH are typical seven-transmembrane domain G protein–coupled receptors. LH interacts with specific high-affinity cell surface receptors on Leydig cells and utilizes a cAMP second messenger (see Chapter 3). Activation of Leydig cell protein kinase via unspecified intermediates eventually results in stimulation of testosterone formation (see above). The rate of testosterone synthesis correlates more closely with the degree of occupancy of the regulatory subunits of the protein kinase by cAMP than with the total amount of cAMP in the cells. Whether the

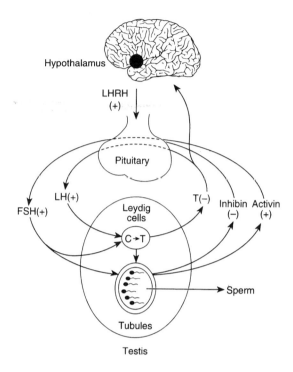

Fig. 10-5 Hypothalamic–pituitary–testicular interrelationships. Schematic diagram to indicate feedback relationship of testosterone, inhibin, and activin produced by testes on gonadotropin secretion by the hypothalamic–pituitary complex, and site of action of FSH and LH on testis. C, cholesterol; T, testosterone; FSH, follicle-stimulating hormone; LH, luteinizing hormone; LHRH, LH-releasing hormone. (From Griffin JE, and Wilson JD: Disorders of the testis. In: *Harrison's Principle of Internal Medicine,* 13th ed., KJ Isselbacher, E Braunwald, JD Wilson, JB Martin, AS Fauci, and DL Kasper, eds., McGraw-Hill, New York, pp. 2006–2017, 1994.)

LH–receptor complex undergoes internalization for degradation or receptor recycling is unclear.

In the intact testis and in cultured Leydig cells, the receptors for LH decrease in number following administration of LH or hCG. This down-regulation of LH receptors is maximal at 24 hours and is followed by return to control levels several days later. It is associated with a decreased responsiveness to subsequent LH administration, but this desensitization is not solely due to decreased receptor number. Rather, the diminished steroidogenic response appears to be due to inhibition of some postreceptor event since cAMP is ineffective in overcoming the desensitization. In fact, the desensitization can be produced by cAMP stimulation of steroidogenesis under conditions that do not alter LH receptor number. The diminished response of the Leydig cell to LH that follows LH administration appears to be a component of an intratesticular control system for regulating testosterone production.

As mentioned above the second messenger for FSH action following its binding to receptors on the basal aspects of Sertoli cells is also cAMP. FSH is known to stimulate the rate of synthesis of androgen-binding protein (ABP) and the aromatase enzyme complex in Sertoli cells. Also, FSH may play a role in steroidogenesis by influencing Leydig cell maturation and modifying effects of LH on steroidogenesis by stimulating paracrine–autocrine factors. Based on *in vitro* studies, IGF-I, TGF-β, epidermal growth factor (EGF), TGF-α, FGF, inhibin/activin, cytokines, GHRH, corticotropin-releasing hormone (CRH), arginine vasopressin (AVP), endothelin, and other agents have been postulated to have effects on Leydig cells. Their physiological significance is unclear.

Regulation of Secretion of LHRH and Gonadotropins

The secretion of LHRH is episodic resulting in the intermittent secretion of both immunoreactive and bioactive LH in 8–14 pulses/24 hours in adult men. Pulsatile secretion of FSH also occurs but is of smaller amplitude, in part because of the longer half-life of FSH in the circulation. The rate of LH secretion is controlled by the action of sex steroids on the hypothalamus and pituitary. The control of LH in men operates primarily by negative feedback since normal levels of gonadal steroids inhibit secretion (Fig. 10-5). Both testosterone and estradiol can inhibit LH secretion. Testosterone and its metabolites act on the central nervous system to slow the hypothalamic pulse generator and consequently decrease the frequency of LH pulsatile release. Testosterone can be converted to estradiol in the brain and pituitary, but the two hormones are thought to act independently. The fact that the testosterone metabolite dihydrotestosterone, which cannot be converted to estrogen, exerts negative feedback on LH secretion suggests that testosterone does not require conversion to estradiol to inhibit LH secretion. Testosterone also appears to have a negative feedback on LH secretion at the pituitary level, since moderate elevations of plasma testosterone levels result in diminished LH response to acute LHRH stimulation in the presence of normal levels of plasma estradiol. In normal men endogenous estrogens also act to restrain tonically the hypothalamic release of LHRH.

The negative feedback inhibition of testicular hormones on FSH secretion is less well understood. Serum FSH levels increase selectively in proportion to the loss of germinal elements in the testis. A nonsteroidal inhibitor of FSH is present in the testis, semen, and cultured Sertoli cells, and a similar material is present in ovarian follicular fluid. The inhibitor is termed *inhibin.* Inhibin is a heterodimeric protein consisting of α- and β-polypeptide subunits connected to disulfide bonds (see Chapter 9). Interestingly, significant structural homology of the β-subunit of inhibin to a subunit of human TGF-β has been found. As discussed in Chapter 12, transforming growth factors may not only affect tumor growth in an autocrine manner but also participate in the regulation of nonneoplastic processes. There are two different forms of the β-subunit of inhibin β_A and β_B. Thus, the α-subunit can combine with either β-subunit to form inhibin A (α-β_A) or inhibin B (α-β_B). Inhibin B is the physiologically important form of inhibin in the human male; an inverse relationship between inhibin B and FSH has been shown across a wide range of FSH concentrations in normal and infertile men. An additional hormone identified during the purification of inhibin, *activin,* is formed by the dimerization of the inhibin β-subunits. Activin A (β_A-β_A), activin B (β_B-β_B), and activin AB (β_A-β_B) stimulate FSH secretion from anterior pituitary cells in culture. Sertoli cells are the site of inhibin production, and inhibin production is enhanced by FSH and androgen.

Studies of pituitary cells cultured with purified bovine inhibin indicate that inhibin acts to block LHRH-stimulated FSH release. Whether inhibin also has effects at the hypothalamic level are not known. Testosterone and estradiol also have direct effects on FSH secretion, and a decrease in the pulse frequency of LHRH release may produce a selective increase in FSH. A primate model has been useful in defining the relative importance of inhibin and gonadal steroids in physiological feedback control of FSH secretion. When episodic gonadotropin secretion was maintained by chronic, intermittent LHRH infusion, neither circulating testosterone nor estradiol could account for the testicular inhibition of FSH, implying by exclusion that inhibin must be the gonadal hormone of greatest importance for feedback control at the level of the pituitary.

DEVELOPMENT AND MAINTENANCE OF REPRODUCTIVE FUNCTION

The development and maintenance of reproductive function in the male can be correlated with alterations in the plasma testosterone. During embryogenesis testosterone levels rise in the late first trimester in association with male sexual differentiation (see Chapter 8). In the first 6 months of life, the testosterone level rises to about half of adult levels, falling back to low levels before age 1 year. This neonatal surge in testosterone secretion results from a rise in plasma LH levels, but the function of the temporary increase in testosterone secretion is not well understood. Temporary inhibition of the pituitary–testicular axis in the neonatal primate is associated with impaired testicular function at puberty. The concentration of testosterone remains low in the childhood years until the onset of puberty when the level rises to adult levels by about age 17. Plasma testosterone concentration remains more or less constant in the adult until it declines somewhat during the later decades of life.

Puberty

Plasma gonadotropins and testosterone are low during the prepubertal years. In boys around age 6 or 7 there is an increased secretion of adrenal androgens termed *adrenarche.* This increased section of dehydroepiandrosterone and androstenedione is probably under the control of corticotropin (ACTH) and is in part responsible for the prepubertal growth spurt and the initial development of axillary and pubic hair. These adrenal androgens are thought to act via the androgen receptor after conversion to testosterone. Total plasma testosterone increases only slightly during this time, and plasma LH levels are low but show some low-amplitude pulsations. However, the low levels of gonadotropins in prepubertal boys are under feedback control by the prepubertal testis and low levels of plasma testosterone (5–20 ng/dl), since castration elevates both gonadotropins. The degree of elevation of gonadotropins in the absence of gonadal feedback is less during the late childhood years than at other times, suggesting that more than exquisite sensitivity of the hypothalamic–pituitary system to feedback inhibition is involved in the low gonadotropin levels of normal prepubertal boys (see also Chapter 9).

The pituitary hormonal changes associated with the onset of puberty are sleep-associated surges in LH secretion. Later, as puberty advances, the increased plasma gonadotropin levels are present throughout the day and are accompanied by increased plasma levels of testosterone. The increase in gonadotropin secretion is thought to result from both increased LHRH secretion and enhanced responsiveness of the pituitary to LHRH. Plasma levels of bioactive LH increase even more than those of the immunoreactive hormone. Thus, it appears that with sexual maturation the hypothalamic–pituitary system becomes less sensitive to the feedback inhibition of testosterone on gonadotropin secretion.

The changes in the testes at puberty include the maturation of Leydig cells and the initiation of spermatogenesis. The anatomical changes characteristic of puberty are a result of testosterone secretion. Usually the first sign of male puberty is testis enlargement with some reddening and wrinkling of the scrotal skin. Pubic hair growth begins first at the base of the penis. On average, this initiation of pubertal development occurs between ages 11 and 12, but occasionally begins as early as age 9 or as late as age 13 or 14. About a year after the onset of testis growth, the penis begins to increase in size. The prostate, seminal vesicles, and epididymis increase in size over a period of several years. Characteristic hair growth includes development of mustache and beard, regression of the scalp line, appearance of body and extremity hair, and extension of pubic hair upward into the upper pubic triangle. The larynx enlarges and the vocal cords become thickened, resulting in a lower pitch of the voice. There is an enhanced rate of linear growth, resulting in a height spurt somewhat later in puberty to a rate of about 3 inches per year. At this time the androgen-sensitive muscles of the pectoral region and the shoulder also increase in their characteristic male pattern, the hematocrit increases, and libido and sexual potency develop. These various maturation processes take place over about 4 years and reach some normal limit for the individual based on genetic and nutritional factors. Linear growth is halted by fusion of the epiphyses, which requires normal estrogen formation and action. Administration of excess exogenous androgens has little effect on the parameters of sexual development once puberty is completed.

Adulthood

At the completion of puberty, usually between ages 16 and 18, plasma testosterone levels are in the adult range of 300–1000 ng/dl, sperm production is normal, and plasma gonadotropins are in the 1–15 mIU/ml range. Most anatomic changes are completed at this time except for androgen-mediated hair growth, which is usually not maximal until the mid- to late 20s. Some effects of androgens, such as the development of the larynx, are permanent and do not reverse if androgen production decreases. Other effects of androgen, such as stimulation of erythropoietin, reverse with androgen deprivation. Beard growth slows following postpubertal androgen deficiency but usually does not completely cease. Two results of postpubertal androgen deficiency are clear-cut. There is a negative nitrogen balance probably resulting from regression of accessory organs of reproduction and to a certain extent skeletal muscle. And complete androgen deficiency is followed by a progressive decline in male sexual drive so that most such men are unable to have intercourse after a few years.

Old Age

Men have a gradual decrease in free plasma testosterone levels and an increase in SHBG levels, beginning around age 40. In elderly men there is a decrease in total plasma testosterone levels, a decrease in the ratio of androgen to estrogen, and some elevation in plasma LH and FSH. Sperm production decreases about 30% between the ages of 50 and 80. It is likely that any decline in sexual activity with age is the result of nonendocrine factors. Healthy elderly men commonly maintain a healthy sex life and reproductive capacity. Whether the changes in body composition that accompany aging—that is, decreased bone density and lean body mass and increased fat mass—are related to the fall in testosterone is under investigation.

CLINICAL ASSESSMENT OF REPRODUCTIVE FUNCTION

History and Physical Exam

The assessment of androgen status should include inquiry about defects of the urogenital tract at birth, sexual maturation at puberty, rate of beard growth, and current libido, sexual function, strength, and energy. If Leydig cell failure occurs before puberty, sexual maturation will not occur, In contrast, the detection of Leydig cell failure beginning after puberty requires a high index of suspicion of androgen deficiency and, usually, laboratory assessment. Many men without hormonal abnormalities complain of decreased sexual function. In addition, even when Leydig cell function is impaired, the rate of beard growth may not decrease for many months or even years.

The prepubertal testis measures about 2 cm in length and increases in size to a range of 3.5–5.5 cm in length in the normal adult. When damage to the seminiferous tubules occurs before puberty, the testes are small and firm. Following postpubertal damage the testes are characteristically small and soft. However, considerable damage must occur before the overall size is decreased below the lower limits of normal. Breast enlargement is the most consistent feature of feminizing states in men and may be an early sign of androgen deficiency.

Gonadotropins and Testosterone

Because of the pulsatile secretion of LH, the consequent pulsatile secretion of testosterone and the need to interpret the LH in light of the testosterone, it is usually appropriate to measure gonadotropins and testosterone on a pool formed by combining equal quantities of blood obtained from three or four samples at 15- to 20-minute intervals. The normal plasma immunoreactive LH and FSH values must be established for each laboratory based on the antibody and standard used. The normal range for plasma testosterone in adult men is 300–1000 ng/dl. Free testosterone concentrations can be estimated by equilibrium dialysis, but as discussed above, a more accurate assessment of available testosterone *in vivo* can be obtained by measuring the non-SHBG-bound fraction (or free plus albumin-bound fraction). The SHBG concentrations can also be measured directly.

Leydig cell function may be assessed before puberty by measuring the response to hCG administration. Single or multiple injections of hCG may be given. The testosterone response increases at the start of puberty, peaking in early puberty.

In certain circumstances the change in plasma LH after the administration of LHRH is measured to assess the functional integrity of the hypothalamic–pituitary–Leydig cell axis. When 100 μg of LHRH is given subcutaneously or intravenously to normal men, there is, on average, a 4- to 5-fold increase in LH, with the peak level at 30 minutes. However, the range of response is broad, some normal men having less than a doubling of LH levels. In general, the peak LH following a single LHRH injection correlates with basal levels. In patients with primary testicular failure, measurement of basal LH is usually sufficient, and measurement of LHRH response adds little to the diagnosis. Men who have either pituitary disease or hypothalamic disease may have either a normal or abnormal LH response to an acute dose of LHRH. Therefore, a normal response is of no diagnostic value, whereas a subnormal response is of value in determining that an abnormality exists, even though the site is not determined. Men with secondary hypogonadism and a subnormal response to an acute infusion of LHRH who develop a normal response to an acute dose after daily infusion of LHRH for a week usually have a hypothalamic cause of the hypogonadism (see Chapter 5 and Fig. 5-4).

Seminal Fluid Examination

Routine evaluation of seminal fluid is largely dependent on tests that do not assess the functional capacity of sperm. Seminal fluid should be obtained after masturbation into a clean glass or plastic container. The volume of the normal ejaculate is 2–6 ml. The specimen should be analyzed within an hour. Estimation of motility is made by examining a drop of undiluted seminal fluid and recording the percentage of motile forms. Normally 60% or more of the sperm should be motile with forward progression. Sperm density can be determined by diluting seminal fluid 20-fold with an appropriate solution and estimating density in a hemocytometer or with the aid of an electronic particle counter. The normal value is usually considered to be greater than 20 million/ml with total sperm per ejaculate of greater than 60 million.

After the first 2 days, the total sperm in the ejaculate per the number of days since the last ejaculation is relatively constant in normal men who ejaculate daily. Random sampling of sperm density in men is complicated by variable extragonadal sperm reserves and by effects of toxic factors such as hot baths, acute febrile illnesses, and unknown medications. The net result is that it is difficult to define the minimally adequate ejaculate. Ordinarily, three ejaculates are required to establish inadequacy of sperm number or cytology.

Seminal cytology is a useful index of fertility, and the seminal fluid smear is prepared in the same way as a blood smear but with special stains. Some abnormal spermatozoa are present in all semen. The best correlations between histological abnormalities and infertility are seen when a single anomaly is found in a large percentage of the sample. It is generally believed that 60% or more of the spermatozoa should have a normal morphology. When it is available the details of sperm structure can be studied by electron microscopy. Such studies are useful in identifying the abnormalities in immotile sperm.

DERANGED REPRODUCTIVE FUNCTION

Abnormalities of male reproductive function may occur at any stage of life from embryogenesis through old age. Disorders of testicular function during embryogenesis result in abnormalities of sexual differentiation (see Chapter 8). This section will consider examples of deranged reproductive function occurring at puberty and in adulthood.

Deficient Puberty: Isolated Gonadotropin Deficiency

Deranged reproductive function related to pubertal events in boys more commonly involves delayed or deficient puberty rather than sexual precocity. This is not so in girls (see Chapter 9). It is often difficult to decide whether puberty is merely being delayed or is actually incomplete or deficient. A common cause of deficient puberty is isolated gonadotropin deficiency, which occurs in both sporadic and familial forms. It is second only to Klinefelter's syndrome (see Chapter 8) as a cause of hypogonadism in men. The disorder was originally described as a familial syndrome associated with an impaired sense of smell (Kallmann's syndrome). The defect in most affected individuals is detected because of a failure to undergo puberty. A subset of patients, particularly familial cases, have associated congenital defects commonly involving midline facial and head structure. There is no sense of smell because of defective development of the olfactory bulbs. Less severely affected individuals may have a negative family history (half of all subjects with the disorder) and only partial defects in FSH and/or LH secretion. Such individuals may undergo partial sexual maturation, develop partial testicular enlargement, and not come to medical attention until adulthood.

The underlying defect is at the hypothalamic level: absence of or inadequate release of LHRH. A defect in a neural adhesion molecule may be responsible for abnormal migration of neurons leading to both the impaired sense of smell and defective LHRH release. Randomly obtained gonadotropin levels might be undetectable, low, or apparently normal in the face of a low testosterone level. The fact that the underlying defect is at the hypothalamic level was established when LHRH became available; following short-term administration of LHRH, plasma LH and FSH increase in about half of subjects. After repetitive infusion of LHRH for 5 days or longer, plasma gonadotropins rise to the normal range in virtually all affected patients but not in individuals with panhypopituitarism.

One group of investigators has attempted to define some of the clinical heterogeneity in patients with isolated gonadotropin deficiency by studying the patterns of LHRH secretion as inferred by frequent measurements of plasma LH. Men with isolated gonadotropin deficiency displayed several abnormal patterns of LHRH secretion. Whereas the majority of men had an apulsatile pattern of LH release, other individuals demonstrated episodic LH secretion only during sleep (as in normal pubertal subjects). In these latter subjects a history of early but arrested pubertal development was often obtained, and testicular size was larger than in those subjects with an apulsatile pattern of LH release. In another family with isolated gonadotropin deficiency, affected men consistently demonstrated a diminished LH pulse amplitude compared to normal men or their unaffected siblings. In yet another family, a diminished frequency of LHRH pulsations was associated with a variably low to low normal testosterone in two affected subjects but not in their normal brother. These findings imply that maintenance of a physiological amplitude and frequency of endogenous LHRH secretion appear to be essential for normal reproductive function.

Adult Reproductive Failure: Infertility

Approximately 15% of couples attempting their first pregnancy are unsuccessful. Couples who have been unable to achieve a pregnancy after 1 year of unprotected intercourse are usually considered to have primary infertility. In approximately one-third of such cases a significant abnormality impairing fertility is thought to be in the man alone, and in an additional fifth of couples both the man and the woman have some abnormality. Thus, in about half of infertile couples some abnormality in the male is in part responsible for the failure to conceive. Any man who has been unsuccessful in achieving fertility with a regularly menstruating woman after 1 year should be considered potentially subfertile.

Infertility in men can be an isolated problem with normal androgen production or one manifestation of an abnormality of testicular function that involves both Leydig cells and seminiferous tubules. In contrast, because sperm production depends on normal Leydig cell function, disorders that primarily affect androgen formation or action are usually associated with infertility. Therefore, it is essential to exclude the presence of subtle Leydig cell dysfunction in every man with infertility.

Adult abnormalities of testicular function can be due to hypothalamic–pituitary defects, testicular disorders, or abnormalities in sperm transport. The hypothalamic–pituitary defects include not only isolated gonadotropin deficiency mentioned above, but also a variety of destructive and infiltrative lesions in the pituitary, and functional impairments of gonadotropin secretion resulting from excess prolactin, glucocorticoids, or endogenous or exogenous androgens.

Testicular disorders known to be associated with infertility can be grouped into several categories. Developmental and structural defects include Klinefelter's syndrome and its variants (see Chapter 8), deletions or mutations in one of the azoospermia factor regions on the long arm of the Y chromosome, abnormal testicular descent, and a structural defect of sperm tails leading to immotile sperm. Acquired testicular defects include viral and other infections, trauma, radiation, drugs including alcohol and marijuana, and self-directed immune responses affecting the entire testis or primarily sperm. Systemic diseases may be associated with testicular abnormalities, as in chronic liver disease, renal failure, and certain neurological disease. Finally, androgen resistance due to a receptor defect may be manifested by underandrogenization with infertility or infertility alone in men with normal development of the external genitalia.

Disorders of sperm transport lead to infertility associated with normal Leydig cell function. The abnormality can be unilateral or bilateral, congenital or acquired. In men with unilateral obstruction, infertility might be due to antisperm antibodies. Obstruction at the level of the epididymis may occur in association with chronic infections of the paranasal sinuses and lungs. Or the vas deferens might be congenitally absent in association with an absence of the seminal vesicles.

Unfortunately, the above elaboration of the known causes and of conditions associated with male infertility does not account for the problem in the majority of men. When a large series of consecutive patients seen by referral groups is evaluated, more than half of such men are classified as having "idiopathic" infertility. Because as many as 1 in 20 men are infertile, this represents a major area for improvement in medical knowledge.

FERTILITY CONTROL

Vasectomy

Other than the condom, the only proven effective means of fertility control in men is surgical interruption of the vas deferens (vasectomy). In the United States about 50% of couples adopting surgical sterilization for fertility control choose vasectomy, and about 1 million vasectomy procedures are performed each year. Bilateral partial vasectomy is a relatively simple operative procedure usually performed with local anesthesia. Vasectomy is considered successful when sperm cannot be demonstrated in the semen on two consecutive specimens. On average, this takes 24 ejaculations following vasectomy. In less than 1% of men, the procedure fails due to recanalization, which occurs at a median time of 6 months. The changes in the testis following occlusion of the vas have been studied in animals. In the primate, spermatogenesis continues following vasectomy, with the sperm being resorbed or stored in distended ducts and cysts. Testicular volume does not change after vasectomy in men. There appear to be no significant changes in peripheral hormone levels following vasectomy as assessed by measuring plasma testosterone and gonadotropins. Moreover, Leydig cell reserve, as assessed by response to hCG, is normal several years later. Although immune complex-mediated atherosclerosis has been described in vasectomized monkeys, no increased prevalence of atherosclerotic cardiovascular disease has been found in vasectomized men. Vasectomy has no deleterious effects on potency or sexual performance. Antisperm antibodies do develop following vasectomy, and the presence of these antibodies may limit the success of attempted vasectomy reversal. Thus, vasectomy reversal (or vasovasostomy) has a success rate for appearance of sperm in the ejaculate of 80%–90%, but the associated pregnancy rate is only 30%–40%.

Search for a Male Contraceptive

Whereas the oral contraceptive is effective and relatively safe in controlling ovulation and fertility in women (see Chapter 9), there is no readily reversible and effective pharmacological contraceptive for men. One explanation for this delay in pharmacological contraception for men is that it intuitively seems easier to prevent the production of only one ovum per month in the female than to prevent the production of millions of sperm each day in the male. In addition, sperm migration, capacitation, fertilization, and implantation all take place in women. Thus, even some measures designed to affect the sperm can be used in women but not in men.

In searching for a male contraceptive, pharmacological and other methods have been directed at inhibiting hypothalamic–pituitary function, directly inhibiting spermatogenesis, or inhibiting epididymal function. It was hoped that the injection of long-acting testosterone esters might suppress gonadotropin secretion, resulting in defective spermatogenesis and at the same time replace endogenous testosterone. However, this proved successful in completely eliminating sperm from the ejaculate in a little over half of men. The inhibition of spermatogenesis in men who responded was reversible. A contraceptive trial of men using weekly testosterone injections who achieved either absence of sperm in the ejaculate or severely decreased numbers (<3 million/ml) found a failure rate no greater than that seen with women using oral contraceptive pills. The requirement for weekly intramuscular injections in this and the regimens below is a hindrance to acceptance. Gonadotropin levels are decreased in men given injections of long-acting analogs of LHRH with a resultant decrease in testosterone levels and associated impaired sexual function. Combining testosterone injections with LHRH agonist treatment results in a return of testosterone levels to normal but inconsistent success in totally inhibiting spermatogenesis. Trials of LHRH antagonists with testosterone gave similar results.

A number of anticancer drugs and other relatively toxic compounds impair sperm production by direct effects on the testes. Most of these compounds produce additional unacceptable side effects. An antifertility agent in cottonseed oil discovered in China is a naphthalphenol termed *gossypol*. It has been given to more than 10,000 men in clinical trials over a decade. Administration of this compound orally for 60 days causes the sperm in the ejaculate to become immotile and to decrease in number. Because the drug affects motility it may not be necessary to have absence of sperm for an antifertility effect. Unfortunately, significant toxicity in regard to lowering the serum potassium has been observed, and the reversibility of the effect of the drug is uncertain. Other drugs with antispermatogenic activity have been studied less extensively. Physical methods such as heat and ultrasound have been tried to a limited extent, and immunological methods with antibodies directed at various testicular components have an uncertain duration of action.

Selective inhibition of epididymal function to cause impairment of sperm maturation would theoretically control fertility without the risk of impaired testicular function. In addition, the time required to achieve an effect on fertility with such agents should be less than the 2 to 3 months necessary for agents affecting the pituitary or testis. Because the epididymis is a target organ for androgens, antiandrogens were used in an attempt to inhibit sperm maturation in the epididymis. Both cyproterone and the nonsteroidal antiandrogen flutamide appear to be ineffective in inhibiting epididymal function. A number of chlorinated sugars have been shown to be effective in producing reversible infertility in animal models by inhibiting glycolysis in sperm and impairing sperm motility. Unfortunately, all such compounds studied thus far have significant toxicity to preclude their trials in men.

In summary, the search for a male contraceptive has not been rewarding.

SUGGESTED READING

Baker HWG: Reproductive effects of nontesticular illness. Endocrinol Metab Clin North Am 27:831–850, 1998.

Baker HWG, Burger HG, de Kretser MD, and Hudson B: Relative incidence of etiological disorders in male infertility. In: *Male Reproductive Dysfunction,* RJ Santen and RS Swerdloff, eds., Marcel Dekker, New York, pp. 341–372, 1986.

Bhasin S, Ma K, Sinha I, Limbo M, Taylor WE, and Salehian B: The genetic basis of male infertility. Endocrinol Metab Clin North Am 27:783–805, 1998.

Carr BR, and Griffin JE: Fertility control and its complications. In: *Williams Textbook of Endocrinology,* 9th ed., JD Wilson, DW Foster, HM Kronenberg, and PR Larsen eds., Saunders, Philadelphia, pp. 901–926, 1998.

DeKretser DM, Risbridger GP, and Kerr JB: Basic endocrinology of the testis. In: *Endocrinology,* LJ DeGroot M, Besser, HG Burger, JL Jameson, DL Loriaux, JC Marshall, WC Odell, JT Potts Jr, and AH Rubenstein, eds., Saunders, Philadelphia, pp. 2307–2335, 1995.

Ewing LL: Leydig cell. In: *Infertility in the Male,* LI Lipshultz and SS Howards, eds., Churchill Livingstone, New York, pp. 43–69, 1983.

Fortunati N: Sex hormone-binding globulin: Not only a transport protein. What news is around the corner? J Endocrinol Invest 22:223–234, 1999.

Griffin JE, and Wilson JD: Disorders of the testes and male reproductive tract. In: *Williams Textbook of Endocrinology,* 9th ed., JD Wilson, DW Foster, HM Kronenberg, and PR Larsen, eds., Saunders, Philadelphia, pp. 819–876, 1998.

Hayes FJ, Hall JE, Boepple PA, and Crowley WF Jr: Differential control of gonadotropin secretion in the human: Endocrine role of inhibin. J Clin Endocrinol Metab 83:1835–1841, 1998.

Hayes FJ, Seminara SB, and Crowley WF Jr: Hypogonadotropic hypogonadism. Endocrinol Metab Clin North Am 27:739–763, 1998.

Johnson L: A reevaluation of daily sperm output of men. Fertil Steril 37:811–816, 1982.

Lieblich JM, Rogol AD, White BJ, and Rosen SW: Syndrome of anosmia with hypogonadotropic hypogonadism (Kallmann syndrome): Clinical and laboratory studies in 23 cases. Am J Med 73:506–519, 1982.

Matsumoto AM, Karpas AE, and Bremner WJ: Chronic human chorionic gonadotropin administration in normal men: Evidence that follicle-stimulating hormone is necessary for the maintenance of quantitatively normal spermatogenesis in man. J Clin Endocrinol Metab 62:1184–1192, 1986.

Matsumoto AM, Paulsen CA, and Bremner WJ: Stimulation of sperm production by human luteinizing hormone in gonadotropin-suppressed normal mem. J Clin Endocrinol Metab 59:882–887, 1984.

McLachlan RI, Wreford NG, O'Donnell L, de Kretser DM, and Robertson DM: The endocrine regulation of spermatogenesis: Independent roles for testosterone and FSH. J Endocrinol 148:1–9, 1996.

Mayo KE: Inhibin and activin. Trends Endocrinol Metab 5:407–415, 1994.

Pardridge WM: Serum bioavailability of sex steroid hormones. Clin Endocrinol Metab 15:259–278, 1986.

Pescovitz H, Srivastava CH, Breyer PR, and Monts BA: Paracrine control of spermatogenesis. Trends Endocrinol Metab 5:126–131, 1994.

Wu FC: Male contraception. Baillieres Clin Obstet Gynaecol 10:1–23, 1996.

11

Fertilization, Implantation, and Endocrinology of Pregnancy

BRUCE R. CARR

The complex and coordinated set of events leading to sperm and egg maturation and transport in the female genital tract that culminates in fertilization is one of the most remarkable phenomena in nature. This set of events is followed by the equally important unique process of implantation, fetal maturation, and parturition. The hormonal changes that regulate these events are dependent upon the close interaction of the fetal–placental–material unit.

FERTILIZATION AND IMPLANTATION

Ovum Maturation and Transport

Just before ovulation, the egg, which has been arrested in the diplotene stage, completes the first meiotic division and forms the first polar body. The second meiotic division starts at the time of ovulation but ends only after fertilization by a sperm.

The process of egg maturation is regulated through a closely interrelated set of hormonal events, most notably involving follicle-stimulating hormone (FSH), luteinizing hormone (LH), and estrogen. At the time of ovulation the fimbria of the oviduct are closely applied to the surface of the ovary. The extruded oocyte and adherent granulosa cells, known as the *cumulus oophorous,* are collected by the ciliated fimbrial end of the fallopian tube. The transport of the egg into the end of the fallopian tube occurs within minutes and is regulated primarily by ciliary action. The cumulus cells are able to communicate with one another via a network of intercellular bridges through the zona to the perivitelline space. The cumulus cells have also been reported to play a role in nutrition and maintenance of the ovum.

There are three different stages of passage of the ovum through the fallopian tube. The first stage includes the transfer of the ovum from the fimbriated end of the fallopian tube until the egg reaches and is retained at the ampullary–isthmic junction. The ampullary–isthmic junction is a functional block but is not a clearly defined anatomical structure. The ovum remains at this junction for 1–2 days during which time fertilization occurs. The second stage begins soon after fertilization when the egg traverses the isthmic portion of the tube where it again is retained at another functional block, the isthmic–utero or utero–tubal junction. The length of time from the process of ovulation until the release of the egg from the isthmus is species dependent and averages 3 days in women. The detection of the egg at the utero–tubal junction appears to be influenced by ovarian steroid hormones, namely estrogen and progesterone. During this stage, estrogen and progesterone also act on the endometrium to prepare it for implantation of the fertilized egg. The final stage of egg transportation occurs during the 3–4 days after ovulation when the fertilized egg leaves the isthmus and arrives in the uterine cavity (Fig. 11-1).

Sperm Transport and Capacitation

The sperm are required to traverse an even greater distance in the female genital tract than is the ovum. Spermatozoa leave the vagina after ejaculation and pass through the cervix, the entire length of the uterine cavity, the utero–tubal junction, the isthmus, and finally the ampullary–isthmic junction where fertilization occurs. The process of sperm transport is very rapid in comparison to egg transport. Spermatozoa have been found in the distal end of the fallopian tube 5 minutes after ejaculation. However, the rate of attrition of sperm is high. Of an estimated 250 million sperm deposited in the vagina, only 50 or less ever reach the oviduct (Fig. 11-1). The principal mechanism controlling sperm transport is flagellar movement; thus, semen characterized by low sperm motility is usually associated with infertility.

In most species, the process of sperm capacitation requires sperm to reside in or be exposed to the female tract before they are capable of fertilizing an ovum. This process is not yet clearly defined, but it includes the acrosome reaction that involves a breakdown and merging of the plasma membrane and acrosomal membrane of the sperm head. This is followed by a release of enzymes thought to play a role

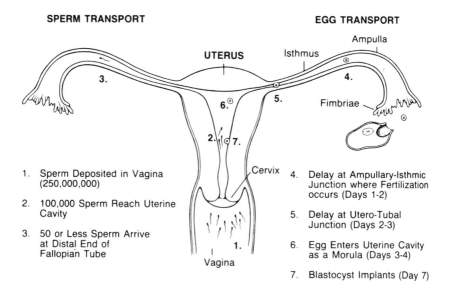

Fig. 11-1   The transport of sperm and the egg in the female reproductive tract.

in sperm penetration. During the process of capacitation, the sperm also become hypermotile.

Process of Fertilization

The first stage of fertilization requires the equitorial region of the sperm head to adhere to the zona pellucida surrounding the egg (Fig. 11-2). The sperm must first penetrate the zona, which requires 15–25 minutes. After passage through the zona pellucida, the sperm moves rapidly across the perivitelline space (in less than 1 second) where it attaches to the perivitelline membrane and penetrates it (in less than 1 minute).

After the sperm head penetrates the vitelline membrane, the male pronucleus is formed. The penetration of the vitelline membrane initiates two important events: the release of cortical granules into the perivitelline space, which prevents further penetration of the egg by other sperm, and the development of polyspermia. The second event is the triggering of the final stage of meiosis of the oocyte. The second polar body is extruded from the egg and a haploid number of chromosomes (23) are present in the egg pronuclei just before fertilization.

The male and female pronuclei are visible about 2–3 hours after the sperm has penetrated the vitelline membrane. Within 4 hours, the sperm tail is incorporated within the egg. Within 24 hours, the two pronuclei have moved toward the center of the egg. Next, their respective haploid chromosomes replicate and a mitotic spindle forms. The fertilized egg then divides and forms two blastomeres.

The initial cleavages of the egg occur in the fallopian tube, and the rate of cleavage remains remarkably constant in mammals. The rate of cleavage of fertilized human eggs has been determined primarily from *in vitro* studies. The timing of cleavage of the human egg is as follows: 2 cells (38 hours), 4 cells (46–48 hours), 8 cells (51–62 hours), morula formation (111–135 hours), and the formation of a blastocyst (123–147 hours).

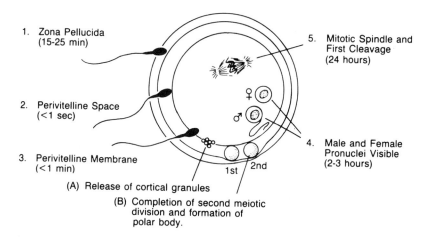

Fig. 11-2 The process of fertilization of a human egg.

The life span of an unfertilized egg is less than 20 hours following ovulation, after which it undergoes cell death and cytolysis. The life span of a sperm is about 24 hours after ejaculation.

In Vitro Fertilization

The initial report of a delivery of a live born infant by the method of *in vitro* fertilization in 1978 stimulated further clinical investigations. The knowledge and methods that were developed from these studies are now available for the treatment of infertile couples with a variety of disorders including damaged or blocked fallopian tubes, male infertility, cervical factors, and even unexplained infertility.

In vitro fertilization and embryo transfer starts with the administration of exogenous human menopausal gonadotropins (hMG) or pure human FSH to stimulate growth and development of multiple ovarian follicles. Follicles are aspirated 32 hours after the injection of human chorionic gonadotropin (hCG), which has LH-like activity. The ova are aspirated from ripe follicles by transvaginal ultrasonographic techniques. The eggs are then transferred to a culture dish containing medium and serum.

Freshly ejaculated semen is washed in buffer and centrifuged to remove the seminal fluid. The sperm are preincubated in defined medium for 1–2 hours to initiate capacitation. Next, approximately 1 million sperm are added to each culture dish containing an ovum. Fertilization occurs within 6–8 hours. During the next 2–3 days, the egg divides and reaches the 4- to 8-cell stage. Then, up to a maximum of 4–6 fertilized, 2- to 8-cell stage eggs are transferred by a catheter to the uterine cavity. The rest of the embryos that are not initially transferred are frozen and placed in the uterus during a subsequent menstrual cycle. If fertilization fails to occur or if the male demonstrates severe impairment in sperm number or motility, direct intracytoplasmic injection (ICSI) is recommended. The pregnancy rate is about 30% of those embryos transferred, with a rate of live births of about 15% worldwide.

Implantation and Placentation

In the human the egg enters the uterine cavity as a morula on the third to fourth day after ovulation. The morula is transformed into a blastocyst during the fifth to sixth day over ovulation. At this stage of development, the embryo appears as a hollow sphere with two clearly distinguishable cell types: the outer cells are the trophectoderm cells that will form the placenta and the inner cell mass from which the fetus will develop.

On the seventh day after ovulation, the blastocyst implants on the endometrial lining of the uterine cavity. The embryo attaches to the endometrium with the embryonic pole facing the uterine cavity. The endometrium, under the influence of progesterone secreted by the corpus luteum, is transformed into a decidua. The decidua consists of large polyhedral endometrial cells that are laden with glycogen and lipid and are often multinucleated. In the absence of progesterone, the development of decidua and implantation fail to occur. Continued progesterone secretion ensures further development of the decidua and maintenance of pregnancy. The corpus luteum is the main source of progesterone during the first 6–8 weeks of pregnancy. During the remainder of gestation, the principal source of progesterone is the placenta. Decidual development also appears to respond to signals from the invading embryo.

Next, endometrial cells begin to interdigitate with the microvilli of the trophectodermal cells. The layer of trophoblast cells develops into an inner cytotrophoblast layer and an outer syncytiotrophoblast layer. The syncytiotrophoblasts secrete proteolytic enzymes that errode the endometrium and allow the syncytiotrophoblast cells to invade further. The human embryo undergoes interstitial implantation in which the embryo is deeply embedded and enclosed by the endometrium by the eleventh day after ovulation (Fig. 11-3).

The placenta develops from the trophoblast. Lacunar spaces form among the syncytiotrophoblasts, and these spaces are contiguous with the maternal capillary circulation. Within these spaces the functional and structural compartment of the placenta, the chorionic villi, develops. In the absence of vascularization of the villi, further development into secondary and tertiary villi do not occur. Instead, the villi become cystic and fill with fluid (hydatidiform mole). The hydatidiform mole is often spontaneously aborted and may result in extensive maternal hemorrhage and shock. This process often precedes the development of invasive trophoblastic disease known as *choriocarcinoma.*

Placental development varies widely between different animal species. The human placenta is hemochorial: fetal endothelium and fetal connective tissues are directly bathed by maternal blood. The maternal side of the placenta is composed of the chorionic villi fused into separate lobes known as *cotyledons.* The cotyledons and their chorionic villi are exposed to maternal blood from the decidual spiral arterioles. The fetal side of the placenta is composed of the amnion and chorion. The amnion is a thin avascular membrane that surrounds the fetus and contains amniotic fluid. Adjacent to the amnion is the chorion tissue layer, and these cells are next to the decidua lining the uterine cavity. It has been proposed that hormones pro-

Fig. 11-3 The early human embryo following implantation.

duced in the fetus, amnion, chorion, and decidua communicate information between each compartment. This information may play a role in the onset of parturition.

ENDOCRINOLOGY OF PREGNANCY

The Fetal–Placental–Maternal Unit

The hormonal change and maternal adaptation that occur during human pregnancy are extensive. During pregnancy the placenta, supplied with precursor hormones from the maternal–fetal unit, synthesizes large quantities of steroid hormones as well as various protein and peptide hormones and in turn secretes these products into the fetal and maternal circulation. Near the end of pregnancy a woman is exposed daily to large quantities of estrogen, progesterone, mineralocorticoids, and glucocorticosteroids. The mother and, to a lesser extent, the fetus are also exposed to large quantities of human placental lactogen (hPL), hCG, prolactin (PRL), relaxin, prostaglandins, and smaller amounts of pro-opiomelanocortin (POMC)-derived peptides such as corticotropin (ACTH) and endorphin, gonadotropin-releasing hormone (GnRH), also called luteinizing hormone–releasing hormone (LHRH), thyroid-stimulating hormone (TSH), corticotropin-releasing hormone (CRH), somatostatin, and other hormones.

Implantation, the maintenance of pregnancy, parturition, and finally lactation depend on a complex interaction of hormones in the maternal–fetal–placental unit. In addition, protein and peptide hormones produced by the placenta act via a paracrine mechanism to regulate the secretion of placental steroid hormones.

Placental Compartment

In mammals, particularly humans, the placenta has evolved into a complex structure that delivers nutrients to the fetus, produces numerous steroid and protein hormones, removes metabolites from the fetus, and delivers them to the maternal compartment.

Progesterone

The main source of progesterone during pregnancy is the placenta. The corpus luteum, however, is the major source of progesterone secretion during the first 6–8 weeks of gestation. It is believed that the developing trophoblast takes over as the major source of progesterone secretion by 8 weeks' gestation, as removal of the corpus luteum before, but not after, this time leads to abortion. After 8 weeks' gestation the corpus luteum of pregnancy continues to secrete progesterone, but the amount of progesterone secreted is only a fraction of that secreted by the placenta. The placenta of a term pregnancy produces approximately 250 mg of progesterone each day. Maternal progesterone plasma levels rise from 25 ng/ml during the late luteal phase to 150 ng/ml at term (Fig. 11-4A). Most of the progesterone secreted by the placenta enters the maternal compartment.

Although the placenta produces large amounts of progesterone, under normal circumstances it has very limited capacity to synthesize cholesterol from acetate.

Fig. 11-4 The range (mean ± 1 SD) of (A) progesterone, (B) estradiol-17β, and (C) estriol in plasma of normal pregnant women as a function of weeks of gestation. (Adapted from Carr BR: In: *Principles and Practice of Endocrinology and Metabolism,* KL Becker, ed., Lippincott, Philadelphia, pp. 887–898, 1990.)

Maternal cholesterol in the form of low-density lipoprotein (LDL) cholesterol is the principal source of precursor substrate for biosynthesis of progesterone in human pregnancy. The LDL cholesterol attaches to its receptor on the trophoblast and is taken up and degraded by the trophoblast to free cholesterol, which then is converted to progesterone and secreted.

A functioning fetal circulation is not important for the regulation of progesterone levels in the maternal unit. In fact, fetal death, ligation of the umbilical cord, and anencephaly, which are all associated with a decrease in estrogen production, have no significant effect on progesterone levels in the maternal compartment.

The physiological role of the large quantity of progesterone produced by the placenta has been an area of great interest. Progesterone binds to receptors in uterine smooth muscle, thereby inhibiting smooth muscle contractility and leading to myometrial quiescence and prevention of uterine contractions. It also inhibits prostaglandin formation, which is known to be critically involved in human parturition. Progesterone is essential for the maintenance of pregnancy in all mammals, possibly owing to its ability to inhibit T lymphocyte cell–mediated responses involved in graft rejection. Because the fetus is a foreign body within the uterus, the high local levels of progesterone can block cellular immune responses to foreign antigens and may be important in giving immunological privilege to the pregnant uterus.

Estrogen

During human pregnancy the rate of estrogen production and the level of estrogens in plasma increase markedly (Fig. 11-4B and C). The levels of urinary estriol have been reported to increase 1000-fold during pregnancy. The corpus luteum is the principal source of estrogen during the first few weeks of pregnancy, but afterward nearly all of the estrogen formed is from the trophoblast of the placenta. However, the mechanism by which estrogen is produced by the placenta is unique. The placenta is unable to convert progesterone to estrogens because of a deficiency of 17α-hydroxylase. Thus, the placenta has to rely on preformed androgens produced in the maternal and fetal adrenal glands. Estradiol-17β and estrone are synthesized by the placenta via conversion of dehydroepiandrosterone sulfate (DHEA-S), which reaches it from both maternal and fetal bloodstreams.

The placenta metabolizes DHEA-S to estrogens in the presence of the following enzymes: placental sulfatase, 3β-hydroxysteroid dehydrogenase, and aromatase enzyme complex. Estriol is synthesized by the placenta from 16α-hydroxydehydroepiandrosterone sulfate formed in fetal liver from circulating DHEA-S secreted by the fetal adrenal gland. At least 90% of urinary estriol is ultimately derived from the fetal adrenal gland. The sources of estrogen biosynthesis in the maternal–fetal–placental until is presented in Figure 11-5. The major source of fetal adrenal DHEA-S is cholesterol circulating in fetal blood. A minor source of fetal adrenal DHEA-S is formed from pregnenolone secreted by the placenta. Only 20% of fetal cholesterol is derived from the maternal compartment. Because amnionic fluid cholesterol levels are negligible, the main source of cholesterol appears to be the fetus itself. As the fetal liver synthesizes cholesterol at a high rate, and if one considers the size of the fetal liver, it can be computed that the fetal liver may supply sufficient cholesterol to the fetal adrenal to maintain steroidogenesis.

The measurement of estrogens, in particular urinary estriol, has been utilized to monitor fetal well-being in high-risk pregnancies. There are several disorders in addition to fetal distress that lead to low urinary excretion of estriol by the mother. The most notable of these conditions to *placental sulfatase deficiency,* also known as *steroid sulfatase deficiency syndrome,* which is an X-linked inherited metabolic disorder characterized during fetal life by decreased maternal estriol production due to deficient placental sulfatase (see Fig. 11-5). In this disorder, the placenta is un-

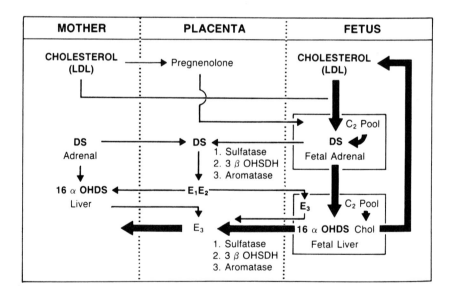

Fig. 11-5 Sources of estrogen biosynthesis in the maternal–fetal–placental unit. LDL, low-density lipoprotein; Chol, cholesterol; C_2 pool, carbon–carbon unit; DS, dehydroepiandrosterone sulfate; E_1, estrone; E_2, estradiol-17β; E_3, estriol; 3β OHSDH, 3β-hydroxysteroidehydrogenase. (Adapted from Carr BR, and Gant NF: The endocrinology of pregnancy-induced hypertension. Clin Perinatol 10:737, 1983.)

able to cleave the sulfate moiety from DHEA-S and, consequently, the levels of maternal estrogens, particularly estriol, are quite low. Placental sulfatase deficiency is also associated with prolonged gestation and difficulty in cervical dilatation at term, often requiring cesarean section. Steroid sulfatase deficiency is thought to occur in 1 of every 2000–6000 newborns. The male offspring are, of course, sulfatase deficient and they have a characteristic skin condition termed *ichthyosis,* which is first apparent after the first few months of life.

The ultimate destination of estrogen and progesterone secretion by the placenta is primarily the maternal compartment. The physiological role of the large quantity of estrogen produced by the placenta of women is not completely understood. It has been proposed that estrogen may regulate or fine-tune the events leading to parturition as pregnancies are often prolonged when estrogen levels in maternal blood and urine are low, as in placental sulfatase deficiency or when associated with anencephaly. Estrogen stimulates phospholipid synthesis and turnover, increases incorporation of arachidonic acid into phospholipids, stimulates prostaglandin synthesis, and increases the number of lysosomes in uterine endometrium. Estrogens are known to increase uterine blood flow and may also play a role in fetal organ maturation and development.

Human Chorionic Gonadotropin (hCG)

Human chorionic gonadotropin is secreted by the syncytiotrophoblast of the placenta into both the fetal and maternal circulation. It is a glycoprotein with a molecular weight of about 38,000 that consists of two noncovalently linked subunits, α and β, and is similar to LH in structure and action. Human chorionic gonadotropin has been used extensively as a pregnancy test and can be detected in serum as early as 6–8 days following ovulation. Plasma levels rise rapidly in normal pregnancy, doubling in concentration every 2–3 days until they reach a peak between 60 and 90 days of gestation. Thereafter, the concentration of hCG in maternal plasma declines, plateauing at about 120 days before delivery. The levels of hCG are higher in multiple pregnancies, in pregnancies associated with Rh isoimmunization, and in pregnant diabetic women; they are highest in pregnancies associated with hydatidiform moles and in women with a tumor known as choriocarcinoma.

There is some evidence that the regulation of the rate of secretion of hCG by the syncytiotrophoblastic cells may be a paracrine mechanism involving the release of LHRH by the cytotrophoblast. Activin and inhibin as well as the transforming growth factors α and β secreted by the trophoblastic cells also appear to regulate hCG secretion. Fetal concentrations of hCG reach a peak at 11–14 weeks' gestation and thereafter fall progressively until delivery.

Various theories have been proposed as to the functional role of hCG in pregnancy. The most widely accepted theory is that hCG maintains the early corpus luteum of pregnancy to ensure continued progesterone secretion by the ovary until this function is replaced by the growing trophoblast. Some investigators have demonstrated that hCG promotes steroidogenesis (namely progesterone) by the trophoblast. It is most likely that a primary role for hCG in the fetus is to regulate the development and the secretion of testosterone by the fetal tests. Male sexual differentiation occurs at an early but critical time in development when fetal serum hCG levels are high and fetal plasma LH levels are low. It has been suggested that hCG may affect

fetal ovarian development as well. An additional role may be to give immunological privilege to the developing trophoblast. Finally, several investigators have demonstrated that the excess thyrotropic activity during the clinical development of
hyperthyroidism observed in some women with neoplastic trophoblast disease results from excessive hCG secretion. Both TSH and hCG have similar structures, and
purified hCG inhibits binding to thyroid membranes and stimulates adenylate cyclase in thyroid tissues.

Human Placental Lactogen (hPL)

Human placental lactogen is a single-chain polypeptide consisting of 191 amino
acid residues that has a molecular weight of about 22,000. As its name suggests,
hPL has both lactogenic and growth hormone-like activity and is also referred to as
chorionic growth hormone or *chorionic somatomammotropin.* Human placental
lactogen mainly exhibits lactogenic activity: it has only 3% or less of the growth-
stimulating activity of human growth hormone (GH). The structure and amino
acid–base residues of hPL, prolactin, and GH are quite similar.

Human placental lactogen is secreted by syncytiotrophoblast and can be detected in serum by radioimmunoassay as early as the third week after ovulation.
The plasma level of hPL continues to rise with advancing gestational age, unlike
hCG, and appears to plateau at term. The concentration of hPL in serum is closely
correlated with increasing placental weight. Its half-life in serum is short. Although
the level of hPL in serum before delivery is the highest of all the protein hormones secreted by the placenta, it cannot be detected in serum after the first postpartum day. The time sequence and peak of hPL secretion are significantly different
from that of hCG, which suggests a different regulation for each hormone. This
is interesting as both are secreted by the syncytiotrophoblast rather than the
cytotrophoblast.

Interestingly, hPL appears to be secreted primarily into the maternal circulation because very low levels are observed in cord blood of newborns. Thus, most
of the proposed physiological roles of hPL have centered around its sites of action
in maternal tissues. Human placental lactogen may have a major sparing influence
on maternal glucose, providing adequate, continued nutrition for the developing fetus. It has been suggested that hPL exerts metabolic effects in pregnancy similar to
those of GH. These effects include stimulation of lipolysis, resulting in increased
circulating free fatty acids (which are available for maternal and fetal nutrition), inhibition of glucose uptake in the mother, resulting in increased maternal insulin levels, development of maternal insulin resistance, and an inhibition of gluconeogenesis
that favors transportation of glucose and protein to the fetus.

A "true" placental growth hormone has been shown to be produced by the syncytiotrophoblast of the placenta and secreted in parallel with hPL. This GH variant
is now recognized to be the product of the hGH-V gene and differs from the major
22-kilodalton (kDa) GH in 13 amino acid residues. A glycosylated variant of this
GH form has also been described in an *in vitro* system, but it is not known if this
form circulates. Because concentrations of the placental GH variant in maternal
plasma correlate with plasma levels of IGF-I, it has been suggested that placental
GH is involved in the control of serum IGF-I levels in normal pregnant women.

Other Placental Peptide and Protein Hormones

In addition to hCG and hPL, several other placental hormones similar or closely related with respect to biological and immunological activity to hypothalamic or pituitary hormones have been reported. These include human chorionic POMC peptides, CRH, growth hormone-releasing hormone (GHRH), human chorionic thyrotropin, and human chorionic gonadotropin-releasing hormone. The regulation of the secretion of these hormones is not well understood, but classical negative feedback inhibition does not appear to exist. Furthermore, the function and significance of these hormones are speculative at best. Most of these hormones are believed to enter primarily the maternal compartment.

Fetal Compartment

The regulation of the fetal endocrine system, as with that of the placenta, is not completely independent but relies to some extent on precursor hormones secreted by the placenta or maternal tissues. As the fetus develops, its endocrine system gradually matures and becomes more independent, preparing the fetus for extrauterine existence. The following section summarizes our present understanding of the fetal endocrine unit and its relationship with the maternal–placental unit.

Fetal Hypothalamic–Pituitary Axis

The fetal hypothalamus begins to differentiate from the forebrain during the first few weeks of fetal life, and by 12 weeks hypothalamic development is well advanced. Most of the hypothalamic-releasing hormones, including LHRH, thyrotropin-releasing hormone (TRH), dopamine, norepinephrine, and somatostatin, as well as their respective hypothalamic nuclei have been identified as early as 6–8 weeks of fetal life. The neurohypophysis is first detected at 5 weeks, and by 14 weeks the supraoptic and paraventricular nuclei are fully developed.

Rathke's pouch first appears in the human fetus at 4 weeks of fetal life. The premature anterior pituitary cells that develop from the cells lining Rathke's pouch are capable of secreting GH, PRL, FSH, LH, an ACTH *in vitro* as early as 7 weeks of fetal life. Recent evidence suggests that the intermediate lobe of the pituitary may be a significant source of POMC hormones. The intermediate pituitary lobe in the human fetus decreases in size after birth, with only remnants remaining in the adult.

The hypothalamo-hypophyseal portal system is the functional link between the hypothalamus and the anterior pituitary. Vascularization of the anterior pituitary starts by 13 weeks of fetal life, but a functioning intact portal system is not present until 18–20 weeks of fetal life. Indirect evidence, however, shows that hypothalamic secretion of releasing hormones may influence anterior pituitary function before 18–20 weeks by simple diffusion as a result of their close proximity in early fetal development.

Fetal growth hormone is detected in the human pituitary as early as 12 weeks; fetal pituitary GH content increases until 25–30 weeks of gestation and thereafter remains constant until term. In contrast, fetal plasma GH levels rise to a peak at 20 weeks of fetal life and thereafter fall rapidly until birth. Fetal plasma concentrations of GH, however, are higher than maternal concentrations at all ages. Maternal levels may be suppressed by the high circulating levels of hPL. The regulation of GH release in the fetus appears to be more complex than in the adult. To explain the high levels of fetal GH at mid-gestation and the fall thereafter, unrestrained release of GHRH or inhibition of somatostatin release leading to excessive release of GH at mid-gestation has been hypothesized. As the hypothalamus matures, somatostatin may increase and GHRH levels decline so that GH release also declines. The role of GH in the fetus is unclear as well. Considerable evidence indicates that GH is not essential to intrauterine somatic growth in primates. In newborns with pituitary agenesis, congenital hypothalamic hypopituitarism or familial GH deficiency, birth weight, and length are usually normal. However, a class of peptides known as *somatomedins,* in particular insulin-like growth factors (IGF-I and IGF-II), increase in fetal plasma and IGF-I and IGF-II levels correlate better with fetal growth than GH levels. Although GH is an important trophic hormone for somatomedin production in the fetus, somatomedin regulation may be independent of GH.

Prolactin is present in pituitary lactotropes by 19 weeks of life. Fetal prolactin content in the pituitary increases throughout gestation. Fetal prolactin plasma levels increase slowly until 30 weeks' gestation, after which the levels rise sharply until term and remain elevated until the third month of postnatal life. Both TRH and dopamine, as well as estrogens, appear to affect human fetal prolactin secretion. Regulation of prolactin secretion by dopamine in the fetus is supported by the observation that the dopamine agonist, bromocriptine, when ingested by the mother, crosses the placenta and inhibits prolactin release from the fetal pituitary gland, lowering prolactin levels in fetal blood. It has been suggested that prolactin influences fetal adrenal growth, fetal lung maturation, and amnionic fluid volume.

Arginine vasopressin (AVP) and oxytocin are found in hypothalamic nuclei and in the neurohypophysis during early fetal development. But there have been relatively few studies of the regulation and secretion of these hormones in the fetus. The levels of AVP have been reported to be high in fetal plasma and newborn cord blood at delivery. The main stimulus to AVP release seems to be fetal hypoxia, although acidosis, hypercarbia, and hypotension also play a role. The elevated AVP level in fetal blood may lead to increased blood pressure, vasoconstriction, and the passage of meconium by the fetus. In contrast, oxytocin levels in the fetus are not affected by hypoxia but appear to increase during labor and delivery.

Fetal Thyroid Gland

Evidence suggests that the placenta is relatively impermeable to TSH and thyroid hormone so that the fetal hypothalamic–pituitary–thyroid axis appears to develop and function independently of the maternal system.

By the end of the first trimester, the fetal thyroid has developed sufficiently to be able to concentrate iodine and synthesize iodothyronines. The levels of TSH and thyroid hormone are relatively low in fetal blood until mid-gestation (Fig. 11-6). At 24–28 weeks' gestation, serum TSH concentrations rise abruptly to a peak and decrease slightly thereafter until delivery. In response to the surge of TSH, thyroxine (T_4) levels rise progressively after mid-gestation until term. During this time, the pituitary becomes more responsive to TRH, and an increase in hypothalamic TRH content occurs. At birth there is an abrupt release of TSH, T_4, and triiodothyronine (T_3), followed by a fall in the levels of these hormones shortly thereafter. This brief

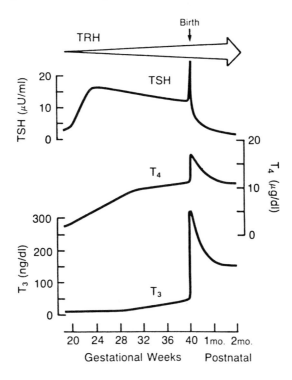

Fig. 11-6 Maturation of serum TSH, thyroxine (T_4), and triiodothyronine (T_3) during the last half of gestation and during early neonatal life. The increase in TRH effect or content is also illustrated. (From Fisher DA: Maternal–fetal thyroid function in pregnancy. Clin Perinatol 10:615, 1983. Reproduced with permission of W. B. Saunders Company.)

thyroid excess is believed to facilitate thermoregulatory adjustments for extrauterine life. The abrupt increases in TSH and T_4 that occur at birth are thought to be stimulated by the cooling process associated with delivery. Finally, 3,3′,5′-triiodothyronine (reverse T_3) levels are high during early fetal life and begin to fall at mid-gestation and continue to fall after birth. The difference between the formation of T_3 and reverse T_3 is thought to be related to maturation of peripheral iodothyronine metabolism.

Fetal Gonads
Biologically active and immunoreactive LHRH has been detected in the fetal hypothalamus by 9–12 weeks of age. The hypothalamic content of LHRH has been reported to increase with fetal age, maximal content being noted between 22 and 25 weeks in females and between 34 and 38 weeks in males. The dominant gonadotropin fraction in the fetal pituitary is the α-subunit. However, the fetal pituitary is capable of secreting intact LH *in vitro* by 5–7 weeks. The plasma concentration of FSH in the human fetal plasma slowly rises and reaches a peak near the twenty-fifth week of fetal life and falls to low levels by term. Plasma FSH levels parallel the pituitary content of FSH with respect to sexual dimorphism, circu-

lating FSH levels being higher in females than in males. The pattern of LH levels in fetal plasma parallels that of FSH. The fall in gonadotropin pituitary content and plasma concentration after mid-gestation is believed to result from the maturation of the hypothalamus. The hypothalamus also becomes more sensitive to sex steroids circulating in fetal blood, originating from the placenta.

In the male, fetal testosterone secretion begins soon after differentiation of the gonad into a testis and formation of Leydig cells at 7 weeks of fetal life. Maximal levels of fetal testosterone are observed at about 15 weeks and decrease thereafter. The early secretion of testosterone is important in initiating sexual differentiation in the male (see Chapter 8). It is believed that the primary stimulus to the early development and growth of Leydig cells and subsequent peak of testosterone is hCG. Thus, it appears that sexual differentiation of the male does not rely solely on fetal pituitary gonadotropins. However, fetal LH and FSH are still required for complete differentiation of the fetal ovary and testes. For example, male fetuses with abnormal brain formation (anencephaly), with low levels of circulating LH and FSH, secrete testosterone normally at 15–20 weeks because of adequate levels of hCG, but they have a decreased number of Leydig cells, exhibit hypoplastic external genitalia, and often have undescended testes. Likewise, male fetuses with congenital hypopituitarism often have small phalluses. These observations suggest that around and after mid-gestation, fetal pituitary gonadotropins affect testosterone secretion from the fetal testes.

The fetal ovary is involved primarily in the formation of follicles and germ cells. Although follicular development in the ovary appears to be relatively independent of gonadotropins, the anencephalic female fetus with small ovaries and a decreased number of ovarian follicles suggests some pituitary involvement (however, the fetal ovaries do not contain hCG [LH] receptors, at least by 20 weeks of gestation). The ovaries appear to be relatively inactive with respect to steroidogenesis during fetal life but are capable of aromatizing androgens to estrogens *in vitro* as early as 8 weeks of gestation.

Fetal Adrenal Gland

Of all the endocrine glands in the human fetus, the adrenal has aroused the greatest interest. The human fetal adrenal glands secrete large quantities of steroid hormones, up to 200 mg of steroid daily near term. This rate of steroidogenesis may be five times that observed in the adrenal glands of adults at rest. The principal steroids found in the fetus are C-19 steroids (mainly DHEA-S), which serve as precursor substrate for estrogen biosynthesis in the placenta.

At the beginning of this century, investigators observed that the human fetal adrenal gland contained a unique fetal zone that accounts for the rapid growth of the fetal adrenal and that this zone disappears during the first few weeks after birth. This fetal zone differs histologically and biochemically from the neocortex (also known as the *definitive* or *adult zone*). The uniqueness of a transient fetal zone has been reported in certain higher primates and some other rare species, but only humans possess the extremely large fetal zone that involutes after birth.

The cells of the adrenal cortex arise from coelomic epithelium. The cells comprising the fetal zone can be identified in the 8 to 10 mm embryo and before the appearance of the cells of the neocortex (14 mm embryo). Growth is most rapid during the last 6 weeks of fetal life. By 28 weeks' gestation, the adrenal gland may be as large as the fetal kidney, and by term may be equal to the size of the adult adrenal. The fetal zone accounts for the largest percentage of growth, and after birth the adrenal gland decreases in size due to involution and necrosis of fetal zone cells (Fig. 11-7).

Studies of the fetal adrenal gland have attempted to determine what factors stimulate and regulate its growth and steroidogenesis and why the fetal zone undergoes atrophy after delivery. All investigations have shown that ACTH stimulates steroidogenesis *in vitro*. Furthermore, clinical evidence shows that ACTH is the major trophic hormone of the fetal adrenal gland *in vivo*. In anencephalic fetuses the plasma levels of ACTH are very low and the fetal zone is markedly atrophic. Maternal glucocorticosteroid therapy effectively suppresses fetal adrenal steroidogenesis by suppressing fetal ACTH secretion. Further evidence that ACTH regulates steroidogenesis early in fetal life is provided by the observation that elevated levels of 17α-hydroxyprogesterone in amnionic fluid are found in fetuses with congenital adrenal hyperplasia due to the absence of 21-hydroxylase activity. Despite these observations, other ACTH-related peptides, POMC derivatives that are formed in the fetal pituitary or placenta, have been proposed as possible trophic hormones for the fetal zone, but the evidence for this proposal is weak. Other hormones or growth factors, including prolactin, hCG, GH, hPL, and epidermal and fibroblast growth factor, have no consistent significant effect on steroidogenesis or adenylyl cyclase activity in preparations of fetal zone organ cultures, monolayer cells, or membrane preparations *in vitro*. However, the role of these or other hormones in promoting growth of adrenal cells is unclear.

After birth the adrenal gland shrinks by over 50% owing to regression of fetal zone cells. This suggests that a trophic substance other than ACTH is withdrawn

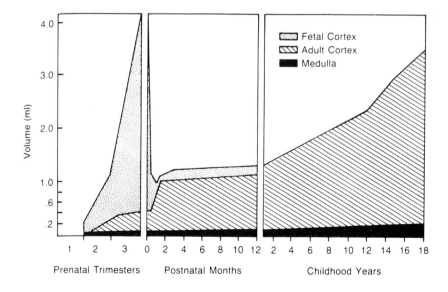

Fig. 11-7 Size of the adrenal gland and its component parts during fetal life, infancy, and childhood. (Adapted from Carr BR, and Simpson ER: Endocr Rev 2:306, 1981.)

from the maternal or placental compartment or that the secretion rates of some other trophic hormone is altered to initiate regression of the fetal zone.

The medulla of the fetal adrenal gland is formed by 10 weeks of gestation. In contrast to the fetal adrenal cortex, the adrenal medulla is relatively immature at term. The secretion of cortisol by the adrenal cortex that surrounds the medulla stimulates the formation of epinephrine from norepinephrine. However, most of the chromaffin tissue in the human fetus is formed in para-aortic paraganglia rather than in fetal adrenal medullary tissue. Both epinephrine and norepinephrine can be detected in the human fetal medulla by 10–15 weeks' gestation. Except for the effect of cortisol, the regulation of catecholamine secretion in the human fetus has not been fully elucidated. In other species, hypoxia and trauma, as well as advancing gestation and maturation, are related to the release of catecholamines by the adrenal medulla.

Fetal Parathyroid Gland and Calcium Homeostasis
The level of calcium in the fetus is regulated largely by the transfer of calcium from the maternal compartment across the placenta. The maternal compartment undergoes a number of adjustments that ultimately allow for a net transfer of sufficient calcium to the fetus to sustain fetal bone growth.

The changes in the maternal compartment that permit fetal accumulation of calcium include an increase in maternal dietary intake, an increase in circulating maternal 1,25-dihydroxyvitamin D [1,25-$(OH)_2$D], and an increase in circulating parathyroid hormone (PTH). No significant changes are observed in maternal calcitonin levels. The levels of total calcium and phosphorus decline in maternal serum, but ionized calcium levels remain unchanged. The "placental calcium pump" allows for a positive gradient of calcium and phosphorus to the fetus. Circulating fetal calcium and phosphorus levels increase steadily throughout gestation. Fetal levels of total and ionized calcium as well as phosphorus exceed maternal levels at term.

The fetal parathyroid gland contains PTH, and the gland is capable of hormone secretion by 10–12 weeks' gestation. Fetal plasma levels at PTH reportedly are low but increase after delivery. The fetal thyroid contains calcitonin, and in contrast to maternal plasma levels, calcitonin levels in the fetus are elevated. Because there is no transfer of PTH or calcitonin across the placenta, the consequences of the observed change in these hormones on fetal calcium are consistent with an adaptation to conserve and stimulate bone growth within the fetus.

Plasma levels of the various forms of vitamin D are lower in the fetus than in the mother. The placenta and decidua are capable of 1α-hydroxylation and of formation of the active metabolite 1,25-$(OH)_2$D. However, the role, if any, of this hormone in the fetus is unknown as its major effect is on intestinal absorption of calcium.

After birth, serum calcium and phosphorus levels fall in the neonate, PTH levels begin to rise 48 hours after birth, and calcium and phosphorus levels gradually increase over the following several days, depending on dietary intake of milk.

Fetal Endocrine Pancreas
The human fetal pancreas appears during the fourth week of fetal life. The α-cells containing glucagon and the δ-cells containing somatostatin develop early, before β-cell differentiation, although insulin can be recognized in the developing pancreas

before apparent β-cell differentiation. Total human pancreatic insulin and glucagon content increase with fetal age and are higher than the concentrations in the adult human pancreas.

In contrast to the pancreatic content of insulin, fetal insulin secretion is low and relatively unresponsive to acute changes in glucose in *in vitro* studies of pancreatic cells, in cord blood at delivery, and in blood samples obtained from the scalp of the fetus at term. In contrast, fetal insulin secretion *in vitro* is responsive to amino acids and glucagon as early as 14 weeks of gestation. Although the acute response to glucose is impaired in the fetal pancreas, β-cells that are chronically exposed to elevated glucose levels, as may occur in maternal diabetes mellitus, undergo hypertrophy so that the rate of insulin secretion increases.

Glucagon has been detected in human fetal plasma as early as 15 weeks' gestation. Although secretion of glucagon is stimulated in late pregnancy by amino acids and catecholamines, acute changes in glucose appear to have little effect on fetal pancreatic glucagon secretion.

Maternal Compartment

Various maternal adaptations involving the endocrine system occur during pregnancy. Many diseases of the maternal endocrine system, if untreated, are associated with infertility and reduced conception rates. If conception occurs, the more serious the disorder, the more likely it will affect the fetus adversely, as in diabetes mellitus. Hormones or drugs used to treat the endocrine disorders may be transported across the placenta and alter the environment and development of the fetus.

Hypothalamus and Pituitary

Little is known about the endocrine alterations of the maternal hypothalamus during pregnancy. Tumors of the hypothalamus or functional disorders of the hypothalamus commonly result in infertility due to amenorrhea and resulting chronic anovulation. The anterior pituitary undergoes a 2- to 3-fold enlargement during pregnancy due primarily to hyperplasia and hypertrophy of the lactotrophs (prolactin-secreting cells) thought to result from estrogen stimulation. Thus, prolactin plasma levels parallel the increase in pituitary size throughout gestation.

In contrast to lactotrophs, the number of somatotropic cells in the pituitary decreases during pregnancy. Maternal levels of GH are low and do not change during pregnancy. Maternal levels of LH and FSH levels are also low during pregnancy. The response of gonadotropins to an infusion of LHRH is severely blunted during pregnancy. The loss of responsiveness to LHRH is thought to be caused by a negative feedback inhibition from the elevated levels of estrogen and progesterone during pregnancy. Levels of TSH are within the normal nonpregnant adult range throughout pregnancy. Furthermore, the response of TSH to a dose of TRH is similar to that in nonpregnant women.

Numerous studies have examined the levels of ACTH- and POMC-related peptides in maternal blood throughout pregnancy. The maternal plasma levels of β-endorphin remain relatively low throughout pregnancy. β-Endorphin levels do increase in maternal blood with advancing labor, but β-endorphin levels in cord blood are similar in infants delivered vaginally and delivered by elective cesarean section from women not in labor. However, fetal hypoxia is associated with significant increases in β-endorphin levels in cord blood. The plasma levels of maternal ACTH have been reported to increase from early to late gestation, but values were either in the normal range or lower than in nonpregnant women, suggesting that ACTH may be suppressed by estrogen and progesterone. The slight increases in ACTH levels that appear to occur during the course of gestation might be explained by the increased secretion of placental ACTH that is not subject to feedback control. Maternal ACTH rises to very high levels during labor and delivery. The levels of ACTH in umbilical cord plasma parallel those of β-endorphin and, because neither crosses the placenta, offer further evidence that in the fetus as in adults these two peptides are processed from a common precursor. CRH increases in maternal serum throughout pregnancy. This is due to an increase of CRH synthesis by the placenta. However, as there is also an increase in carrier protein, which binds CRH, CRH probably exhibits little biologic activity.

Maternal plasma AVP levels remain low throughout gestation and are not believed to play a role in human parturition. Maternal oxytocin levels are reported to be low and do not vary throughout pregnancy but increase during the later stages of labor.

Thyroid

The thyroid gland increases slightly in size during pregnancy as a result of increased vascularity and mild glandular hyperplasia, but a true goiter is not present. There is a modest increase in oxygen consumption (basal metabolic rate) during pregnancy secondary to fetal requirements.

During pregnancy the mother is in a euthyroid state. Serum total T_4 and T_3 increase markedly but do not indicate a hyperthyroid state as there is a parallel increase in thyroxine-binding globulin (TBG). The elevation of total T_4 and T_3 is due to increased TBG from estrogen exposure. A similar finding is observed in women on oral contraceptives. A reduced T_3-resin uptake is also observed in pregnancy and in women on oral contraceptives. The levels of free T_3 and T_4, however, are not increased in pregnancy. There is little if any transfer of T_4, T_3, or TSH across the placenta. TRH is capable of crossing the placenta, but under normal physical conditions there is little TRH circulating in peripheral maternal plasma.

Adrenal

Compared to changes in the fetal adrenal, the maternal adrenal gland does not change morphologically during pregnancy. During pregnancy plasma adrenal steroid hormones increase with advancing gestation.

The increase in total plasma cortisol is due principally to a concomitant increase in cortisol-binding globulin (CBG), also known as *transcortin*. There is a slight increase in free plasma cortisol and urinary-free cortisol, but pregnant women do not exhibit any overt signs of hypercortisolism.

Aldosterone levels increase with advancing gestation, reflecting an increased secretion rate of aldosterone by the zona glomerulosa. The levels of renin and angiotensinogen rise in pregnancy, which leads to elevated angiotensin II levels and markedly elevated levels of aldosterone.

Parathyroid

Calcium and parathyroid hormone changes during normal pregnancy were discussed in the fetal parathyroid section of this chapter.

Endocrine Pancreas

The metabolic adaptation of pregnancy in which glucose is spared for the fetus is related to an appropriate bihormonal secretion by the maternal endocrine pancreas. In response to a glucose load, there is a greater release of insulin from the β-cells and a greater suppression of glucagon release from the α-cells compared to the non-pregnant state. In association with the increased release of insulin, the maternal pancreas undergoes β-cell hyperplasia and islet cell hypertrophy, accompanied by an increase in blood flow to the endocrine pancreas. During pregnancy, fasting blood glucose levels fall, but rise more in response to a glucose load than in nonpregnant women. The increased release of insulin is related to a relative insulin resistance. The insulin resistance is due to hormones secreted by the placenta that spare transfer of glucose to the fetus. Glucagon levels are suppressed in response to a glucose load, with the greatest suppression occurring near term.

Endocrinology of Parturition

The mechanism by which labor is initiated in women is not completely understood. It is of vital importance that the etiology of the onset of parturition is clarified so as to eventually prevent preterm birth. The sequelae of prematurity includes not only increased fetal and neonatal mortality, but significant morbidity that can result in severe physical and mental impairment of the newborn. Several theories involving endocrine changes in the fetal–placental unit have been proposed to explain the onset of labor. However, our present knowledge in human pregnancy is fragmented.

Oxytocin

Oxytocin has been used in clinical obstetrics for years to induce or augment labor. When sensitive radioimmunoassays became available to detect low levels of oxytocin in maternal and fetal blood, it was determined that oxytocin levels do not rise before the onset of labor. The role of oxytocin is believed to be the regulation of the expulsive phase of labor and contraction of the uterus to reduce blood loss following delivery.

Relaxin

Relaxin is a large polypeptide that is synthesized by the corpus luteum and the decidua. Relaxin ripens the cervix in various animal species. In many mammals, a significant increase in circulating level of relaxin occurs prior to parturition. In humans, the level of plasma relaxin is highest in the first trimester of pregnancy but declines and thereafter remains constant until delivery. Relaxin has been reported to decrease myometrial contractility *in vitro*.

Progesterone Withdrawal

In most, if not all mammalian species, a decline in maternal levels of progesterone precedes the onset of parturition. In both primates and humans, however, there is no significant decrease in plasma progesterone levels before labor. Some investigators have reported a decrease in the number of myometrial progesterone receptors just prior to delivery.

Fetal Adrenal

The cause of labor in certain mammalian species, such as sheep, appears to be regulated by signals first occurring in the fetal pituitary (ACTH), which lead to increased cortisol secretion by the fetal sheep adrenal gland. In turn, increased fetal cortisol levels stimulate 17α-hydroxylase activity in sheep placenta leading to decreased progesterone and increased estrogen production, which triggers the onset of labor. Administration of corticoids or ACTH to the sheep fetus stimulates labor and the removal of the fetal pituitary or adrenal prolongs labor.

In the human, however, the role of fetal adrenal steroid secretion on the onset of labor is less clear. For example, cortisol or ACTH administration to mother or fetus does not stimulate parturition. Fetal plasma levels of cortisol do not increase markedly before labor. In contrast, conditions that result in low levels of estrogen in the maternal compartment are often accompanied by prolonged or postdate pregnancy, failure of cervical ripening, or poor cervical dilation during labor. Such conditions include anencephaly or failure of brain development, congenital absence or hypoplasia of the fetal adrenal, and steroid sulfatase deficiency. In each of these cases, inadequate fetal adrenal hormone precursor is available for placental aromatization to estrogen. In addition, local application of estrogen to the cervix leads to ripening.

It is believed that estrogen derived from fetal adrenal precursors does not directly cause the onset of labor, but instead may modify or fine-tune other events leading to the onset of parturition. One of the effects of estrogen is the stimulation of prostaglandin synthesis in the tissues of the uterus and fetal membranes.

Prostaglandin

Because of the complexities and discrepancies of parturition in different mammalian species, a paracrine mechanism has been proposed to explain the onset of parturition in humans. This mechanism is related to the close proximity of the fetus, amnionic fluid, fetal membranes (amnion and chorion), and contiguous layer of uterine decidua and myometrium. Signals not yet identified, originating in the fetus, may by a paracrine mechanism be transmitted to fetal membranes and uterine tissues, leading to increased production of prostaglandin. Accumulating evidence suggests that prostaglandins and prostanoids play a crucial role in human parturition. The trigger for release of prostaglandins is unknown, but is thought to be of fetal origin and regulated by hormone changes in the fetal–placental–maternal unit.

Prostaglandins, when administered to pregnant women, cause cervical ripening, softening, dilation, and the onset of uterine contractions resulting in labor. The administration of prostaglandin inhibitors to pregnant women prevents or averts preterm labor. Moreover, marked increases occur in the levels of prostaglandins in amnionic fluid and in fetal membranes before the onset of labor. Injury to the fetal membranes resulting in increased prostaglandin release results from uterine infections, stripping of the membranes from the cervix, and the installation of hypertonic saline into the amnionic sac.

SUGGESTED READING

Brody SA, and Ueland K: *Endocrine Disorders in Pregnancy,* Appleton & Lange, Norwalk, CT, 1989.

Byrd W: Fertilization, embryogenesis, and implantation. In: *Textbook of Reproductive Medicine, 2nd ed.,* BR Carr and RE Blackwell, eds., Appleton & Lange, Stamford, CT, pp 1–20, 1998.

Carr BR: The endocrinology of pregnancy: The maternal–fetal–placental unit: In: *Principles and Practice of Endocrinology and Metabolism,* 3rd ed., KL Becker, ed., Lippincott, Philadelphia, 2000 (in press).

Carr BR, and Rainey WE: The adrenal. In: *Infertility and Reproductive Medicine Clinics of North America,* Vol. 5, JP Bruner, ed., Saunders, Philadelphia, pp. 749–764, 1994.

Carr BR, and Simpson ER: Lipoprotein utilization and cholesterol synthesis by the human fetal adrenal gland: Endocr Rev 2:306–326, 1981.

Casey ML, and MacDonald PC. Endocrine changes of pregnancy. In: *Williams Textbook of Endocrinology,* 9th ed., JD Wilson, DW Foster, HM Kronenberg, and PR Larsen, eds., Saunders, Philadelphia, pp. 1259–1271, 1998.

Cunningham FG, MacDonald PC, Gant NF, Leveno KJ, Gilstrap LC, Hankins GDV, and Clark SC: *Williams Obstetrics,* Appleton & Lange, Stamford, CT, pp. 69–226, 1997.

Fisher DA: Endocrinology of fetal development. In: *Williams Textbook of Endocrinology,* 9th ed., JD Wilson, DW Foster, HM Kronenberg, and PR Larsen, eds., Saunders, Philadelphia, pp. 1273–1301, 1998.

Harper MJK: Gamete and zygote transport. In: *The Physiology of Reproduction,* Vol. 1, E Knobill and JD Neill, eds., 2nd ed., Raven Press, New York, pp. 127–188, 1994.

Knobil E, and Neill JD. *Encyclopedia of Reproduction,* Vols. 1–4. Academic Press, San Diego, 1998.

Laufer N, Gunfeld L, and Garrise C: In-vitro fertilization. In: *Infertility,* MM Seibil, ed., Appleton & Lange, Norwalk, CT, pp. 481–511, 1990.

Meldrum DR, Chetkouski R, Steingold KA, de Zeigler D, Cedars MI, and Hamilton M: Evolution of a highly successful in vitro fertilization embryo transfer program. Fertil Steril 48:86–93, 1987.

Parker CR Jr: The endocrinology of pregnancy. In: *Textbook of Reproductive Medicine,* 2nd ed., BR Carr and RE Blackwell, eds., Appleton & Lange, Stamford, CT, pp. 19–44, 1998.

Pederson RA, and Burdsal CA: Mammalian embryogenesis. In: *The Physiology of Reproduction,* 2nd ed., Vol. 1, E Knobil and JD Neill, eds., Raven Press, New York, pp. 319–390, 1994.

Steinkampf MP, Davis OK, and Rosenwaks Z: Assisted reproductive technology. In: *Textbook of Reproductive Medicine,* B Carr and R Blackwell eds., Appleton & Lange, Stamford, CT, pp. 665–678, 1998.

Tulchinsky D, and Little AB, eds: *Maternal–Fetal Endocrinology,* Saunders, Philadelphia, 1994.

Veech LI: *Atlas of the Human Oocyte and Early Conceptus,* Williams & Wilkins, Baltimore, 1986.

Wassarman PM: Fertilization in mammals. Sci Am 259:78–84, 1988.

Weitauf HM: Biology of implantation. In: *The Physiology of Reproduction,* 2nd ed., Vol. 1, E Knobil and JD Neill, eds., Raven Press, New York, pp. 391–440, 1994.

Word RA: Parturition. In: *Textbook of Reproductive Medicine,* 2nd ed., BR Carr and RE Blackwell, eds., Appleton & Lange, Stamford, CT, pp. 45–56, 1998.

Yanagimachi R: Mammalian fertilization. In: *The Physiology of Reproduction,* 2nd ed., Vol. 1, E Knobil and JD Neill, eds., Raven Press, New York, pp. 189–318, 1994.

12

Growth Regulation

PINCHAS COHEN
RON G. ROSENFELD

ENDOCRINE REGULATION OF GROWTH

Growth Hormone Secretion and Action

Although multiple hormones influence somatic growth, the main regulator of post-natal growth is growth hormone (GH), which is secreted in a pulsatile manner from the anterior pituitary primarily as a 22-kilodalton (kDa) molecule (although other forms may be found). GH gene expression is regulated by the pituitary transcription factors *Pit-1* and *Prop-1*. Under normal waking conditions, GH levels are often low or undetectable, but several times during the day, and particularly at night during phase 3 of sleep, surges of GH secretion occur. GH secretion is mainly under hypothalamic control, which in turn is regulated by catecholamin-ergic neurotransmitters from higher cortical centers. The hypothalamic hormones, growth hormone releasing hormone (GHRH) and somatostatin, stimulate and in-hibit GH secretion, respectively (see Chapter 6). In addition, growth hormone re-leasing peptides (GHRP) also stimulate GH secretion. Many other factors influence this interaction, notably glucose, which inhibits, and certain amino acids, which stimulate GH secretion. Exogenous physiological and pharmacological factors are known to stimulate GH secretion. Indeed, some of these agents, which include clonidine, L-dopa, and the amino acid arginine, are used in GH stimulation tests. In plasma the majority of GH is bound to a carrier protein termed *GH-binding protein,* which is the extracellular domain of the GH receptor. GH binds to its re-ceptor and mediates a cascade of cellular events. First, dimerization of the GH re-ceptor occurs, followed by the activation of a specific kinase, JAK-2 linked to signal transducers and activators of transcription (STAT) signaling. These events lead to the activation of insulin-like growth factor (IGF)-I gene transcription and modulation of gene expression of other metabolic and growth-regulatory molecules.

The Somatomedin Hypothesis

In the liver and other target cells (such as bone), through interaction with its re-ceptor, GH induces the production of *somatomedins,* or *insulin-like growth factors* (IGF-I and IGF-II). The IGFs are found in plasma bound to a family of proteins

most important

called *IGF-binding proteins* (IGFBPs). The majority of IGFs are bound to IGFBP-3, which, together with a third protein known as the *acid labile subunit* (ALS), form a ternary complex in serum. The somatomedins, particularly IGF-I (previously known as SM-C), are thought to interact with target organs, such as growing cartilage to induce growth; they may also feed back on the pituitary to inhibit GH secretion. Both IGFs and their main serum binding proteins (IGFBP-3 and ALS) are reduced in GH deficiency and elevated in conditions of GH excess. As IGF therapy of humans has shown, however, not all of the anabolic actions of GH are mediated by the somatomedins. This cascade of growth control, known as the *somatomedin hypothesis,* is summarized in Figure 12-1

Additional Growth Regulators

Other endocrine factors that are involved in the regulation of growth include thyroid hormone, which is essential for normal linear skeletal growth, and glucocorticoids, which can stunt growth when present in excess. Sex steroids, through several direct and indirect mechanisms, can accelerate growth and normally facilitate the pubertal growth spurt. When these are present in excess at an earlier age, the resulting acceleration of growth is associated with premature closure of the epiphysis and reduced adult height. This effect has been demonstrated as being mediated by estrogen, regardless of the gender of the individual. Parathyroid hormone and vita-

Fig. 12-1 Diagram showing regulation of growth. Growth hormone (GH) secretion is regulated by growth hormone–releasing hormone (GHRH), growth hormone-releasing peptides (GHRP), and somatostatin (SMS). In plasma, GH is bound to the GH-binding protein (GHBP). In the liver, GH mediates secretion of insulin-like growth factor (IGF)-I, IGF-binding protein (IGFBP)-3, and the acid labile subunit (ALS). IGFs mediate growth by binding to the IGF receptor (IGF-R).

min D are essential for normal skeletal ossification, and the absence of or resistance to these agents is associated with abnormal growth patterns. Nonendocrine factors affecting growth are many and incompletely understood; by far the most important are genetic factors, which determine the growth rate, the age of puberty, and adult height. Psychological and social influences can prevent the genetic potential for growth from being fully expressed. Malnutrition, either through dietary deficiencies, malabsorption, or as a manifestation of chronic illness, can interrupt normal growth. Interestingly, GH levels are often elevated in these conditions, but somatomedin levels are depressed.

One critical growth period is the pubertal growth spurt, which is regulated by changes in GH secretion and by modulation of GH action, both related to the effects of sex steroids. Puberty is associated with an increase in the number and amplitude of nightly GH surges and a rise in serum IGF-I, both of which parallel the increase in the growth velocity of puberty (see Chapter 9). This peak height velocity occurs earlier in girls than in boys. Similarly, growth arrest due to epiphyseal fusion occurs earlier in girls. This, and the fact that puberty begins about 6–12 months earlier in girls, accounts for much of the difference in adult heights between men and women. It is interesting that peak height velocity does not parallel the levels of estrogen (which rise later in girls) or testosterone (which rises earlier in boys).

THE IGF AXIS

[handwritten annotation: Causes closure of epiphyseal plate]

Insulin-Like Growth Factors (IGFs) and Their Role in Somatic Growth

Both IGF-I and IGF-II are two closely related peptide hormones of approximately 7 kDa molecular weight. The IGFs were first identified in 1956 and were originally named *sulfation factors* or *somatomedins.* The IGFs belong to a family of peptide hormones that includes relaxin and insulin, and they share a high degree of structural similarity with proinsulin. Like proinsulin, they are composed of A, B, and C domains but also include a D domain, which together form the mature IGF peptide. Both IGF-I and IGF-II are synthesized with an additional extension peptide known as the *E peptide.* In the liver and most other sites of IGF production this peptide is removed as part of the posttranslational processing of IGF-I and IGF-II. Both IGF-I and IGF-II have a complex gene structure, with the IGF-I gene spanning 95 kb (containing 6 exons) at the long arm of chromosome 12, and the IGF-II gene being made up of 9 exons and having a total genomic size of 35 kb. Both genes are subject to multiple splicing, and their mRNA species exist in several different sizes.

The IGFs are important metabolic and mitogenic factors involved in cell growth and metabolism. Produced in the liver, in bone cells, and in other tissues, IGFs are at least partially under GH control. Circulating IGFs have direct (endocrine) effects on somatic growth and on the proliferation of many tissues and cell types, both *in vivo* and *in vitro.* However, the IGFs are also thought to be significant autocrine–paracrine factors involved in cellular proliferation. Locally produced IGFs have been demonstrated in bone, brain, prostate, muscle, mammary tissue, and other sites where they are considered to be responsible for tissue growth and differentiation. About

80% of serum IGF-I levels are hepatic in origin, as evident from specific liver targeting of IGF-I.

The cardinal role of IGF-I and IGF-II in somatic growth has been elegantly determined by gene-targeting models. Mice in which the IGF-II gene has been eliminated by targeted disruption are severely growth retarded *in utero,* being less than half the normal size at birth. After birth, however, IGF-II–lacking mice grow at a near-normal rate, although their size remains small relative to normal littermates. This illustrates the role of IGF-II as a fetal growth factor, with an unclear postnatal role. The IGF-I gene–targeted mice are also very small (40% of normal) at birth but display dramatic growth arrest postnatally. It appears that IGF-I is critical for growth at all stages of development. In comparison, GH deficiency results in normal growth *in utero* and postnatal growth arrest. This indicates that IGF-I is not regulated by GH until the postnatal period, and its expression appears to be under genetic, rather than endocrine, control in the prenatal period. Conversely, IGF-I transgenic mice are larger than normal, as are GH transgenic mice. However, IGF-II transgenic mice do not exhibit rapid growth after birth. The IGFs and their cell surface receptors are depicted schematically in Figure 12-2.

IGF Receptors (IGF-R)

The IGFs interact with specific receptors, designated as *type I* and *type II IGF receptors,* as well as with the insulin receptor. The type I IGF receptor binds IGF-I with high affinity, IGF-II with slightly lower affinity, and insulin with low affinity. The insulin receptor can bind IGF-I and IGF-II, but with much lower affinity than insulin. The type II IGF receptor binds only IGF-II with high affinity (in addition to being a mannose-6-phosphate receptor).

Fig. 12-2 Overview of the insulin-like growth factors (IGF) receptors. The IGFs bind to the type I IGF receptor and similar heterotetramer receptors containing α- and β-subunits and activate a tyrosine kinase (TK), which in turn phosphorylates the insulin-responsive substrates (IRS)-1 and -2. IR, insulin receptor; M6P, mannose-6-phosphate.

The type I IGF receptor and the closely related insulin receptor are heterotetramers composed of two pairs of α- and β-subunits, which result from posttranslational processing of a single gene product that encodes for the entire receptor. The two α-subunits are linked by disulfide bonds and are primarily extracellular; they are involved in ligand binding. The β-subunits are connected to the α-subunit by disulfide bonds and function as intracellular tyrosine kinases. They undergo autophosphorylation after the interaction of the receptors with their ligands, associated by a series of conformational changes.

Subsequently, these kinases appear to phosphorylate cytoplasmic molecules known as the *insulin-responsive substrates* (IRS-1 through -4, of which IRS-1 and IRS-2 are the most important), which are involved in mediating many of the effects of insulin and IGFs. Gene targeting of the type I IGF receptor results in severe *in utero* growth retardation (to 30% of normal) similar to that seen in a double IGF-I/IGF-II gene targeting. These mice and multiple *in vitro* models demonstrate that the mitogenic effects of IGFs are mediated primarily through the type I IGF receptor. The metabolic effects of IGFs are probably mediated through the interactions of IGFs with the insulin receptor, as well as the type I IGF receptor, or may involve insulin-IGF hybrid receptors. Gene targeting of IRS-1 and IRS-2 resulted in an impairment of both growth and carbohydrate metabolism, which are compatible with their role in mediating both insulin and IGF-I effects.

Recent evidence indicates that there is a class of receptors for the IGF family that has biological properties characterized between those of the insulin and the type I IGF receptors. Analysis of tissues where these receptors appear to be common (such as placenta), as well as transfection experiments, revealed that these receptors are composed of one insulin receptor α-β dimer and one type I IGF receptor α-β dimer. This receptor has been labeled the *hybrid receptor* and appears to have high affinity for insulin as well as for IGFs. The physiological role of the hybrid receptor remains elusive, but it may explain the potent insulin-like effects seen with intravenous administration of IGF-I to humans. While IGF-I binds to the insulin receptor with only 1%–2% of the affinity of insulin, it mediates hypoglycemia *in vivo* with 7%–10% the effectivity of insulin.

The cDNA for a newly described member of this family of receptors has been cloned and, owing to the high homology it shares with the insulin receptor, has been designated the *insulin receptor-related receptor* (IRR). There are no known ligands for the IRR, and both IGFs and insulin bind to it very poorly. It appears, however, to be expressed in a specific manner in renal and neural tissues and may have a role in fetal development. In chimeric transfection experiments, it has been documented as a very potent mediator of cellular proliferation.

Although the type II IGF receptor is structurally distinct and binds primarily IGF-II, it also serves as a receptor for mannose-6-phosphate–containing ligands. It is not a member of the insulin receptor family but rather displays homology to certain cytokine receptors. The receptor is 270 kDa in size and has 15 repeat extracellular domains. The type II IGF receptor has a very short intracellular domain and an unknown mechanism of signal transduction. It has been associated with changes in calcium influx and has been reported to mediate cell motility. It has been suggested that the type II IGF receptor serves as a targeting mechanism to mediate lysosomal destruction of excess IGF-II during fetal life. Gene targeting of the type II receptor results in mice that are larger than littermates, which is compatible with its negative growth-modulating effect.

Insulin-Like Growth Factor Binding Proteins (IGFBPs)

An important class of proteins with high affinities for the IGFs, the IGFBPs, have been shown to be involved in the modulation of the proliferative and mitogenic effects of IGFs on cells. These molecules appear to regulate the availability of free IGFs for interaction with the IGF receptors, as well as to directly interact with cell function. The human IGFBP family consists of six proteins. The IGFBP-1 is a 25-kDa protein found in high concentrations in amniotic fluid and is also secreted by hepatocytes under negative control by insulin. The IGFBP-2 has a molecular weight of 31 kDa, is found in serum, cerebrospinal fluid (CSF), and seminal plasma, is secreted by many cell types, and is expressed in many fetal and adult tissues. The IGFBP-3 is the major binding protein in postnatal serum and is synthesized by hepatocytes and other cells. In plasma, IGFBP-3 is found as part of a 150-kDa complex, which also includes the acid labile subunit and an IGF molecule, all of which are GH dependent. The IGFBP-4 is a 24-kDa protein that has been identified in serum and in seminal plasma, as well as in numerous cell types. The IGFBP-5 is found in CSF and, in smaller amounts, in serum; it is also observed in rapidly growing fetal tissues. The IGFBP-6 is found in CSF and is produced by transformed fibroblasts; IGFBP-6 has relative specificity for IGF-II over IGF-I. A high degree of structural homology among the six cloned cDNAs for the binding proteins and remarkable sequence conservation across species have been demonstrated. The IGFBPs are tightly regulated by various endocrine factors and are uniquely expressed during ontogeny. The IGFBPs are schematically depicted in Figure 12-3.

The molecular mechanisms involved in the interaction of the IGFBPs with the

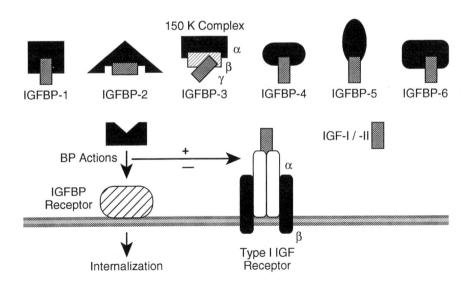

Fig. 12-3 The insulin-like growth factor binding proteins (IGFBP-1 through -6) are shown at the cellular environment.

IGFs and their receptors are now emerging, with three possible models for their actions having been suggested. The first mechanism suggested for IGFBP action is that these molecules regulate the availability of free IGFs for interaction with the IGF receptors. Indeed, the additions of IGFBPs to many *in vitro* cell culture systems results in the inhibition of IGF actions within these experimental systems. Additionally, several trophic hormones have been shown to suppress IGFBP production by their target cells. These include TSH inhibiting IGFBP-2 in thyroid cells, FSH inhibiting IGFBP-3 in Sertoli cells, and FSH inhibiting the elaboration of IGFBP-5 produced by granulosa cells.

In contrast, $1,25$-$(OH)_2$ vitamin D, which is inhibitory for bone cells, stimulates the production of IGFBP-4. In these models, it has been assumed that the suppression or stimulation of an inhibitory IGFBP stimulates or inhibits cell growth, respectively. Of great interest is the recent observation that IGFBP-3 can be internalized into cells and is localized in the nucleus of certain cells. The roles of nuclear IGFBP-3 are currently unknown, but it may play a role in gene transcription.

In other systems, however, IGFBPs have been demonstrated to enhance IGF action under circumstances that may involve cellular processing of the IGFBPs. These IGF-enhancing actions of IGFBPs have been demonstrated for IGFBP-1, IGFBP-3, and IGFBP-5. It appears that a processing step, such as an affinity change involving proteolysis or phosphorylation, may be required for the activation of this function.

Finally, as recently shown in several *in vitro* systems, IGFBPs have an IGF-independent mechanism of cell inhibition. The mechanism by which IGFBPs independently interact with cells has not yet been fully elucidated. Both IGFBP-1 and IGFBP-2 contain a unique recognition sequence, which may allow them to interact with a class of cell surface receptors known as *intergrin receptors*. The IGFBP-3 does not contain such a sequence but has recently been shown to bind to specific receptors on the cell membrane. It appears that IGFBP-3 mediates an IGF-independent growth inhibitory effect via its own receptors.

IGFBP Proteases
Also recognized as potential modulators of IGF action is a group of enzymes that are capable of cleaving IGFBPs. First identified in pregnancy serum, IGFBP-3 proteolytic activity is responsible for the disappearance of intact IGFBP-3 from the serum of pregnant individuals, with no change in IGFBP-3 immunoreactivity. Also, IGFBP proteases have been reported in the serum of severely ill patients in states of cachexia, in patients with growth hormone receptor deficiency, in prostate cancer patients, and in patients with other malignancies. Seminal plasma contains an IGFBP-3 protease that has been identified as *prostate-specific antigen* (PSA). This IGFBP protease belongs to the kallikrein family. The CSF from patients with malignancies and urine from patients with renal failure also contain IGFBP proteases. The IGFBP proteases have been described for all six IGFBPs, and both acid and neutral activities have been detected. It has been speculated that the IGFBP proteases are important modulators of IGF bioavailability and bioactivity through their modification of the IGF carrier proteins. The proteolytic activity may play a role in regulating IGF availability at the tissue level by altering the affinity of the binding proteins for the growth factors, releasing free IGFs, and allowing increased receptor binding. A theoretical model of such interactions is illustrated in Figure 12-4.

Fig. 12-4 Mechanism of action of insulin-like growth factor binding proteins (IGFBP) proteases. The proteases cleave IGFBPs and release free IGFs to interact with the IGF receptors.

IGFBP-Related Proteins

Recently recognized as part of the IGFBP superfamily are several IGFBP-related proteins (IGFBP-rPs), which bind IGFs with low affinity. The IGFBPs and IGFBP-rPs share the highly conserved and cysteine-rich N-terminus, which appears to be crucial for several biological actions, including their binding to IGFs. The IGFBP-rP1 (first named mac25) is a 31-kDa protein cloned originally from leptomeninges and more recently from breast cancer cells. The IGFBP-rP1 mRNA is down regulated in several tumor cell lines and highly expressed in senescent mammary epithelial cells, suggesting that IGFBP-rP1 has growth-suppressing activity. The IGFBP-rP2 (previously called *connective tissue growth factor;* CTGF) is involved in human atherosclerosis and fibrotic disorders and can be identified in serum-free conditioned media of human breast cancer cells and in human biological fluids such as normal sera, pregnancy sera, and cerebrospinal, amniotic, follicular and peritoneal fluids. Recent studies indicate that IGFBP-rP2 appears to be an important endocrine factor and one of the critical downstream effectors of TGF-β. The IGFBP-rPs designated 3, 4, 5, and 6 have been proposed though few reports of their structures and functions have been published to date. Clearly, the IGFBP-rPs are critical to cellular growth and may operate primarily in an IGF-independent manner, as discussed above.

ADDITIONAL GROWTH-REGULATING PEPTIDES

The FGF Family of Peptides and Receptors

Fibroblast growth factors (FGFs) constitute an important and rapidly expanding family of peptide cytokines, which are important in the regulation of many tissues. Initially it was suggested that these factors may be specific for cells of stromal lineage, but it appears that many other cells respond to FGFs as well. There are at least seven different FGFs (FGF-1 through -7) that have been identified, including the best characterized acidic FGF (aFGF or FGF-1), basic FGF (bFGF or FGF-2), and keratinocyte growth factor (KGF or FGF-7). The FGFs mediate their actions by binding to at least three receptors, FGFR1, FGFR2, and FGFR3, which have distinct tissue distributions. For the most part, FGFs appear to be autocrine–paracrine growth factors that participate in organ growth and differentiation as well as in carcinogenesis but not in somatic growth. An exception to this rule is the observation that the genetic form of dwarfism known as *achondroplasia* is caused by a mutation in the FGFR3 gene, suggesting that normal FGFR3 signaling is essential for the normal growth of long bones. A human mutation in the FGFR2 gene causes craniosynostosis, a disease characterized by abnormal closure of the bones in the skull but normal long bone growth. So far, targeted disruptions of several murine FGF and FGF-R genes have been reported, and the phenotypes associated with them include various developmental abnormalities. Future studies will further define the role that different components of the FGF systems play in somatic and tissue growth.

The EGF System

Epidermal growth factors (EGFs) and their receptors are ubiquitous in many tissues and participate in developmental processes in mice such as precocious eyelid opening and tooth eruption. The mitogenic actions of EGF have been extensively explored in cell culture systems, and the receptor for EGF was characterized as a prototype model for signal transduction involving tyrosine kinases. The extensive *in vitro* data indicate multiple cellular functions of EGF. In addition, EGF has been identified in most body fluids of several mammalian species; however, neither EGF antibody administration to newborn animals nor gene targeting of EGF has caused major deleterious effects as might be expected from the *in vitro* studies. The EGF family of growth factors appears to be important in mammalian development and function, although the precise roles and significance are not yet clear. Members of the EGF family may have a role in embryogenesis and fetal growth as receptors have been identified in fetal tissues. It has been proposed that abnormal EGF–EGF receptor interactions may be instrumental in the development of cancer, but it appears that they are not involved in somatic growth.

Other Growth-Promoting Peptides

An ever-growing number of growth factors are being recognized, and multiple hormones and peptides are being characterized as having growth-promoting activities in certain cell types. In general, these molecules appear to lack somatic growth-promoting effects but play important autocrine–paracrine as well as endocrine roles. Notable among these are groups of growth factors that have tissue-specific effects. Endothelin, platelet-derived growth factor (PDGF), and vascular-epithelial growth factor (VEGF) regulate angiogenesis and other vascular processes in addition to modulating the function of numerous cultured cells. A variety of hematopoetic growth factors such as the granulocyte and macrophage colony stimulating factors (GCSF, MCSF), erythropoetin, and thrombopoetin promote the growth of the different lineages of the hematopoetic cells. The growth of various cells of the immune system is stimulated by an array of cytokines including interleukins and interferons (see Chapter 4). The complex array of cells comprising the nervous system is under the regulatory influence of specific growth factors such as nerve growth factor (NGF), the neurotrophins, and brain- and glial-derived neurotrophic factors (BDNF,

GDNF). Other growth factors that have been attributed to specific tissues (such as hepatocyte growth factor, HGF) are being recognized as having a general growth-promoting effect in numerous tissues. Additional organ-specific growth regulatory processes are being described in the gastrointestinal tract, kidneys, and other organs.

Growth Inhibitory Peptides

Of particular interest are a class of cytokines that can negatively modulate cellular growth. The transforming growth factor-β (TGF-β) can act both as an agent that mediates cellular growth and malignant transformation and as a growth inhibitory substance that has the potential of arresting the growth of both normal and neoplastic cells. Tumor necrosis factors (TNF) and other compounds have been described to have similar effects. These molecules may regulate the entry of cells into programmed cell death (apoptosis). The growth inhibitory processes of TGF-β and other cytokines may prove to be of great importance in the development of cancer treatments. A family of genes/proteins, of which the most important is p53, is also critical for both growth and tumor suppression. These tumor suppressors are often involved in fetal growth.

DISORDERS OF GROWTH

Growth Curves and Growth Patterns

The growth of an individual is a dynamic function of height increment over time. Accordingly, to evaluate growth accurately, one must obtain serial and accurate measurements of a child's height and plot them on a growth curve. Growth curves are based on normative population data, and the ones commonly available reflect the North American means compiled by the National Center for Health Statistics of the U.S. Public Health Service. It is preferable to use those growth curves, which show the standard deviations (SD) from the mean or Z score. These types of curves allow a more precise estimation of the degree of short stature, when it exists. However, it must be emphasized that such growth curves are cross-sectional rather than longitudinal, and they are particularly nonrepresentative during adolescence, when growth acceleration may normally occur at widely divergent ages. Consequently, it is preferable to perform consecutive measurements of height that are then used to calculate growth velocity and are plotted on a growth velocity chart.

Definition and Epidemiology of Short Stature

Because height is a normally distributed function, it is simple to provide a statistical definition of normal height as that falling between 2 SD (Z scores) above and below the mean for each age group. This will include those individuals between the 2nd and 98th percentiles but will exclude approximately 4% of the population, many of whom represent variants of the normal state. Prediction of adult height is helpful in determining the diagnosis and prognosis of short children. Factors influencing adult height include mean parental height, the patient's current height and sexual maturation rating, the chronological age, and the bone age. Many methods have been developed for calculating estimated adult height. A simple method of predicting adult height is to determine the mean parental height and add or subtract (for males and females, respectively) 6.5 centimeters or 2.5 inches (genetic potential). The use of a bone age radiograph allows for a much more accurate prediction. The most commonly used method for the determination of bone age is the Greulich and Pyle (GP) method, which relies on an atlas of left hand and wrist radiographs of healthy children at various ages. Likewise, the simplest and most common method for adult height prediction is the Bayley-Pinneau (BP) method. This method assigns to each bone age a percentage of the adult height that has already been achieved, and the adult height can then be calculated by dividing the present height by the fraction given in the table. The confidence limits of the above predictions are usually within 2 inches of the actual achieved height.

Causes of Short Stature

A height greater than 2.5 SD below the mean for age during adolescence can have many causes, including, as shown in Table 12-1, multiple endocrine and systemic disorders. Of these, the normal variants are by far the most common. When normal variant short stature is associated with delayed puberty, skeletal maturation, and growth, it is termed *normal variant constitutional delay* (NVCD). When it is found in individuals with normal progression through puberty and normal skeletal maturation, it is termed *normal variant short stature* (NVSS). NVSS is a growth pattern

Table 12-1 Causes of Short Stature

Normal variants
   Normal varient short stature (NVSS)
     familial
     sporadic
   Normal varient constitutional delay (NVCD)
Abnormal variants
   Chromosomal disorders
     Turner's syndrome
     Down's syndrome (trisomy 21)
     Other chromosomal conditions
   Dysmorphic syndromes
   Skeletal dysplasias (primary and secondary)
     Achondroplasia (FGFR3 deficiency)
   Systemic disease
     Malnutrition
     Eating disorders
     Malabsorption
     Other occult chronic disease
   Psychosocial dwarfism
   Endocrine disorders
     Growth hormone deficiency (GHD)
     Hypothyroidism
     Glucocorticoid excess
     Congenital abnormalities of bone metabolism

representing the genetic potential for growth of that individual and is not associated with any endocrine or systemic pathology of any kind.

Often, but not always, NVSS is associated with a family history of short stature in at least one parent. These patients commonly have normal birth weights, and in the first few years of life their growth pattern usually settles at or just below the 3rd percentile and then follows this percentile with a pubertal growth spurt at a normal age. The adult height achieved by these patients is typically below the 3rd percentile and is predictable by bone age measurements. Criteria for the diagnosis of NVSS include the exclusion of organic or emotional pathology by history, physical exam, and simple laboratory tests outlined later. NVCD occurs in both sexes, although males are more likely to present to a physician with this condition. A family history of delayed maturation is usually present in at least one parent.

The growth patterns typically observed in this condition consist of one of three forms. The delay in growth could occur in the first 3 years of life followed by growth at or slightly below the 5th percentile throughout childhood. Growth can gradually fall below the norm during the course of childhood. Finally, the deviation from the normal growth curve could occur at the time puberty should normally occur. Some children present with a combined picture. Puberty develops late in all of these patients, but when it does it is associated with a near normal growth spurt, and the adult height achieved is entirely normal. The diagnosis of NVCD is made by exclusion. Systemic and endocrine causes must be ruled out by the appropriate tests before NVCD is diagnosed.

Other causes of growth failure may be the result of chromosomal disorders; among these, the most common are Down's syndrome (trisomy 21) and Turner's syndrome, which is caused by a monosomic 45,X state or other abnormalities of the X chromosome. Short stature is the most common finding in Turner's syndrome, with primary ovarian failure being the other important feature (see Chapter 8). Additional findings include typical dysmorphic features, and cardiac and renal anomalies. Nevertheless, short stature may be the only presenting sign in a girl with Turner's syndrome, and even this finding may only manifest itself late in childhood. It is therefore imperative to consider this condition in the evaluation of any short female.

Growth failure associated with systemic disease or malnutrition is usually characterized by normal or elevated growth hormone, but depressed somatomedin levels. During adolescence, these conditions are often associated with delayed puberty as well as a delayed bone age and must be differentiated from NVCD. In underdeveloped countries, overt protein calorie malnutrition is the most common form of malnutrition, but in developed countries, self-inflicted malnutrition (anorexia nervosa and bulimia) or malnutrition associated with chronic disease is also common. Specific mineral deficiencies, especially of iron and zinc, can also be associated with growth delay.

Gastrointestinal disease can also cause growth retardation, often with little or no appreciable symptoms, usually as a result of malabsorption. Insulin-dependent diabetes mellitus, when not adequately controlled, is associated with depressed somatomedin levels and poor growth. Adequate control of the diabetic state and regulation of the nutritional intake can restore growth rate in diabetics back to the normal range. Poverty, depression, and neglect can lead to a form of growth delay referred to as *psychosocial dwarfism*. Although nutritional factors may play a role in the etiology of this condition, defective GH secretion has also been documented.

Endocrine Causes of Short Stature

It is helpful to bear in mind that chronic illness frequently tends to retard weight to a greater degree than height, whereas endocrinopathies tend to do the opposite. Endocrine abnormalities account for only about 10% of the cases of short stature; it is, however, imperative to diagnose these children promptly, because adequate therapy can normalize the growth and correct the other abnormalities associated with these disorders.

Hypothyroidism in childhood is generally associated with poor linear growth. Indeed, poor growth and/or delayed puberty may be the presenting signs of chronic hypothyroidism. It is important to note that hypothyroidism may coexist with GH deficiency and that it may also cause false negative results on provocative GH testing. It is therefore imperative to consider hypothyroidism as the first step of short stature evaluation. Glucocorticoid excess, either iatrogenic or due to Cushing's disease or primary adrenal hypercortisolism, is associated with attenuation of the growth rate (see Chapter 14).

Growth Hormone Deficiency

A classification of growth hormone (GH) abnormalities is given in Table 12-2. Familial GH deficiency (GHD) displays a variety of hereditary patterns, ranging from autosomal recessive (type I), to autosomal dominant (type II) and X linked (type III). Hereditary GHD may also be caused by deficiencies of the pituitary transcrip-

Table 12-2 Classification of Growth Hormone Abnormalities

Growth hormone deficiency (GHD)
    Familial
        Type IA (complete, autosomal recessive)
        Type IB (nearly complete, autosomal recessive)
        Type II (autosomal dominant)
        Type III (X-linked GHD)
        Prop1 deficiency (panhypopituitarism)
        Pit1 deficiency (hypopituitarism)
    Sporadic/idiopathic
    Peri-sellar tumors
    CNS irradiation and chemotherapy
    Postinfectious/post-traumatic

Growth hormone insufficiency
    Partial GH deficiency
    Neurosecretory dysfunction

Biologically inactive GH

GH resistance
    Genetic (Laron syndrome)
    Acquired (liver diseases)

tion factor *Pit1* (in which case it may be associated with additional pituitary hormone deficiencies including prolactin and TSH) or the pituitary transcription factor *Prop1* (in which case it may be associated with deficiency of all anterior pituitary hormones). Congenital GHD is usually recognized early in life, with the constellation of hypoglycemia, small phallus, relative adiposity, and subnormal length. Type I GHD is divided into two types. Type IA GHD has complete GHD secondary to gene deletion or point mutations and is associated with development of GH antibodies when treatment is initiated. Type IB patients have splice-site mutations in the GH gene, have very low levels of endogenous GH, and do not develop GH antibodies. Sporadic GHD can be either idiopathic (which is most common) or secondary to pathological processes at the level of the pituitary or hypothalamus. Space-occupying lesions of the brain are the second-most frequent cause of GHD. Infiltrative processes and posttraumatic and postinflammatory conditions can all cause GHD and growth failure.

A growing number of children presenting with GHD and growth failure in adolescence are survivors of central nervous system (CNS) irradiation and chemotherapy treatments for malignancies. Although some short children may successfully pass provocative GH testing, they may nevertheless respond to GH therapy. Integrated GH levels have been shown to be low in a subset of these children, and the term *neurosecretory dysfunction* (of GH secretion) has been used to describe their condition. Regardless of the etiology, children with characteristic GHD display short stature, decreased growth velocity, delayed bone age, and low serum IGF-I and IGFBP-3 levels. Failure to adequately secrete GH in two stimulation tests is currently required for the diagnosis of classical GHD, but abnormal serum levels of GH-dependent markers, such as IGF-I, IGFBP-3, and ALS, may soon replace it as the diagnostic tests of choice.

Biologically inactive GH is another potential cause of short stature. Patients with this disorder would be expected to have a normal response to exogenous GH, but no convincing cases of this condition have been documented.

Laron-type dwarfism (or GH receptor deficiency; GHRD) is caused by mutations or deletions of the GH receptor gene and is associated with elevated GH levels and depressed IGFs and IGFBP-3 levels. This condition can now be diagnosed by assays of the plasma GH-binding protein. Treatment with recombinant IGF-I is efficacious in this condition.

Evaluation of Short Stature

Historical features that aid in the evaluation of short stature include the pregnancy and perinatal history, the growth pattern from infancy to adolescence (for both height and weight), the general medical history, and any symptoms of systemic disease. Particular emphasis should be placed on the review of systems for the presence of neurological, visual, or gastrointestinal disturbances and any symptom of hypothyroidism. The family history should be probed for parental heights and for growth and maturation patterns, as well as for any short stature in the family background.

The complete physical exam should include accurate auxological measurements of height, weight, arm span, upper-to-lower segment ratios, and an exam of the thyroid and sexual maturity rating. Any abnormality in the physical exam, especially those suggesting systemic disease, or evidence of dysmorphism, should be carefully noted.

In the child with clinically significant short stature, where a systemic disease is not the obvious cause of the growth problem, laboratory evaluation is frequently necessary. The presence of occult chronic disease causing short stature can usually be ruled out with a complete blood count, erythrocyte sedimentation rate, a urinalysis, and a blood chemistry panel that includes serum electrolytes, blood urea nitrogen (BUN), creatinine, calcium, phosphorus, and alkaline phosphatase. Thyroid function can be evaluated with a TSH and free thyroxine (T_4). In girls, a karyotype is often necessary to rule out Turner's syndrome, even if no other stigmata exist. A bone age is essential for the diagnostic evaluation and prognosis of all short children. Measurements of serum IGF-I and IGFBP-3 levels can predict the presence of GHD. Although IGF-I levels may be low in malnutrition, systemic disease, and hypothyroidism, the IGFBP-3 levels are commonly normal in the absence of GHD. The clinical utility of serum growth factor levels is mainly as an adjunct or an alternative for GH stimulation tests. The serum levels of the third component of the IGF complex, the ALS (acid labile subunit) are also GH dependent and may soon become part of the diagnostic evaluation of GHD. Finally, in the adolescent male suspected to have NVCD and considered for therapy, a serum testosterone level is often helpful.

If the child being evaluated for possible GHD is growing poorly (i.e., is shorter than 2.5 SD below the mean for age and has a low growth velocity and low serum IGF-I and IGFBP-3 concentrations), GH testing is often performed. In normal children random, unstimulated GH levels are typically under 5 ng/ml; therefore, if GHD is suspected, GH should be measured after appropriate pituitary stimulation. Pharmacological agents, which stimulate GH, include L-dopa, clonidine, propranolol, glucagon, insulin, and arginine. Levels of less than 10 ng/ml (by a polyclonal GH assay) are diagnostic of GHD, and levels greater than 10 are considered normal (although neurosecretory dysfunction of GH secretion remains a possibility). Priming the pituitary with estrogen will sometimes augment the GH response. An MRI of the head is recommended in patients with documented GHD to evaluate possible local pathology.

Management of Short Stature

After the evaluation of short stature has been completed, the physician must balance the needs of the child and the family, the severity of the growth retardation, and the expected adult height in deciding upon a therapeutic plan. It is important to appreciate both the potential of growth-enhancing therapy to affect these issues and the cost and possible complications of therapy. For some of the above-mentioned disorders, particularly the normal variants, reassurance and support for the patient and the family, coupled with close follow-up, are all that might be required. In contrast, for some of the pathological causes of short stature, as well as for selected severe cases of the normal variants, medical therapy is prudent. NVCD is associated with normal predicted adult height and, in the case of the socially well adjusted adolescent, reassurance is the most important aspect of therapy, as these patients will all enter puberty eventually and will experience a growth spurt at that time. Counseling the patient and the family should center around the expected growth that comes with puberty. If, however, the patient feels that he has become so stigmatized by the combination of short stature and sexual immaturity that reassurance alone is insufficient, a course of androgenic steroids (such as intramuscular testosterone) should be considered in male patients older than 14 years who have normal thyroid and GH evaluation and low testosterone levels.

Turner's syndrome patients have been shown to benefit from growth-enhancing therapy, and the currently recommended regimen for their management involves initiation of GH, regardless of the response to provocative testing. Combining GH with low-dose anabolic steroids such as oxandrolone enhances the early growth response. Other chromosomal and genetic syndromes do not respond to therapy quite as well and have not yet been adequately studied with regard to GH treatment.

Growth hormone deficiency of any type requires GH therapy, and, with the unlimited availability of recombinant GH, therapy can be provided to all these patients. If the diagnosis of GHD is made, GH therapy should be started immediately. Growth hormone is best given daily, at bedtime, as a subcutaneous injection at a dose ranging from 0.025–0.05 mg/kg/day. The cost of GH may be a significant burden on the average family budget, with current costs ranging between $10,000 and $30,000 a year. All of the above considerations should be weighed and discussed before embarking on therapy.

In patients with GH unresponsiveness, as is found in GHRD (Laron syndrome), therapy with IGF-I has been documented to be beneficial in improving growth velocity and adult height prediction.

In patients in whom a growth disorder is being managed around the time of puberty, closure of the epiphysis (either prematurely or at an appropriate age) may hamper the effects of the growth-promoting therapy employed. As the closure of the epiphysis has recently been demonstrated to be an estrogen effect, inhibition of puberty (with GnRH analogs) or estrogenic blockade (with estrogen receptor antagonists or aromatase inhibitors) can enhance and prolong the growth treatment and result in taller adult stature.

CONCLUSION

Over the last decade, the medical and scientific literature has witnessed an explosion of information regarding the physiology of growth and growth factors in general and the various components of the IGF axis in particular. Undoubtedly, the coming years will bring even more new information on the physiology and pathology of these key cellular regulators. Furthermore, these discoveries are likely to lead to the increasing use of diagnostic tests as well as to therapeutic applications of these agents.

SUGGESTED READING

Baserga R: Oncogenes and the strategy of growth factors. Cell 79:927–930, 1994.

Cohen P, and Rosenfeld RG: Growth problems in adolescence. In: *Textbook of Adolescent Medicine*, RE MacAnarney, ER Kreipe, DP Orr, and GD Comerci, eds., Saunders, Philadelphia, pp. 495–508, 1992.

Cohen P, and Rosenfeld RG: The IGF axis. In: *Human Growth Hormone, Basic and Scientific Aspects,* AL Rosenbloom ed., CRC Press, Boca Raton, FL, pp. 43–56, 1995.

Ferry RJ Jr, Cerri RW, and Cohen P: Insulin-like growth factor binding proteins: New proteins, new functions. Horm Res 51:53–67, 1999.

Liu JP, Baker J, Perkins AS, Robertson EJ, and Efstratiadis A: Mice carrying null mutations of the genes encoding insulin-like growth factor I (Igf-1) and type 1 IGF receptor (Igf1r). Cell 75:59–72, 1993.

Metzger RJ, Krasnow MA: Genetic control of branching morphogenesis. Science 284:1635–1639, 1999.

Rajah R, Katz L, Nunn S, Solberg P, Beers T, and Cohen P: IGFBP proteases—functional regulators of cell growth. Prog Growth Factors Res 6:273–284, 1996.

Rosenfeld RG: An endocrinologist's approach to the growth hormone—insulin-like growth factor axis. Acta Paediatr Suppl 423:17–19, 1997.

Wilson DM, Kraemer HC, Ritter PL, and Hammer LD: Growth curves and adult height estimation for adolescents. Am J Dis Child 141:565–570, 1987.

Wu W, Cogan JD, Pfaffle RW, Dasen JS, Frisch H, O'Connell SM, Flynn SE, Brown MR, Mullis PE, Parks JS, Phillips JA III, and Rosenfeld MG: Mutations in PROP1 cause familial combined pituitary hormone deficiency. Nat Genet 18:147–149, 1998.

13

The Thyroid

JAMES E. GRIFFIN

Thyroid hormones are important for the normal growth and development of the maturing human. In the adult, thyroid hormones maintain metabolic stability by regulating oxygen requirements, body weight, and intermediary metabolism. Thyroid function is under hypothalamic–pituitary control, and thus like the gonads and adrenal cortex, it serves as a classical model of endocrine physiology. In addition, the physiological effects of thyroid hormones are regulated by complex extrathyroidal mechanisms resulting from the peripheral metabolism of the hormones. These mechanisms are not under hypothalamic–pituitary regulation.

SYNTHESIS AND SECRETION OF THYROID HORMONES

Iodide Kinetics

Adequate iodide intake is necessary for normal thyroid hormone synthesis as thyroid hormones are the only substances in the body that have iodine in their structure. The major sources of dietary iodide are iodated bread, iodized salt, and dairy products. Individuals may also be exposed to iodide in medications, disinfectants, and radiographic contrast agents. The minimum dietary requirement of iodide is about 75 μg/day. This amount, or half of the recommended daily allowance of iodide (150 μg/day), could be obtained from 10 g of salt alone if iodized at the recommended World Health Organization rate of 1 part KI in 100,000 parts NaCl. In the United States, iodized salt contains 1 part KI in 10,000 parts NaCl.

Dietary iodine intake in the United States ranges from 200 to 500 μg/day. The higher number is used in Figure 13-1 to depict normal iodine metabolism. Iodine is ingested in both inorganic and organically bound forms, and the organically bound form is converted to inorganic iodide. Iodide itself is efficiently absorbed; little is lost in the stool. Absorbed iodide is largely confined to the extracellular fluid, and its concentration in extracellular fluid is normally about 1 μg/dl and the total extracellular fluid pool about 250 μg. The major sites of removal of iodide from the extracellular fluid are the thyroid and the kidneys. The renal clearance of iodide—30–40 ml/minute—results from complete glomerular filtration and passive reabsorption. Iodide clearance in humans appears to be largely independent of serum iodide concentration. Total renal iodide excretion approximates intake. Iodide re-

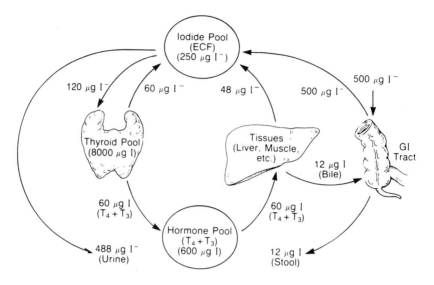

Fig. 13-1 Normal pathways of iodine metabolism in a state of iodine balance. T$_4$, thyroxine; T$_3$, 3,5,3'-triiodothyronine; ECF, extracellular fluid. Arrows indicate daily flux from one compartment to another. Numbers in parentheses indicate pool sizes. (Redrawn from Larsen PR, and Ingbar SH: In: *Williams Textbook of Endocrinology,* 8th ed., JD Wilson and DW Foster, eds., Saunders, Philadelphia, p. 361, 1992.)

moved from the serum by the thyroid is returned to the circulation as iodothyronines (thyroid hormones), whose iodine is largely returned to the extracellular fluid after peripheral deiodination. The hormone pool of iodide includes that in the circulation as well as thyroid hormones in the tissues. The largest pool of iodine is in the thyroid, which contains about 8000 μg, virtually all in iodinated amino acids (Fig. 13-1). The thyroid iodine pool has a slow turnover of about 1% daily.

Iodide Transport and Organification

An overall scheme of thyroid hormone biosynthesis, secretion, and metabolism is depicted in Figure 13-2. The thyroid concentrates inorganic iodide from the extracellular fluid by an active, saturable energy-dependent process. This iodide carrier is a 643-amino acid transport protein termed the *sodium iodide symporter.* It is located on the cell surface of the acinar cell and has the typical multiple membrane spanning domains of transport proteins. Under normal conditions the rate of inward clearance of iodide by the thyroid exceeds the rate of incorporation of iodide into amino acids (organification) and back-diffusion so that the thyroid to plasma (T:P) ratios of iodide are greater than unity, usually about 20 to 40. Both thyroid-stimulating hormone (TSH) and an internal autoregulatory system influence this sodium iodide symporter. TSH stimulates iodide transport; in general, an increasing glandular content of organic iodine diminishes iodide transport and its response to TSH. Iodide transport is inhibited by certain anions, notably perchlorate and thiocyanate. Perchlorate both inhibits trapping of iodide by the gland and facilitates back-diffusion out the gland. Thiocyanate mainly increases iodide efflux. Other tissues such

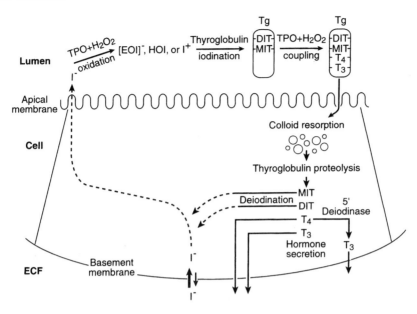

Fig. 13-2 Diagram of the steps of thyroid hormone biosynthesis and release. TPO, thyroid peroxidase; MIT, monoiodotyrosine; DIT, diiodotyrosine; T_4, thyroxine; T_3, 3,5,3'-triiodothyronine; I^+, activated iodide; ECF, extracellular fluid. Redrawn from Taurog A: In: *Werner and Ingbar's The Thyroid*, 6th ed., LE Braverman and RD Utiger, eds., Lippincott, New York, p. 87, 1991.)

as the salivary glands and gastric mucosa are known to be able to concentrate iodide, and the human sodium iodide symporter has been identified in the breast, colon, and ovary.

The two principal thyroid hormones are thyroxine (3,5,3',5'-tetraiodo-L-thyronine), or T_4, and 3,5,3'-triiodo-L-thyronine, or T_3 (see Fig. 13-3 for chemical structure). These hormones are produced from the precursor amino acids diiodotyrosine and monoiodotyrosine. These iodoamino acids are formed by the iodination of tyrosine residues within the matrix of thyroglobulin (Fig. 13-2), a large protein molecule unique to the thyroid. The iodination is catalyzed by thyroid peroxidase, a membrane-bound heme-protein enzyme. The source of the hydrogen peroxide is not known. The active iodinating agent is probably I^+ or hypoiodous acid (HOI) formed by peroxidase-catalyzed oxidation of I^-.

The thyroid has a limited capacity to utilize excess iodides in hormonogenesis. Progressive increases in the concentration of iodide in extracellular fluid are associated with progressively decreasing values of the T:P ratio, while the amount of iodide actively transported into the gland and organified rises progressively until reaching a maximum followed by a sudden decrease, termed the *acute Wolff–Chaikoff effect*. The increasing iodination occurs despite a falling percentage uptake of circulating iodide. The serum iodide level beyond which iodination decreases is 15–20 μg/dl. The inhibitory effect of excess iodide upon iodination in thyroid glands requires iodide organification. Inhibition is of brief duration and escape from or adaptation to iodide inhibition occurs after a few days.

Fig. 13-3 Structures of the principal thyroid hormones, thyroxine, and 3,5,3'-tri-iodothyronine and part of the pathway of metabolism by deiodination. (Reprinted from Griffin JE: *Manual of Clinical Endocrinology and Metabolism,* McGraw-Hill, New York, p. 50, 1982.)

Both T_4 and T_3 form within thyroglobulin (Fig. 13-2) by a coupling reaction involving two diiodotyrosyl residues or a monoiodotyrosyl and diiodotyrosyl residue, respectively. This coupling reaction occurs separately from iodination and also is catalyzed by thyroid peroxidase. The specific tertiary structure of thyroglobulin is thought to be important for efficient coupling since disruption of its native structure or substitution of other proteins for thyroglobulin results in very low levels of T_4 formation. Thyroglobulin is a large molecule with a molecular weight of 660,000 Da. Almost all of the thyroglobulin in the normal thyroid gland is present as a soluble protein in the lumen of the thyroid follicle. Only three or four molecules of thyroxine are formed in each molecule of thyroglobulin, and certain tyrosines such as the one at position 5 from the amino-terminus appear to be favored for sites of thyroxine formation. The thyroid normally makes much more T_4 than T_3 if iodine intake is adequate, and the T_4 to T_3 ratio of normal thyroglobulin is 10:1.

Storage and Release of Thyroid Hormones

In contrast to most endocrine glands, which do not store appreciable amounts of hormone, the thyroid contains several weeks' supply of thyroid hormones in the thyroglobulin pool. Thyroglobulin must be hydrolyzed to release T_4 and T_3. This cleavage of iodothyronines from thyroglobulin is accomplished by lysosomal proteases within the follicular cell (Fig. 13-2). In response to TSH stimulation, colloid droplets are formed at the apical surface of the follicular cells by endocytosis of adjacent luminal colloid. Lysosomes migrate from the basal end of the follicular cell to fuse with the colloid droplets and release their hydrolytic enzymes. Digestion of thyroglobulin apparently releases all iodinated amino acids in the free form. Iodotyrosines are largely prevented from being released into the circulation by the action of an intracellular deiodinase that is specific for iodotyrosines and not active on iodothyronines (Fig. 13-2). The iodide released from monoiodotyrosine and diiodotyrosine is then available for reutilization in the thyroid gland. The free T_4 and T_3 diffuse from the cell into the circulation.

Although the thyroid is capable of deiodinating T_4 to T_3, the contribution of this pathway of T_3 formation to overall T_3 production is considered small (see below).

Thyroglobulin itself is not normally released into the circulation in significant quantities. Some small quantities of thyroglobulin can be measured by sensitive immunoassays in peripheral blood of most normal subjects. It appears that this thyroglobulin reaches the blood via lymphatics. When the thyroid gland is damaged by disease processes, such as the inflammation associated with thyroiditis, significant quantities of thyroglobulin may leak into the circulation.

Release of thyroid hormones is inhibited by excess iodide. This effect of iodide is used in the treatment of severe hyperthyroidism. It may involve inhibition of adenylyl cyclase activity that increases as part of the normal response to thyroid stimulators.

TRANSPORT OF THYROID HORMONES AND TISSUE DELIVERY

Iodothyronines in the circulation are largely bound to thyroid hormone-binding globulin (TBG), transthyretin, and albumin. Under normal conditions at equilibrium, about 70% of both T_4 and T_3 is bound to TBG. About 10% of T_4 is bound to transthyretin and 15% to albumin. In contrast, very little T_3 is bound to transthyretin and about 25% is bound to albumin. About 3% of T_4 and 6% of T_3 are bound to lipoproteins. Only about 0.03% of T_4 and 0.3% of T_3 is "free" or dialyzable in *in vitro* studies. T_4 binds more tightly to serum-binding proteins than T_3, resulting in a lower metabolic clearance rate and longer serum half-life. The serum half-life of T_4 is about 7 days whereas the half-life of T_3 is less than 1 day.

As discussed in Chapter 5, we recognize that the capillary exchangeable or bioavailable thyroid hormone, as assessed by *in vivo* studies, is greater than the free fraction as assessed by *in vitro* analysis. Measured bioavailable T_3 in brain tissue (as an example of peripheral nonhepatic tissues) was found to equal 10% of the albumin-bound T_3, whereas bioavailable T_3 in liver tissue was equal to all of the albumin-bound fraction and more than half of the TBG-bound fraction. The bioavailable T_4 in brain is similar to T_3, whereas bioavailable T_4 in liver is primarily the albumin-bound fraction. Thus, like steroid hormones, the capillary exchangeable fraction of thyroid hormones more closely approximates the sum of the free plus the albumin-bound fraction than it does the free fraction.

THYROID HORMONE METABOLISM

Kinetics of Thyroid Hormone Production and Turnover

As mentioned above, the primary iodothyronine secreted by the thyroid gland is thyroxine. Most circulating T_3 is produced by monodeiodination of T_4 in peripheral tissues. About 80% of T_4 is monodiodinated either in the 5' or 5 positions to form either T_3 or reverse T_3 (Fig. 13-3). About 40% of the 80 μg of T_4 secreted each day is peripherally metabolized via 5'-deiodination to produce about 80% of the 30 μg of T_3 produced each day (Fig. 13-4). Most of this conversion occurs in liver and kidney, and the T_3 that is formed is released into serum. The remaining 20% of T_3 production comes from direct secretion by the thyroid gland. In most systems, T_3 has about 10 times the potency of T_4 (see below). Because under physiological conditions most of the activity of T_4 can be accounted for by the T_3 formed from it, T_4 can be considered a prohormone.

The alternate monodeiodination product of T_4, formed by removal of an inner ring iodine, is 3,3',5'-triiodo-L-thyronine or reverse T_3 (rT_3) (Fig. 13-3). Nearly all rT_3 is produced extrathyroidally and a little more than a third of secreted T_4 is converted to this metabolite (Fig. 13-4). Serum rT_3 concentrations are lower than T_3

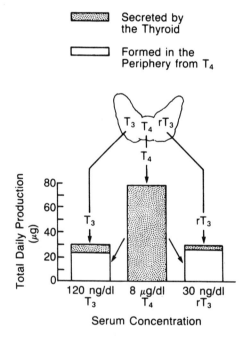

Fig. 13-4 Dynamics of thyroid hormone production and mean serum concentrations. The total daily production and distribution into the components of directed secretion by the thyroid and peripheral conversation of secreted thyroxine are shown. T_4, thyroxine; T_3, 3,5,3'-triiodothyronine; rT_3, reverse triiodothryonine or 3,3',5'-triiodothyronine. (Adapted with permission from Schimmel M, and Utiger RD: Thyroidal and peripheral production of thyroid hormones. Review of recent findings and their clinical implications. Ann Intern Med 87:760, 1977.)

concentrations because of its more rapid metabolic clearance. Reverse T_3 has little or no thyroid hormone biological activity. Both T_3 and rT_3 are further deiodinated to 3,3′-diiodothyronine (Fig. 13-3) as well as other diiodothyronines and mono-iodothyronines that are biologically inactive. Both T_4 and T_3 also form glucuronide conjugates that are excreted via the bile into the feces.

DEIODINASE ENZYMES INVOLVED IN THYROID HORMONE ACTIVATION AND INACTIVATION

There are three distinct iodothyronine deiodinases (Table 13-1). They all have the uncommon amino acid, selenocysteine, in their active site and make use of the structure formed as a result of a selenocysteine insertion sequence to insert selenocysteine at codon UAG, which is normally a stop codon.

Type 1 deiodinase (D1) has both outer ring (5′) and inner ring (5) actively. It is thought to be the primary deiodinase providing T_3 to the circulation with locations in the liver, kidney, thyroid, and brain. It converts T_4 to T_3 and rT_3 to 3,3′-diiodothyronine. It has a relatively low affinity for T_4 (Table 13-1) and thus would not be saturated at normal or elevated T_4 concentrations. It is sensitive to inhibition by propylthiouracil, a drug that competes with the thiol co-factor involved with regeneration of the enzyme. Reverse T_3 is actually the preferred substrate for 5′ deiodination, and inner ring deiodination of T_4 and T_3 (or preferably their sulfates) is also accomplished by this same enzyme. Fasting may be associated with lowered D1 actively by depletion of co-factors. Thyroid hormone excess enhances and thyroid hormone deficiency decreases D1 activity.

Type 2 deiodinase (D2) has outer ring activity and is thought to be an important source of intracellular T_3 in certain tissues as well as a source of circulatory T_3.

Table 13-1 Characteristics of the Human Iodothyronine Deiodinases

	Type 1	Type 2	Type 3
Deiodination site	5′ and 5	5′	5
Physiologic roles	Provide T_3 for the circulation, Inactivate T_4 and T_3 Degrade rT_3	Provide intracellular T_3 in pituitary, brain, and brown adipose tissue; provide T_3 for the circulation	Inactivate T_4 and T_3
Tissue location	Liver, kidney, thyroid, brain	Pituitary, brain, brown adipose tissue, placenta, thyroid, skeletal and cardiac muscle	Brain, placenta, skin
Substrate preference	$rT_3 \gg T_4 > T_3$	$T_4 \geq T_3$	$T_3 > T_4$
Km	$\sim 10^{-7}\,M\,(rT_3)$ $\sim 10^{-6}M\,(T_4)$	$\sim 10^{-9}M\,(T_4)$ $\sim 10^{-8}M\,(rT_3)$	$\sim 10^{-9}M\,(T_3)$ $\sim 10^{-8}M\,(T_4)$
Inhibition by propylthiouracil	sensitive	resistant	resistant
Response to thyroid hormone excess	increase	decrease	increase

Adapted from Larsen PR, Biochemical Society Transactions 25:589, 1997.

In humans it is found in the pituitary, brain, brown adipose tissue, thyroid, placenta, and both skeletal and cardiac muscle. It has a much higher affinity for T_4 and rT_3 than does D1 and prefers T_4. The regulation of D2 activity by thyroid status is opposite to that of D1; thyroid hormone deficiency enhances and thyroid hormone excess decreases D2 activity. The T_3 formed by intracellular conversion of T_4 by D2 is important for providing more than half of the T_3 occupying the nuclear receptors in the pituitary, brain, and brown adipose tissue. The T_3 formed in the anterior pituitary is necessary for physiological feedback inhibition of T_4 on TSH secretion. In contrast, the majority of nuclear T_3 in the liver and kidney is derived from circulating T_3. D2 is not sensitive to inhibition by propylthiouracil, perhaps because of slower turnover of D2 compared with D1.

Type 3 deiodinase (D3) has an inner ring (5-deiodinase) activity and is thought to be important for inactivation of T_4 and T_3. It is present in the brain, placenta, and skin. It has higher affinity for T_3 than T_4 and may serve to protect the fetus from maternal thyroid hormones. It is not sensitive to propylthiouracil. The D3 is enhanced in the brain by thyroid hormone excess, and it is decreased by thyroid hormone deficiency. The opposite regulation of D2 and D3 activities in the brain may work to keep brain T_3 levels constant in conditions of thyroid hormone excess or deficiency.

Effects of Illness and Drugs on Thyroid Hormone Metabolism

The majority of patients hospitalized with nonthyroidal illness have serum T_3 levels below the normal range. These low values are not usually appreciated because serum T_3 levels are not measured. The routine screening tests (free T_4 estimates, see below) are within the normal ranges in these patients. Both TSH levels and the TSH response to thyrotropin-releasing hormone (TRH, see below) are also usually normal. However, serum rT_3 levels are elevated, and the depressed T_3 and elevated rT_3 levels return to normal upon recovery from illness. These changes are due to a temporary decrease in 5'-deiodinase activity (D1). A decrease in 5'-deiodinase would not only impair T_4 to T_3 conversion but would also impair further deiodination of rT_3, in effect, decreasing its clearance. A model for the low T_3 levels of illness is starvation. Total caloric deprivation results in a greater than 50% decrease in serum T_3 levels without major changes in T_4 or TSH. As in nonthyroidal illness, serum rT_3 levels increase about 50% with starvation.

A major question about the low T_3 state is whether patients with significantly reduced T_3 levels have thyroid hormone deficiency at the tissue level. Although the fact that TSH values are not usually increased would seem to argue against it, it could be postulated, however, that impaired hypothalamic TRH secretion might mask actual thyroid hormone deficiency. When fasted subjects with decreased serum T_3 levels are given exogenous T_3 replacement, muscle protein catabolism is enhanced, as evidenced by increased urinary urea, ammonia, and 3-methylhistidine excretion. This has been taken as evidence of a protein-sparing effect of the low T_3 levels in starvation. In clinical observations of patients with low T_3 levels associated with illness, basal metabolic rate and the cardiac measurement of thyroid status—pulse wave arrival time—are normal, again suggesting adequate thyroid effects at the tissue level. Dynamic tests of feedback at the hypothalamic–pituitary level, though normal in fasted subjects, may be subtly abnormal in some patients with illness and

Thyroxine

Iopanoic Acid

Amiodarone

Fig. 13-5 Structures of thyroxine, the oral cholecystographic agent iopanoic acid, and the antiarrhythmic agent amiodarone. The similarities of iodine substitutions on the benzene rings and aliphatic side chains are shown. (Reprinted from Griffin JE: Am J Med Sci 289:86, 1985, with permission.)

low T_3 levels. In general, however, there is little evidence for significant thyroid hormone deficiency at the tissue level, and the impaired T_4 to T_3 conversion is probably beneficial in sparing protein catabolism.

Two iodine-containing drugs given to patients with nonthyroidal illness inhibit 5′-deiodinases in all tissues and result in elevated T_4 levels (Fig. 13-5). They are iopanoic acid, a drug used for radiographic visualization of the gallbladder, and amiodarone, a drug used to treat cardiac arrhythmias. These compounds appear to mimic the structure of T_4 in the iodine substitutions on the benzene ring and the presence of an aliphatic side-chain (Fig. 13-5). The evidence for inhibition of D2 is that these drugs result in an elevation of TSH levels. Upon discontinuing the amiodarone or waiting for the elimination of iopanoic acid, the alterations in thyroid function tests return to normal.

REGULATION OF THYROID FUNCTION

The Hypothalamic–Pituitary–Thyroid Axis

The function of the thyroid gland is regulated mainly by TSH, an anterior pituitary glycoprotein hormone with an α- and β-subunit and a molecular weight of about 28,000 (see Chapter 5). The α-subunit of TSH is identical to the α-subunit of gonadotropins, whereas the β-subunit is distinct and confers on the intact TSH mole-

cule its biological activity. The TSH stimulates the thyroid by interacting with specific cell surface, G protein–linked receptors on thyroid follicular cells to enhance
the activity of adenylyl cyclase and thus stimulate the generation of cyclic AMP as
a second messenger inside the cell. All of the intracellular effects of TSH stimulation can be mimicked by cyclic AMP in the absence of TSH.

The regulation of TSH secretion by the pituitary is primarily under the dual
control of the hypothalamic tripeptide TRH and thyroid hormones (Fig. 13-6). TRH
is derived from a pro-TRH peptide. Like other hypothalamic-releasing hormones,
TRH reaches the anterior pituitary via the hypothalamic–pituitary portal circulation
(see Chapter 6). The TRH interacts with specific receptors on pituitary thyrotrophs
to release TSH and on mammotrophs to release prolactin. TRH belongs to the category of stimulating factors whose action starts with the hydrolysis of phosphatidylinositol 4,5-bisphosphate (PIP_2) (see Chapter 3). The hydrolysis of PIP_2 in
the cell surface membrane generates two second messengers, inositol trisphosphate
(IP_3) and 1,2-diacylglycerol. This hydrolysis is catalyzed by the membrane-bound
enzyme phospholipase C and is associated with the rapid elevation of the concentration of free ionized calcium in the cell cytoplasm. The released calcium is thought
to stimulate exocytosis. Together with these effects of IP_3 there is a parallel activation of protein kinase C by diacylglycerol that leads to phosphorylation of proteins
involved in exocytosis and that mediates the sustained phase of secretion.

The release of TRH is controlled by central nervous system mechanisms (see
Chapter 6). TRH is probably released in a pulsatile fashion, as pulsatile TSH secretion has been identified. The release of TSH is not absolutely dependent on TRH because low residual secretion of TSH persists even after the secretion of TRH has been
stopped. Thus, the decrease in thyroid activity is more severe following hypophy-
sectomy, which eliminates the source of TSH, than following hypothalamic lesions.

The ability of the thyrotroph to respond to TRH with increased TSH release is

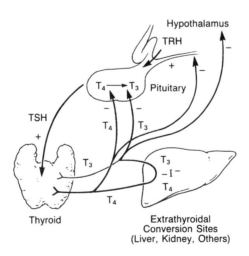

Fig. 13-6   The regulation of thyrotropin (TSH) secretion by the anterior pituitary. Positive effects of thyrotropin-releasing hormone (TRH) from the hypothalamus and negative effects of circulating 3,5,3'-triiodothyronine (T_3) and T_3 from intrapituitary and
hypothalamic conversion of thyroxine (T_4).

controlled by the feedback inhibition of thyroid hormones (Fig. 13-6). Either T_4 or T_3 is capable of inhibiting TSH secretion; however, as previously discussed, T_3 formed in the pituitary by 5'-deiodination (D2) of circulating T_4 appears to be a more important source of thyroid hormone to occupy nuclear receptors and mediate this feedback inhibition than is circulating T_3. Negative feedback by T_3, formed by D2, occurs at both the pituitary and the paraventricular nucleus of the hypothalamus. Negative feedback involves decreased transcription of TSH-α and -β genes and also the pro-TRH gene. It is not known whether thyroid hormones also inhibit TRH release. Studies in which exogenous TRH was administered to normal subjects and patients with thyroid hormone deficiency or thyroid hormone excess indicate that feedback at the level of the pituitary is sufficient to explain the regulation of TSH secretion. The TSH response to administered TRH is enhanced in patients with thyroid hormone deficiency compared to normal subjects. In contrast, thyroid hormone excess diminishes or abolishes the TSH response to TRH. Also, TRH receptors on thyrotrophs are increased in hypothyroidism and decreased in hyperthyroidism.

In addition to TRH and thyroid hormone, other substances of hypothalamic origin play some role in regulating TSH secretion. Somatostatin, another hypothalamic hormone (see Chapter 6), can inhibit TSH secretion. Because injection of antisomatostatin antiserum into normal animals increases TSH levels, somatostatin may be a tonic inhibitor of TSH secretion. The neurotransmitter dopamine may also be responsible for tonic inhibition of TSH release as dopamine antagonists cause elevation of serum TSH levels in normal subjects. It is not known by what mechanism dopamine inhibits TSH; it may act via effects on somatostatin. Finally, glucocorticoids, when present at supraphysiological levels, lead to partial inhibition of TSH secretion.

Thyroid Autoregulation

Although TSH is the primary regulator of thyroid function, the thyroid is also capable of some degree of autoregulation (as discussed above in relation to iodide transport and organification). The autoregulatory responses appear to operate in a manner to maintain thyroid hormone stores in the thyroid gland. Thus, in a state of iodide deficiency the efficiency of iodide transport is enhanced, with the opposite occurring in the presence of iodide excess. This response occurs without a detectable change in TSH levels. Proof of the autoregulatory nature of the inverse effect of iodide availability on iodide transport is found in the persistence of the phenomenon in the hypophysectomized animal. As previously mentioned, the mediator of the autoregulatory effect appears to be organic iodine rather than inorganic iodine in the gland.

EFFECTS OF THYROID HORMONES

Mechanism of Thyroid Hormone Action

Thyroid hormones, like steroid hormones, are thought to enter target cells by passive diffusion. However, there is now evidence to support the concept of a carrier system for both steroid and thyroid hormones to enter cells. The carrier system for iodothyronines is saturable and requires energy. Decreases in cellular uptake in fasting and illness may contribute to the decreased deiodination of iodothyronines in these settings.

Although there is some evidence to support cell surface and mitochondrial sites of action of thyroid hormones, most of the characteristic biological effects of thyroid hormones are thought to be mediated by an interaction of T_3 with specific nuclear receptors. The mechanism of action of thyroid hormones is quite similar to that of steroid hormones in that the binding of the hormone is to a nuclear receptor with resultant alteration of transcription of specific messenger RNAs (see Chapter 3). In contrast to steroid hormone receptors that may not be firmly anchored in the nucleus before hormone binding (and thus are found in cytosol fractions following cell disruption), thyroid hormone receptors are thought to be tightly associated with acidic nonhistone nuclear proteins.

This nuclear thyroid hormone receptor has a low capacity (about 1 pmol/mg DNA) and a high affinity for T_3 (about 10^{-10} M). The affinity of the receptor for T_4 is an order of magnitude less. Initial studies of the nuclear receptor demonstrated a correspondence of receptor number and known responsiveness to thyroid hormones in a number of tissues. In the normal animal, about 85% of the total iodothyronine bound to liver and kidney nuclei is T_3 and the remaining 15% is T_4. Among the tissues examined for T_3 receptors, the anterior pituitary was notable for having the highest number of binding sites and greater than 50% of tissue T_3 bound to receptor sites. In contrast to the liver and kidney, in which most of the nuclear T_3 is derived from serum T_3, only about 40%–50% of nuclear T_3 in the pituitary appears to originate from serum T_3. The remaining 50%–60% of nuclear T_3 in the pituitary is derived from local conversion from T_4 by D2. As a consequence of this extra quantity of intracellular T_3, the nuclear receptors of the pituitary are about 80% saturated, compared to only 50% in the liver and kidney.

All of the major effects of thyroid hormones appear to be mediated by the nuclear receptor. The production of many major classes of messenger RNA rises in response to thyroid hormones. Thyroid hormones stimulate the cell membrane enzyme Na^+, K^+-ATPase and thus increase oxygen consumption. That this stimulation of ATPase activity is mediated through the nuclear receptor is indicated by the observation that the increased enzyme activity is due to an increased number of "pump units" rather than an alteration in preexisting enzyme molecules. Likewise, in studies of the effects of thyroid hormones on myocardial β-adrenergic receptors, the number but not the affinity of the receptors increased in response to thyroid hormones. The stimulation of uncoupling proteins in the inner mitochondrial membrane (see below) is also thought to be mediated by the nuclear receptor.

The thyroid hormone receptor has been resistant to attempts to isolate it in a purified form using methods applied to other intracellular receptors. Thyroid hormone receptors were identified as being 50,000-Da nonhistone proteins. The actual description of the thyroid hormone receptor was achieved when two separate groups of investigators reported that c-*erb*-A, the product of the cellular homologue of the viral oncogene v-*erb*-A, has the ability to bind T_3 with high affinity and specificity. Because v-*erb*-A had been shown to be structurally related to steroid receptors, this confirmed that the thyroid receptor belonged to the same family of intracellular receptors (see Chapter 3). The most fascinating aspect of this story is that multiple thyroid hormone receptors exist. These different thyroid receptors (TR) are divided into α- and β-forms on the basis of sequence similarities and chromosomal location (Fig. 13-7). A TRβ2 cDNA has been found in rat, mouse, and chicken but not in frogs or humans. The TRβ gene is on human chromosome 3. TRβ2 differs from TRβ1 in that it is not widely distributed and thus far appears to be specific to pituitary and brain. TRα1 has been localized to human chromosome 17 and is widely distributed like TRβ1. Alternative splicing of the TRα gene transcripts yields a species called c-erb-Aα2, which is identical to TRα1 for the first 370 amino acids, including the DNA-binding domain, then diverges completely (Fig. 13-7). This latter c-erb-Aα does not bind T_3 and is thus not a TR. However, it is widely distributed and demonstrates regulation by T_3, as do the true TRs.

In addition to binding T_3, a true TR must also be able to bind to a thyroid hormone response element (TRE), a specific DNA sequence in the promoter region of thyroid-responsive genes. Generally, binding of T_3 and the TRE by TRs results in alteration (either activation or suppression) of gene transcription. TRβ1, TRβ2, and TRα1 all bind T_3 in a similar manner. The transcriptional activation of the rat growth hormone gene by T_3 is due to a TRE. The binding of TRs to TREs is independent of T_3. All three TRs are able to confer T_3 responsiveness when expressed in cells that normally do not respond to T_3. In contrast, c-erb-Aα2 does not produce a T_3 dependency of transcription of genes bearing TREs. Instead, it appears to inhibit the action of TRs in a concentration-dependent manner. Although it may regulate thyroid hormone action, the exact *in vivo* functions of c-erb-Aα2 have not been defined. The v-erb-A protein has a similar dominant negative effect by means of its DNA-binding domain. In the absence of T_3, a TRE-bound TR may actually decrease basal T_3-responsive gene expression.

Based on evidence of heterodimer formation of TRs with the closely related retinoid X receptor (RXR), a dimerization domain has been identified in TRs. The TRs can form homodimers or heterodimers with each other or form heterodimers

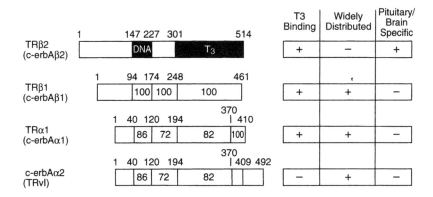

Fig. 13-7 Thyroid hormone receptors and the carboxy-terminal variant c-erb-Aα2. The sequences deduced from rat cDNAs are depicted with the amino acids numbered above. Putative DNA- and T_3-binding domains are indicated. Numbers in boxes indicate percent identity with TRβ2.

with one of the RXRs. When TRs bind T_3, they undergo a conformational change that can cause TR dimers to dissociate. The TR:RXR heterodimer may be the most important complex *in vivo* because (*1*) TR:RXR heterodimers bind with much higher affinity than TRs to each other; (*2*) binding of TR:RXR heterodimers to most TREs is more stable than binding of TR monomers or homodimers; and (*3*) transcriptional activation by TRs is enhanced by the presence of RXRs. Mutations in TRβ can cause thyroid hormone resistance.

Physiological Effects

Thyroid hormones have effects in almost all tissues of the body. In many respects, thyroid hormones may be viewed as tissue growth factors. Indeed, normal overall whole body growth does not occur in the absence of thyroid hormones despite adequate levels of growth hormone. In amphibians the effects of thyroid hormones on differentiation are dramatically evidenced by the failure of metamorphosis to occur in their absence.

Thyroid hormones have specific tissue effects that are perhaps best exemplified by the effects of thyroid hormone deficiency and excess (see below). These effects are mediated by the action of thyroid hormones on the concentration and activity of enzymes, the metabolism of substrates, vitamins, and minerals, and the function of other endocrine systems. The earliest recognized physiological effect of thyroid hormones is its ability to stimulate the basal metabolic rate or calorigenesis. Thyroid hormones stimulate oxygen consumption in the whole animal and in isolated tissues *in vitro*.

The stimulation of synthesis of membrane Na^+,K^+-ATPase is thought to contribute to the increased energy expenditure in going from the thyroid-deficient to the normal (euthyroid) state. This effect of thyroid hormones to enhance ATPase activity can be detected in many but not all tissues. Spleen and testes have very low concentrations of nuclear thyroid hormone receptors and fail to show increased calorigenesis in response to thyroid hormones. Thyroid hormones exert effects on thermogenesis and temperature regulation that are related to their effects on energy metabolism. Rats deficient in thyroid hormones are unable to survive in a cold environment.

Uncoupling protein (UCP1) was initially described in the brown adipose tissue of the rodent as a molecule that allowed the return of protons to the mitochondrial matrix, bypassing ATP synthase, and therefore uncoupling oxidative phosphorylation. Thus, fatty acids can be oxidized with generation of heat but not ATP. Because thyroid hormone stimulates uncoupling protein, this was considered a potential site of regulation of energy metabolism. However, very little brown adipose tissue is present in humans. Recently, two additional uncoupling proteins, UCP2 and UCP3, have been identified in rodents and humans. The UCP2 is widely distributed, including most tissues examined, especially skeletal muscle, lung, spleen, thymus, leukocytes, and macrophages. In rodents it is present in white and brown adipose tissue and liver. The UCP3 is present in high levels only in skeletal muscle in humans. The overall contribution of these uncoupling proteins to thyroid hormone regulation of energy metabolism is yet to be determined.

Protein synthesis and degradation are stimulated by thyroid hormones. Stimulation of protein synthesis may be responsible for a portion of the calorigenic effect of thyroid hormones. The positive influence of thyroid hormones on normal body growth is derived largely from stimulation of protein synthesis. In the presence of a large excess of thyroid hormones there is accelerated protein catabolism, leading to increased nitrogen excretion.

Thyroid hormones affect most aspects of carbohydrate metabolism. They appear to enhance the actions of epinephrine in stimulating glycogenolysis and gluconeogenesis and to potentiate the actions of insulin on glycogen synthesis and glucose utilization. As with thyroid hormone effects on protein metabolism, a biphasic action of thyroid hormones on carbohydrate metabolism can be detected. Thus, low doses of thyroid hormones given to animals enhance glycogen synthesis in the presence of insulin, whereas large doses stimulate glycogenolysis. Thyroid hormones also enhance the rate of intestinal absorption of glucose and its rate of uptake by adipose tissue and muscle.

Thyroid hormones have multiple effects on lipid metabolism. Cholesterol synthesis and its metabolic conversions are depressed in thyroid hormone deficiency. However, as degradation is affected to a greater extent than synthesis, serum cholesterol levels increase in the thyroid-deficient state, and serum levels of cholesterol, phospholipids, and triglycerides decrease with thyroid hormone excess. One mechanism that may partially account for enhanced cholesterol metabolism in response to thyroid hormones is the ability of thyroid hormones to increase the number of low-density lipoprotein receptors on the cell surface (see Chapter 16). Fatty acid metabolism is affected by thyroid hormones that enhance lipolysis in adipose tissue.

Effects of Thyroid Hormone Deficiency

Severe thyroid hormone deficiency in infancy is termed *cretinism* and is characterized by mental as well as growth retardation. The developmental milestones of the infant such as sitting and walking are delayed. Linear growth impairment may lead to dwarfism, characterized by limbs that are disproportionately short compared with the trunk. When the onset of thyroid hormone deficiency is later in childhood mental retardation is less prominent, and impairment of linear growth is the major feature. The result is a child who appears younger than his or her chronological age. Epiphyseal development is delayed so that bone age is less than chronological age.

The onset of thyroid hormone deficiency in the adult is usually insidious; the symptoms and signs gradually appear over months or years. The early symptoms are nonspecific. Tiredness and lethargy are common, and constipation may develop or worsen. Eventually there is an overall slowing of mental function and motor activity. Although some weight gain usually occurs, appetite is usually decreased so that gross obesity is rare. Cold intolerance may be the first manifestation of thyroid hormone deficiency, the individual complaining of feeling cold in a room in which others are comfortable. Women may experience abnormalities of menstrual function, with increased menstrual flow being more common than cessation of menses. Decreased clearance of adrenal androgens may facilitate extraglandular estrogen formation leading to anovulatory cycles with infertility. Hair loss may occur, as may brittle nails and dry, coarse skin. The voice may become hoarse.

When thyroid hormone deficiency is long-standing and severe, there is an accumulation of mucopolysaccharides in subcutaneous tissues and other organs, termed *myxedema*. Dermal infiltration results in thickened features, periorbital edema, and swelling of the hands and feet that does not indent with pressure. Stiffness and aching of muscles may be followed by muscle swelling as an early manifestation. Delayed muscle contraction and relaxation lead to slow movement and delayed tendon reflexes. Both stroke volume and heart rate are reduced so that cardiac output decreases. The heart may enlarge and a pericardial effusion develops. Pleural and peritoneal fluid rich in protein and mucopolysaccharides may accumulate. The slowing of mental function is characterized by impaired memory, slow speech, decreased initiative, and eventually somnolence. Mild hypothermia may lead to more severe hypothermia if there is environmental exposure. Eventually, coma may develop in conjunction with hypoventilation.

Effects of Thyroid Hormone Excess

The earliest manifestations of thyroid hormone excess are usually nervousness, irritability or emotional instability, a feeling that the heart is pounding, fatigue, and heat intolerance. As with thyroid hormone deficiency, this latter manifestation may be manifested as altered comfort in a room in which others are comfortable and lead to resetting the thermostat or requiring lighter clothing. Increased sweating is commonly noticed. Although fatigue invariably occurs, the nervousness and irritability may give the impression of increased energy. Weight loss despite normal or increased food intake is one of the most common manifestations. The increased food intake occasionally can be so great as to overcome the hypermetabolic state and result in weight gain. Interestingly, most patients relate that their increased caloric intake is predominantly in the form of carbohydrates. Women have decreased or absent menstrual flow. The number of bowel movements per day often increases, but true watery diarrhea is rare. Physical findings may include warm, moist skin of a velvety texture often compared to that of a newborn, a change in the fingernails, termed *onycholysis,* involving separation of the nail from the nail bed, and proximal muscle weakness, often making it difficult for the patient to rise form a sitting or squatting position. In contrast to thyroid hormone deficiency, the hair has a very fine texture, but hair loss may similarly occur. On extending the fingers of an outstretched hand a fine tremor may be seen. The eyelids may retract, leading to the impression that the patient is staring. Tachycardia that persists during sleep is characteristic, and atrial arrhythmias and congestive heart failure may develop.

CLINICAL ASSESSMENT OF THYROID STATUS

To assess thyroid status one must search the medical history for symptoms of thyroid hormone deficiency or excess and examine the patient for thyroid enlargement as well as other physical findings typical of thyroid disease (see above). Because thyroid disease is relatively common and the clinical manifestations may be subtle, laboratory tests are widely used to screen for the presence of thyroid dysfunction and to confirm the suspected diagnosis.

Measurement of Serum TSH

With the development of immunometric assays (see Chapter 5), measurement of the serum TSH has become the best initial test in clinical assessment of thyroid status in most situations. The previous (or first-generation) TSH assays were radioimmunoassays that did not have sufficient sensitivity to differentiate low values from normal values. The current second- and third-generation TSH assays have increased sensitivities (0.1 and 0.01 μU/ml, respectively). The typical range of serum TSH in a normal population is 0.4–4.5 μU/ml. Because the overwhelming majority of patients with thyroid disease have primary disease of the thyroid rather than abnormalities of the hypothalamus or pituitary (see below), the usual clinical laboratory second-generation TSH assay can distinguish thyroid hormone deficiency or excess by the response of the hypothalamic–pituitary axis. Thyroid hormone deficiency results in increased serum TSH levels if the axis is intact, and thyroid hormone excess results in low TSH levels (Fig. 13-8). If hypothalamic–pituitary function is not normal—as in the patient with hypopituitarism or a TSH-producing pituitary tumor (see Chapter 6)—the TSH is not a reliable indicator of thyroid status. The serum TSH may also be unreliable in some patients with nonthyroidal illness (see below). The reason that the serum TSH is particularly useful in assessment of thyroid status is the log-linear relationship that exists between serum TSH and the free thyroid hormone estimate (Fig. 13-9). A small change in the free thyroid levels results in a much greater proportional change in TSH levels. For example, a 2-fold change of the free T_4 concentration results in a 160-fold change in the serum TSH level (Fig. 13-9).

Measurement of Circulating Thyroid Hormones

Measurement of total T_4 and T_3 concentrations in the plasma is accomplished by immunoassay. As discussed above, both hormones are largely bound to serum

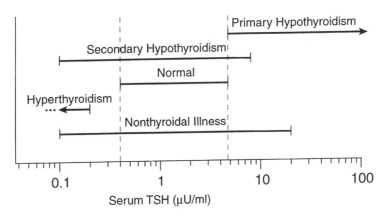

Fig. 13-8 The range of serum TSH values encountered in various thyroid states and nonthyroidal illness. The usual sensitivity of the second-generation immunometric TSH assay of 0.1 μU/ml is shown. Patients with hyperthyroidism are shown as having values that may be undetectable not only in this assay but also in more sensitive assays.

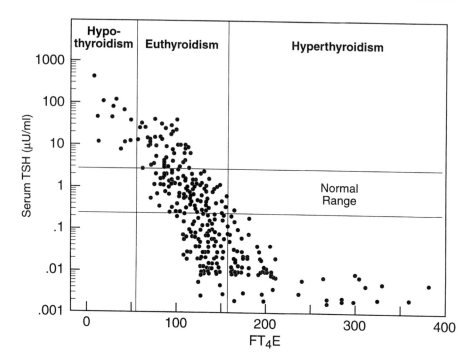

Fig. 13-9   The physiologic log/linear relationship of TSH to the free T_4 estimate (FT_4E). The FT_4E is given in arbitrary units. A 2-fold change in the serum FT_4E results in a 160-fold change in serum TSH. (Redrawn from Spencer C, New roles for TSH measurement in thyroid testing. Kodak Thyroid Information Service 1992, p. 17.)

proteins, and the bioavailable component would appear to be the most desirable fraction to measure. However, the bioavailable fraction is different for T_4 and T_3 and varies in different tissues.

Although the actual bioavailable thyroid hormone fraction is greater than the free or unbound fraction in the plasma (see above), clinical states of thyroid hormone deficiency and excess correlate reasonably well with the free iodothyronine concentrations. Thus, attempts have been made to assess the free T_4 and T_3 concentrations. The reference test for free thyroid hormone levels is *equilibrium dialysis.* In this test radiolabeled iodothyronine is added to the patient's serum, and the percent that is able to pass through a dialysis membrane is determined. This percentage is then multiplied by the total iodothyronine concentration measured by immunoassay to obtain a free iodothyronine concentration. The free T_4 concentration by dialysis in a normal population is about 0.8–1.5 ng/dl.

Because determination of the free T_4 by equilibrium dialysis is laborious and not routinely available in clinical laboratories, several approaches in obtaining an approximation of the free T_4 (or T_3) have been developed. These free T_4 and T_3 estimates are primarily important for correcting for variations in the concentration of TBG (see below).

Until recently, the most commonly used method for estimating free T_4 and T_3 level was the correction of the measured total T_4 or T_3 by an *in vitro* test to assess total available binding sites for thyroid hormone in the serum and calculate a free T_4 or T_3 index. The ranges for the total T_4 and T_3 concentrations in a normal population are 5–12 μg/dl and 60–180 ng/dl, respectively. The *in vitro* test used to adjust the total iodothyronine concentrations is termed the T_3-*resin uptake* or T_3-*uptake ratio* and is performed by incubating a serum sample with radioactive T_3. After equilibration a resin or other substance is added to the mixture to bind the radioactive T_3 not bound to serum proteins. The percentage of the total radioactive T_3 bound to the resin is related in a reciprocal manner to the thyroid hormone-binding capacity in the sample. There are two possible interpretations of both an increased and a decreased T_3-resin uptake. An increased T_3-resin uptake (i.e., more T_3 bound to the resin and less to the serum-binding proteins) could be due to greater saturation of a normal amount of TBG secondary to increased thyroid hormone production (i.e., thyroid hormone excess). Alternatively, because of a decreased concentration of TBG with normal thyroid hormone production, there could be fewer available binding sites, resulting in more T_3 being bound to the resin.

Conversely, a decreased T_3-resin uptake (i.e., less T_3 bound to the resin and more to the serum-binding proteins) could be due to decreased saturation of a normal amount of TBG because of decreased thyroid hormone production (i.e., thyroid hormone deficiency). Alternatively, because of an increased concentration of TBG with normal thyroid hormone production, there could be more available binding sites, resulting in less T_3 being bound to the resin. The value of the T_3-resin uptake is either reported as a percentage or compared to the T_3-resin uptake of a normal serum pool and reported as a T_3-uptake ratio, with the normal being unity. The free T_4 index is the product of the serum total T_4 and the T_3-resin uptake. This calculation is usually made only for the total T_4, but it can also be done for the total T_3.

The effect of pregnancy and other conditions that alter the level of TBG (Table 13-2) is to increase or decrease total T_4 and T_3 concentrations without changing the level of free, unbound hormone in the steady state. For example, if TBG increases in concentration, the amount of free hormone decreases temporarily until compensatory mechanisms result in a new steady state with increased total hormone concentration but normal free hormone. The correction of the increased total T_4 by the decreased T_3-resin uptake results in a normal free T_4 index. Thus, changes in the T_3-resin uptake are reciprocal to the changes in the number of available binding sites on TBG and the total T_4 when the primary abnormality is a change in binding pro-

Table 13-2 Conditions and Hormones That Alter the Level of Thyroid Hormone–Binding Globulin (TBG)

Increased TBG	Decreased TBG
Pregnancy	Androgens and anabolic steroids
Newborn state	Large dose of glucocorticoids
Oral contraceptives and other sources of estrogens	Chronic liver disease
Infectious and chronic active hepatitis	Severe systemic illness
Genetically determined	Active acromegaly
	Kidney disease with proteinuria
	Genetically determined

teins. When there is a primary alteration in thyroid hormone production, the change in the T_3-resin uptake is in the same direction as the change in the total T_4 level.

An alternative to calculation of the free T_4 index as an estimate of the free T_4 concentration is one of the newer assays to measure the free T_4 either indirectly or directly. In the *indirect approach,* a two-step method of preincubation of the serum with an anti-T_4 antibody coated tube is followed by addition of labeled T_4. In the *direct approach* a one-step incubation of a labeled T_4 analog is incubated with an anti-T_4 antibody coated tube. In each assay the amount of labeled iodothyronine bound is inversely proportional to the free T_4 level in the test specimen. In persons with marked alteration of TBG, these free T_4 estimates may correlate better than the free T_4 index with the clinical thyroid state. However, these free T_4 assays are still subject to spurious results in the setting of extreme alterations in serum proteins, confounding antibodies, and nonthyroidal illness (see below).

In normal individuals there are variations in the concentration of thyroid hormones with age. In the fetus the T_3 level is decreased as it is in euthyroid individuals who are fasted or who have acute or chronic illnesses (see above). Shortly after birth the T_3 level rises. The mean T_3 level declines slightly with advanced age, but the lower limit of normal does not fall until after age 70 in men and age 80 in women. The T_4 level does not decline with age.

Effect of Nonthyroidal Illness on Thyroid Function Tests

Abnormal results on thyroid function tests are frequently encountered in the evaluation of patients without obvious thyroid disease. Some of these abnormal results are caused by altered levels of TBG (see above). In the remainder it is necessary to decide whether subtle thyroid hormone deficiency or excess exists or whether the abnormal values are somehow spurious. The T_4 and free T_4 estimate may be either decreased or increased in subjects who are actually euthyroid but suffer from acute or chronic nonthyroid illness. As discussed in the section on thyroid hormone metabolism, the most common effect of nonthyroidal illness on thyroid function tests is to lower T_3 levels.

In addition to the low T_3 levels, some patients with nonthyroidal illness have a decreased total T_4 and free T_4 estimate. These are often the more critically ill patients. Studies have shown that the decreased level of T_4 is due to a circulating inhibitor of thyroid hormone binding to serum-binding proteins and that this inhibitor likely comes from tissue breakdown associated with severe illness. Because the inhibitor is not detected in the T_3-resin uptake test, the decreased total T_4 is not adjusted in calculations of the free T_4 index. These inhibitors of the thyroid hormone binding can also result in spuriously low levels of direct free T_4 estimates. The free T_4 concentrations by equilibrium dialysis are not usually decreased in such patients with nonthyroid illness, and the T_4 production rate is usually normal. All of the abnormalities of iodothyronine levels revert to normal on recovery from the illness.

The serum TSH may be helpful in confirming that the thyroid status of an ill individual with a low free T_4 estimate is normal. However, current sensitive TSH assays have also been found to be temporarily abnormal in patients with nonthyroidal illness, especially acutely ill hospitalized patients (Fig. 13-8). In some instances administration of high-dose glucocorticoids or dopamine lowers TSH levels below the lower reference range with a brief rebound elevation above the upper reference range once the drug is discontinued. In other patients the nonthyroidal illness itself, perhaps by cytokines inhibiting TRH synthesis, lowers TSH levels. During recovery from the illness, the patient's TSH levels may transiently rise above normal.

DERANGED THYROID PHYSIOLOGY

Deranged thyroid physiology may involve altered thyroid growth, in either a diffuse or a nodular pattern, while thyroid hormone production remains normal. Although this simple increase in thyroid size, termed *euthyroid goiter,* is common in the population, the physiological derangement(s) leading to its development in areas of iodide sufficiency are poorly understood. Thus, to illustrate the effects of thyroid hormones and pathophysiological mechanisms of thyroid hormone secretion, only hypothyroidism and hyperthyroidism will be considered here.

Hypothyroidism

Hypothyroidism is a clinical state resulting from decreased production of thyroid hormones. It may begin *in utero,* or later in life, resulting in a different set of clinical features as we saw in the discussion of thyroid hormone deficiency.

Hypothyroidism is relatively common, occurring in about 2% of adult women in a clinically overt form. It is much less common in men. Spontaneous hypothyroidism may be due to disorders of the thyroid (primary hypothyroidism), of the anterior pituitary or hypothalamus (secondary hypothyroidism), or, rarely, of peripheral target tissues (severe generalized thyroid hormone resistance). Primary hypothyroidism accounts for over 95% of patients with hypothyroidism. In rare congenital forms of hypothyroidism, enzyme defects in thyroid hormone formation or mutations in the sodium iodide symporter may result in hypothyroidism with goiter, or inactivating mutations in the TSH receptor may cause congenital hypothyroidism without thyroid enlargement.

Primary hypothyroidism developing later in life also may be associated either with a decrease in thyroid tissue or with thyroid enlargement. Both the nongoitrous and goitrous forms are commonly the result of an autoimmune thyroiditis leading to destruction of thyroid parenchyma. In those who have goiters, lymphocytic infiltration of the thyroid is seen and the condition is termed *Hashimoto's disease.* This autoimmune destruction of the thyroid may be part of a polyglandular endocrine deficiency syndrome in which the adrenals, parathyroids, gonads, pancreatic islets, and stomach parietal cells are variably involved, but the hypothyroidism is usually an isolated finding. The most common cause of primary hypothyroidism in adults is destruction of the thyroid tissue by prior surgery or radioactive iodine treatment for hyperthyroidism.

In areas in which iodine is not sufficient, goitrous hypothyroidism may be due to endemic iodine deficiency. This is rare in North America but quite common in many other parts of the world. The incidence of endemic goiter has been greatly reduced in many areas by the introduction of iodized salt.

Secondary hypothyroidism is due to decreased TSH secretion. Although an isolated abnormality of TSH release has been described, most secondary hypothyroidism is due to pituitary insufficiency involving multiple anterior pituitary hormones (see Chapter 6). The pituitary may be affected directly or indirectly as a result of hypothalamic disease inhibiting the delivery of releasing factors.

As with almost all hormones, resistance to the action of thyroid hormones has been described as a disease mechanism. In more severely affected individuals the resistance is present in all target tissues. This leads to increased thyroid hormone production in the absence of symptoms of thyroid hormone excess and occasionally in the face of symptoms of thyroid hormone deficiency (delayed bone age, epiphyseal stippling, and decreased hydroxyproline excretion). In such patients the serum TSH is normal. The defect in most instances is due to a $TR\beta$ mutation.

Most patients with clinical hypothyroidism have a free T_4 estimate below the lower range of normal. Because the normal range is relatively broad, some hypothyroid patients may have T_4 levels that are within the low normal range. As most patients with hypothyroidism have primary disease of the thyroid gland rather than secondary hypothyroidism resulting from hypothalamic or pituitary disease, the serum TSH is the most useful screening test (see above). The serum TSH in patients with primary hypothyroidism can range from values just slightly above the normal range in patients with mild disease to values ranging from 20 to greater than 100 μU/ml in patients with more severe and long-standing thyroid deficiency (Fig. 13-8).

Although the TSH response to TRH stimulation is enhanced in primary hypothyroidism, such testing is not necessary for the detection of hypothyroidism because the basal TSH is elevated. The TSH level is usually inappropriately normal in the presence of a low free T_4 estimate in patients with hypothalamic or pituitary disorders resulting in secondary hypothyroidism. However, the TSH is occasionally low or even elevated in such patients (Fig. 13-8). Altered glycosylation of TSH resulting in a prolonged half-life and reduced biological activity is thought to account for the mildly increased TSH levels observed in some patients with hypopituitarism. Usually, TSH levels are only undetectable in patients with secondary hypothyroidism who are receiving exogenous thyroid hormone.

The thyroid radioactive iodine uptake (RAIU) is a direct test of thyroid function; a tracer dose of ^{123}I is given orally, and the percentage accumulation in the thyroid is measured, usually at 24 hours. The RAIU varies directly with the functional activity of the thyroid. However, this test is not useful in suspected hypothyroidism because many normal subjects have RAIUs in the range observed in patients with hypothyroidism.

Hyperthyroidism

Hyperthyroidism is the clinical state resulting from increased circulating levels of available thyroid hormones. The manifestations are, in general, an exaggeration of the normal physiological actions of thyroid hormones. In fact, except for the specific form of eye changes, termed *ophthalmopathy,* certain skin changes (which may or may not be present depending on the cause of the hyperthyroidism), and goiter, all of the clinical manifestations can be related to excess thyroid hormone. In contrast to hypothyroidism, which tends to be insidious in onset and slowly progressive in course, hyperthyroidism usually results in recognized symptoms and may (in the case of the most common cause, Graves' disease) undergo periods of exacerbation and remission. The clinical manifestations common to all forms of hyperthyroidism were described in the section on thyroid hormone excess.

As is true for hypothyroidism, hyperthyroidism is relatively common, occurring in 2% of women but only one-tenth as many men. The predominant cause is diffuse toxic goiter, usually termed *Graves' disease*. The mechanism of the autonomous thyroid hormone secretion in Graves' disease is stimulation of the gland by an IgG immunoglobulin that interacts with the TSH receptor. In contrast to most antireceptor antibodies, this antibody does not inhibit but profoundly activates the receptor. Most patients with Graves' disease have a palpably enlarged thyroid gland. A specific infiltrative ophthalmopathy is seen only in Graves' disease. The eyes become protuberant due to infiltration of the extraocular tissues with mucopolysaccharides. Trapping of extraocular muscles in the confined space of the orbit may result in paralysis of eye movement and double vision. In some patients the ophthalmopathy may be the most severe manifestation of Graves' disease. The specific cause of the infiltrative ophthalmopathy of Graves' disease is unknown.

Other causes of hyperthyroidism such as toxic uninodular or multinodular goi-

NORMAL

HYPERTHYROIDISM

Fig. 13-10 Hypothalamic–pituitary–thyroid interactions and the serum thyrotropin (TSH) response to thyrotropin-releasing hormone (TRH) injection in normal subjects and patients with hyperthyroidism. The increased thyroid hormone levels in the hyperthyroid patients inhibit the TSH response to TRH. T_4, thyroxine; T_3, 3,5,3'-triiodothyronine. (Adapted from Kaplan MM, and Utiger RD: Diagnosis of hyperthyroidism. Clin Endocrinol Metab 7:97, 1978.)

ters or inflammation of the thyroid gland (thyroiditis) account for only 10%–15% of patients. Recently, patients with toxic uninodular and multinodular goiters have been found to have somatic mutations in the TSH receptors in the hyperfunctioning nodules, which result in constitutive activation of the receptor. Similar germline mutations cause familial nonautoimmune diffuse toxic goiter. Excess dietary or medication iodide may lead to a low RAIU form of hyperthyroidism, and ingested thyroid hormones may mimic endogenous hyperthyroidism.

The appropriate initial test in patients with suspected hyperthyroidism is the serum TSH. In patients with mild thyroid hormone excess, as in the older individual with autonomous function of a multinodular goiter or a patient slightly overmedicated with thyroid hormone, the TSH level may be below the lower limit of a reference population but still detectable. However, in almost all subjects with symptomatic thyroid hormone excess, the serum TSH is below the limit of detection (less than 0.1 μU/ml in the usual second-generation assay) (Fig. 13-8). Before the availability of sensitive TSH assays, which can distinguish low from normal values, the TRH test was used to identify some patients with subtle thyroid excess and equivocal clinical findings (see Fig. 13-10). Inhibition of the response of serum TSH to an intravenous injection of TRH was consistent with thyroid excess.

After finding a low serum TSH, it is necessary to assess whether there are elevations in thyroid hormone levels to confirm overt hyperthyroidism. Because the average increase in circulating T_4 in patients with the common form of hyperthyroidism is approximately 2-fold, whereas T_3 levels increase 3-fold or 4-fold, the measurement of the total serum T_3 concentration is useful in patients in whom the free T_4 estimate is not clearly elevated.

Finally, although the thyroid RAIU is of limited value in the evaluation of suspected hypothyroidism, it has a role in the assessment of hyperthyroidism. Elevation of the RAIU above the normal range indicates thyroid hyperfunction. However, some patients with endogenous thyroid hormone excess have RAIUs in the normal or low range.

SUGGESTED READING

Abramowicz MJ, Duprez L, Parma J, Vassart G, and Heinrichs C: Familial congenital hypothyroidism due to inactivating mutation of the thyrotropin receptor causing profound hypoplasia of the thyroid gland. J Clin Invest 99:3108–3124, 1997.

Bodenner DL, and Lash RW: Thyroid disease mediated by molecular defects in cell surface and nuclear receptors. Am J Med 105:524–538, 1998.

Freake HC: Uncoupling proteins: Beyond brown adipose tissue. Nutr Rev 56:185–189, 1998.

Gershengorn MC: Mechanism of thyrotropin releasing hormone stimulation of pituitary hormone secretion. Annu Rev Physiol 48:515–526, 1986.

Griffin JE: Hypothyroidism in the elderly. Am J Med Sci 299:334–345, 1990.

Gruters A, Schoneberg T, Biebermann H, Krude H, Krohn HP, Dralle H, and Gudermann T: Severe congenital hyperthyroidism caused by a germ-line neo-mutation in the extracellular portion of the thyrotropin receptor. J Clin Endocrinol Metab 83:1431–1436, 1998.

Hamburger JI: The various presentation of thyroiditis: Diagnostic considerations. Ann Intern Med 104:219–224, 1986.

Klee GG, and Hay ID: Biochemical testing of thyroid function. Encodrinol Metab Clin North Am 26:763–775, 1997.

Larsen PR: Update on the human iodothyronine selenodeiodinases, the enzymes regulating the activation and inactivation of thyroid hormone. Biochem Soc Trans 25:588–592, 1997.

Larsen PR: The thyroid gland. In: *Williams Textbook of Endocrinology,* 9th ed., JD Wilson, DW Foster, HM Kronenberg, and PR Larsen, eds., Saunders, Philadelphia, pp. 389–575, 1998.

Larsen PR: Tyroid-pituitary interaction. Feedback regulation of thyrotropin secretion by thyroid hormones. N Engl J Med 306:23–32, 1982.

Lazar MA: Thyroid hormone receptors: Multiple forms, multiple possibilities. Endocr Rev 14:184–193, 1993.

Motomura K, and Brent GA: Mechanisms of thyroid hormone action. Endocrinol Metab Clin North Am 27:1–23, 1998.

Nicoloff JT, and Spencer CA: The use and misuse of the sensitive thyrotropin assays. J Clin Endocrinol Metab 71:553–558, 1990.

Pisarev MA: Thyroid autoregulation. J Endocrinol Invest 8:475–484, 1985.

Ribeiro RCJ, Aprilette JW, Wagner RL, West BL, Fend W, Huber R, Kushner PJ, Nilsson S, Scanlan T, Fetterick RJ, Schaufele F, and Baxter JD: Mechanisms of thyroid hormone action: Insights from x-ray crystallographic and functional studies. Recent Prog Horm Res 53:351–394, 1998.

Schmutzler C, and Kohrle J: Implications of the molecular characterization of the sodium-iodide symporter (NIS). Exp Clin Endocrinol Diabetes 106 Suppl 3:S1–S10, 1998.

Spitzweg Christine, and Heufelder AE: The sodium iodide symporter: Its emerging relevance to clinical thyroidology. Eur J Endocrinol 138:374–375, 1998.

St Germain DL, and Galton VA: The deiodinase family of selenoproteins. Thyroid 7(4):655–668, 1997.

Taurog A: Hormone synthesis: Thyroid iodine metabolism. In: *Werner and Ingbar's The Thyroid: A Fundamental and Clinical Text,* 7th ed., LE Braverman and RD Utiger, eds., Lippincott, New York, pp. 47–81, 1996.

14

The Adrenal Glands

NORMAN M. KAPLAN

The adrenal glands, weighing only 6–10 g, are essential for life. In their absence, death occurs in a few days.

The overall function of the adrenals is to protect the organism against acute and chronic stress, a concept popularized by Walter Cannon in 1929 as the "fight-or-flight" response for the medulla and by Hans Selye in 1936 as the "alarm" re-action for the cortex. The steroid hormones of the cortex and the catecholamines of the medulla probably developed as protection against immediate stress or injury and more prolonged deprivation of food and water. In acute stress, catecholamines mobilize glucose and fatty acids for energy and prepare the heart, lungs, and muscles for action. Glucocorticoids protect against overreactions from the body's responses to stress, which themselves threaten homeostasis. In the more chronic stress of food and fluid deprivation, the cortical steroid hormones stimulate gluconeogenesis to maintain the supply of glucose and increase sodium reabsorption to maintain body fluid content.

Diseases associated with adrenal hypofunction are relatively rare; those associated with adrenal hyperfunction are slightly more common. However, subtle increases in cortisol secretion or tissue sensitivity to glucocorticoids may be involved in many of the devastating effects of chronic stress, including visceral obesity, hypertension, diabetes, dyslipidemia, and depression. Beyond these possible contributions of endogenous glucocorticoids to multiple diseases, exogenous steroids are widely used to treat numerous diseases. When used in such super-physiologic doses, adrenal steroids may induce many serious adverse effects.

ANATOMY

The adrenals are located on top of the kidneys (ad-renal) (Fig. 14-1). In keeping with their essential function, they are well supplied with arterial blood from branches of the aorta, the renal arteries, and the phrenic arteries. Per gram of tissue, they have about the highest rate of blood flow in the body. Arterial blood enters from the outer cortex, flows through fenestrated capillaries between the cords of cells, and drains inwardly into venules in the medulla. On the right, the adrenal vein directly enters the inferior vena cava; on the left, it usually drains into the left renal vein. Awareness of this arrangement is important when attempts are made to obtain blood from

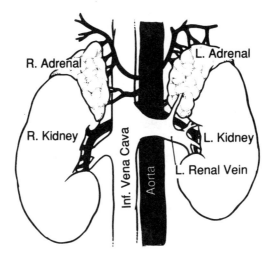

Fig. 14-1   Gross anatomy of the adrenal glands.

or inject radiographic dye into the adrenals in the diagnosis of various primary adrenal diseases.

Anatomical Zonation

The cortex is derived from mesodermal tissue and comprises 90% of the gland. It consists of three zones below its fibrous capsule: the outer zona glomerulosa, the middle zona fasciculata, and the inner zona reticularis (Fig. 14-2). The major secretions of the three zones differ as do the mechanisms primarily responsible for the modulation of their activity (Table 14-1).

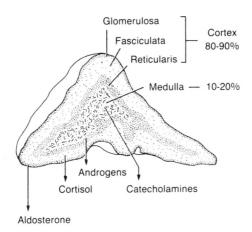

Fig. 14-2   Secretion of adrenocortical hormones by the different zones of the adrenal cortex. (From Guyton AC: *Textbook of Medical Physiology,* Saunders, Philadelphia, p. 909, 1986.)

Table 14-1 Functional Zonation of the Adrenal Cortex

Zone	Major secretion	Major control mechanism
Z. glomerulosa	Aldosterone (mineralocorticoid)	Renin–angiotensin
Z. fasciculata	Cortisol (glucocorticoid)	ACTH
Z. reticularis	Dehydroepiandrosterone (androgen)	ACTH

The medulla, which is derived from neuroectodermal cells from the neural crest, synthesizes and secretes catecholamines. Whereas norepinephrine is the primary neurotransmitter secreted from sympathetic ganglia and neurons, the adrenal medulla secretes mainly epinephrine, reflecting the presence of the N-methyltransferase enzyme, which converts norepinephrine into epinephrine only within the adrenal medulla.

In the fetus, the adrenal glands are much larger relative to body size than in the adult. In absolute size, they are almost as large at term as the fetal kidneys. The fetal gland has an outer subcapsular zone, the precursor of the three zones of the postnatal cortex, and a much larger inner zone, comprising about 80% of the fetal cortex. The cells of the inner fetal cortex are very active but, since the enzyme 3β-hydroxysteroid dehydrogenase needed to convert the early precursors into either glucocorticoids or mineralocorticoids is not active, they produce instead large quantities of dehydroepiandrosterone, which serves as a precursor for the synthesis of estrogens by the placenta (see Chapter 11). After birth, the fetal zone rapidly involutes and the outer subcapsular zone differentiates into the three zones of the postnatal gland.

Functional Zonation

The arrangement of blood flow from the outer cortex into inner medulla may be involved in the differentiation of secretions from the various anatomical zones. Subcapsular cells are capable of generating all three cortical zones. One theory for their differentiation is that the youngest cells are beneath the capsule, forming the zona glomerulosa, and over time the cells migrate downward. The inner zona reticularis cells, being the oldest, have lower rates of cell division and more pigmentation and other signs of a progressive loss of functional activity.

The arrangement of blood flow from the outer cortex into inner medulla also appears to serve the function of maintaining high levels of synthesis and secretion of the major catecholamine required for the response to acute stress, epinephrine. The enzyme responsible for the conversion of norepinephrine to epinephrine, N-methyltransferase, is specifically induced by cortisol, the major steroid secreted by the cortex. Therefore, after the immediate response to stress by release of stored epinephrine, the secretion of cortisol will ensure a continued supply of the hormone.

The traditional view of a simple separation of adrenal zones and secretions shown in Figure 14-2 and Table 14-1, which largely reflected *in vitro* study of adrenal tissue, has been challenged by recent *in vivo* research. As reviewed by Bornstein and Vaudry, adrenal tissues produce a large number of regulatory peptides, neuro-transmitters, cytokines, and growth factors that enable adrenal cells to communicate with each other and adapt hormonal secretions to various circumstances. As the investigators note: "The integrated control of adrenocortical function involves direct innervation, regulation of the blood supply and intraglandular cell-to-cell interaction. These systems influence each other and form complex intra-adrenal regulatory circuits." Among these influences are multiple secretory products of chromaffin cells, now known to be interspersed throughout the adrenal cortex rather than being sequestered only within the medulla.

With the rich blood supply to the adrenals, virtually every cell is adjacent to an endothelial cell, thereby exposing adrenal cells to the multiple endothelium-derived secretions including nitric oxide, adrenomedullin, and endothelin (see Chapter 7). Moreover, an intra-adrenal renin–angiotensin system likely is involved in stimulation of aldosterone synthesis from the zona glomerulosa.

As complicated as the control of adrenal function may turn out to be, the basic concepts of the regulation of adrenal steroidogenesis remain valid.

ADRENAL CORTEX

The three major secretory products of the adrenal cortex will be considered separately, but first the biosynthetic pathways for all steroidogenesis will be examined.

Steroidogenesis

All adrenal steroids are derived from cholesterol by various enzymatically mediated modifications of its structure (Fig. 14-3). Cholesterol can be synthesized within the adrenal from acetyl CoA, but most is taken up from the blood by specific plasma membrane receptors that bind low-density lipoproteins (LDL) that are rich in cholesterol. The LDL–cholesterol is transferred into the cell by endocytosis, the cholesterol split from the lipoprotein, esterified, and stored in cytoplasmic vacuoles. Stimulation by corticotropin (ACTH) activates the cholesterol esterase, which releases free cholesterol from its storage depots, providing the substrate for steroid synthesis. Transfer of the substrate cholesterol from the outer mitochondrial membrane to the inner mitochondrial membrane, the site of the cholesterol side chain cleavage enzyme system, is the rate-limiting step in steroid biosynthesis and is mediated by the steroidogenic acute regulatory protein (StAR) [see Chapter 9], whose *de novo* synthesis is also stimulated by ACTH.

The synthesis of the various adrenal hormones involves cytochrome P450 enzymes, which are mixed function oxygenases that catalyze steroid hydroxylations. Cytochrome P450 side-chain cleavage enzyme, 20,22-desmolase, converts cholesterol into pregnenolone. All stimuli of steroidogenesis, including ACTH, increase the interaction of cholesterol with the side-chain cleavage enzyme.

Once pregnenolone is available, it is rapidly removed from mitochondria and sequentially modified by dehydrogenases and hydroxylating enzymes within the endoplasmic reticulum and mitochondria to form the three major types of adrenal hormones.

Fig. 14-3 Pathways of adrenal steroidogenesis. Gene products mediating each biosynthetic step are boxed with the corresponding enzymatic activity listed in parentheses. Note that one enzyme may have more than one activity. The planar structures of cholesterol, the mineralocorticoid aldosterone, the glucocorticoid cortisol, and the androgen androstenedione, are shown. 3β-HSD, 3β-hydroxysteroid dehydrogenase. 18-Hydroxylase and 18-oxidase are also called *corticosterone methyloxidase I and II* or *aldosterone synthase.* (From White PC, and Speiser PW: Steroid 11β-hydroxylase deficiency and related disorders. Endocrinol Metab Clin North Am 23:325–339, 1994.)

An Example of Aberrant Steroidogenesis

As seen in Figure 14-3, human adrenal cells have two different 11β-hydroxylase isozymes, CYP11B1 (also called *P450c11* or *11β-hydroxylase*) and CYP11B2 (also called *P450c18* or *aldosterone synthase*), that are responsible for cortisol and aldosterone biosynthesis, respectively. CYP11B2 first 18-hydroxylates and then 18-oxidizes corticosterone to aldosterone; these activities are also referred to as *corticosterone methyloxidase I and II.*

These two enzymes are encoded by two genes on the long arm of chromosome 8 (8 q21-q22). A form of familial hypertension has been shown to be caused by an unequal crossing over of the 5′ end of CYP11B1 (11-OHase), including regulatory sequences, with the 3′ end of CYP11B2 (aldosterone synthase) yielding a chimeric hybrid gene (Fig. 14-4) that is regulated like the 11β-hydroxylase located in the zona fasciculata by ACTH but which leads to increased secretion of 18-hydroxylated derivatives with mineralocorticoid activity. Thus, the crossover empowers the zona

Fig. 14-4 Diagram depicting unequal crossing over between aldosterone synthase and 11-OHase genes. Each gene is represented by a wide bar, with the location of exons indicated by either black (11-OHase) or stipled (aldosterone synthase) bands. One of the two products of unequal crossing over will have a chimeric gene fusing sequences of the normal AldoS and 11-OHase genes. In this example, unequal crossing over is depicted as occurring in the intron between exons 3 and 4. (From Lifton RP, Dluhy RG, Powers M, Rich GM, Cook S, Ulick S, and Lalouel JM: A glucocorticoid-remediable aldosterone synthase gene causes glucocorticoid-remediable aldosteronism and human hypertension. Nature 355:262–265, 1992.)

fasciculata to produce mineralocorticoids whose origin is normally only from the zona glomerulosa. Though rare, this syndrome provides a fascinating picture of normal physiology gone slightly awry.

Because production of these mineralocorticoids is under the influence of ACTH, administration of glucocorticoids will stop the entire process, giving rise to the name *glucocorticoid remediable aldosteronism.*

Adrenal Steroid Secretion

As noted, the major hormones secreted from the adrenal are cortisol, aldosterone, and dehydroepiandrosterone (DHEA) (Table 14-2). Small amounts of these hormones are stored in the adrenal. When more is needed, the biosynthetic pathway must be activated, particularly at the rate-limiting STAR protein. Most of the DHEA is sulfated, and plasma levels of DHEA sulfate are much higher than that of the free hormone.

Syndromes of Congenital Enzymatic Deficiency
Some precursors of the major end products are also secreted from the adrenal gland. They tend to be less active and present in smaller concentrations. However, congenital deficiencies of various adrenal enzymes may block the normal biosynthetic path and cause the progressive buildup of whichever precursors can be formed. This buildup tends to be progressive since, when cortisol synthesis is severely limited by the enzyme deficiency, there is insufficient circulating cortisol to inhibit the release of more ACTH. The high levels of ACTH continue to stimulate the gland to syn-

Table 14-2 Secretion Rates and Plasma Concentrations of Major Adrenocortical Hormones

Class	Steroid	Secretion rate (mg/day)	Plasma concentration (ng/ml)[a]
Glucocorticoid	Cortisol	8–25	40–180
	Corticosterone	1–4	2–6
Mineralocorticoid	Aldosterone	0.05–0.20	0.05–0.20
	Deoxycorticosterone	0.1–0.6	0.05–0.20
Androgen[b]	DHEA	7–15	2–8
	DHEA-S		400–1200
	Androstenedione	2–3	1–2

[a]Plasma concentrations vary with time of day and, in women, with phase of menstrual cycle.
[b]Secretion rates vary with gender.

thesize as much as possible in the presence of an enzymatic deficiency. The resulting hyperplasia of the gland gives these relatively rare congenital syndromes their name: *congenital adrenal hyperplasia.*

The most common form of adrenal enzymatic defect, responsible for about 95% of all cases, involves the 21-hydroxylase enzyme. This enzyme is needed to convert both 17-hydroxyprogesterone to 11-deoxycortisol, the precursor of cortisol, and progesterone to 11-deoxycorticosterone, the precursor of aldosterone (Fig. 14-5). Because cortisol is deficient, increasing amounts of ACTH stimulate the gland to produce more and more of the precursors formed prior to the 21-hydroxylation step, precursors that can be converted into androgens. The excess androgens lead to virilization. This is usually obvious at birth in girls, who display enlargement of the clitoris and fusion of the labia. The enzymatic deficiency is variable. In some girls, the defect is less complete, leading only to excessive hair growth with menstrual irregularities in adult life. In others, the defect may be so severe as to cause misassignment of sex at birth, since the external genitalia may be completely virilized, with a penile urethra and a "scrotum" (see also Chapter 8).

In affected males, the virilization usually does not become clinically obvious until after age 2 and sometimes not until age 10. The manifestations include a rapid spurt in body height along with early maturation of the genitalia.

Much less common are those congenital adrenal enzyme deficiencies involving other portions of the biosynthetic pathway. Their manifestations vary. If the defect is early, as with lack of functional steroidogenic acute regulatory protein, all steroids may be deficient, the syndrome of *congenital lipid adrenal hyperplasia.* If the defect involves the 17-hydroxylase enzyme, mineralocorticoid levels may be high. If it involves the 18-hydroxylase enzyme, aldosterone may be deficient with cortisol normal. With knowledge of the normal pathway, the clinical expression of each enzyme deficiency can be easily determined.

Glucocorticoids

Cortisol is the primary glucocorticoid for humans and most mammals. Corticosterone serves this function in some rodents.

NORMAL STEROID SYNTHESIS

21-HYDROXYLASE DEFICIENCY

Fig. 14-5 Schematic representation of normal adrenal steroid biosynthesis and of the 21-hydroxylase deficiency from congenital adrenal hyperplasia. Wide arrows denote pathways with increased synthesis proximal to the block. Dashed arrows denote pathways with decreased or absent steroid synthesis. The box shows the deficient enzyme. (From Baxter JD, and Tyrrell JB: In: *Endocrinology and Metabolism,* 2nd ed., P Felig, JD Baxter, AE Broadus, and LA Frohman, eds., McGraw-Hill, New York, p. 625, 1987.)

Regulation of Glucocorticoid Secretion

As described in Chapter 6, the hypothalamic–pituitary axis controls adrenal cortical function through the release of ACTH. After it binds to its adrenal plasma membrane receptor, ACTH activates adenylyl cyclase, increasing cyclic AMP and thereby activating protein kinases that convert cholesterol esters to free cholesterol. In concert with this and other effects, ACTH stimulates the rate-limiting transport of cholesterol by STAR, increasing the conversion of cholesterol to Δ^5-pregnenolone and starting the biosynthetic cascade to cortisol (Fig. 14-3).

Plasma levels of cortisol rise within minutes of the intravenous infusion of ACTH, increasing two to five times by 30 minutes. With chronic ACTH stimulation, the mass of adrenal tissue increases, so that cortisol secretion may rise to 200–250 mg/day, some 10 to 20 times the basal levels.

Secretion. Under ordinary circumstances, the daily secretion of cortisol is both episodic and variable (Fig. 14-6). The episodes follow by 15–30 minutes those of plasma ACTH, and there is a major burst of activity in the early morning hours be-

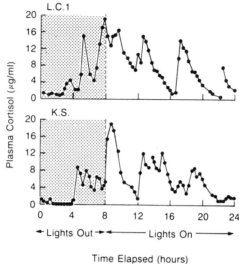

Fig. 14-6 A typical pattern of cortisol secretion during the 24-hour day. Note the oscillations in secretion as well as a daily secretory surge an hour or so after waking in the morning. (From Weitzman ED, Fukushima D, Noseire C, Roffwarg H, Gallagher TF, and Hellman L: Twenty-four-hour pattern of the episodic secretion of cortisol in normal subjects. J Clin Endocrinol Metab 33:14, 1971.)

fore awakening. Thereafter, the release of ACTH from the pituitary and of cortisol from the adrenal generally occur only for brief bursts, 7–15 episodes per day. After each episode, plasma cortisol rises enough to suppress further ACTH release. Circulating levels of cortisol then progressively fall, and after variable periods reach the set point of hypothalamic–pituitary negative feedback control so that more corticotropin-releasing hormone (CRH) and ACTH are then released.

The normal fine-tuning of hypothalamic–pituitary control of cortisol secretion may be interrupted by administration of supraphysiologic doses of glucocorticoids, usually to control serious inflammatory or immune reactions, in keeping with their actions as described in the next section. Various steroids are available, derivatives of cortisol with substitutions that enhance the glucocorticoid and reduce the mineralocorticoid effect (Table 14-3).

Exogenous glucocorticoids are initially administered in doses far beyond the normal physiologic levels, usually enough to provide the equivalent of 200–300 mg of cortisol per day, the maximal secretory capacity of the adrenal. When that amount is given, or any amount beyond the equivalent of the 20–30 mg of cortisol per day that is normally secreted, the hypothalamic–pituitary axis remains suppressed. With no stimulation by ACTH, the adrenal atrophies both in function and in structure.

As long as the patient receives exogenous steroid, suppression of the hypothalamic–pituitary–adrenal system is irrelevant. However, when the exogenous steroid is discontinued, the release of ACTH for a short time, and the release of cortisol for a longer time, may remain suppressed (Fig. 14-7). The levels of ACTH return rather quickly, and, because the adrenal remains unresponsive, they rise above

Table 14-3 Relative Glucocorticoid and Mineralocorticoid Potency of Natural Adrenal Steroids and Some Derivatives

	Glucocorticoid	Mineralocorticoid
Cortisol	1.0	1.0
Prednisone (1,2 double bond)	4	<0.1
6α-Methylprednisone	5	<0.1
9α-Fluoro-16α-hydroxyprednisolone (triamcinolone)	5	<0.1
9α-Fluoro-16α-methylprednisolone (dexamethasone)	30	<0.1
Aldosterone	0.25	500
Deoxycorticosterone	0.01	30
9α-Fluorocortisol	10	500

normal. The levels of cortisol take considerably longer to return to the normal range. Obviously, after prolonged adrenal suppression the patient remains susceptible to the development of adrenal insufficiency if stressed when the adrenal is not capable of normal responsiveness.

Metabolism. Once in the circulation, cortisol is largely bound to a specific glucocorticoid-binding α_2-globulin, transcortin. The normal level of transcortin, 3–4 mg/dl, is saturated at a level of cortisol of about 28 μg/dl. Of that which is not bound to transcortin, 15%–20% is bound less tightly to albumin, leaving only about 5% of circulating cortisol as unbound.

The hepatic synthesis of transcortin is increased by estrogen, in a manner similar to that of thyroid-binding globulin (TBG) and other hormone carrier proteins. With more transcortin, more cortisol is bound. Therefore, women taking exogenous

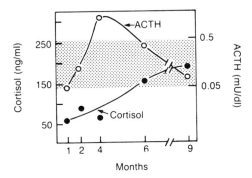

Fig. 14-7 Recovery of the hypothalamic–pituitary–adrenocortical axis after exposure to a long-term elevated concentration of glucocorticoids. All measurements were made at 0600 hours and closed circles represent median values from 14 patients. The dotted area represents the range for normal subjects. (Based on original data of Graber AL, Ney RL, Nicholson WE, Island DP, and Little GW: J Clin Endocrinol Metab 25:11, 1965.)

estrogen or with high endogenous levels during pregnancy have high total plasma cortisol levels but, since their free cortisol levels are normal, they have no manifestations of cortisol excess. In contrast, transcortin levels are lower in diseases with reduced blood protein concentrations, for example, cirrhosis of the liver; here again, free cortisol levels are normal.

The half-life of exogenous cortisol is about 70–90 minutes. Cortisol can be interconverted to its 11-keto analogue cortisone (Figure 14-8). Most cortisol, sometimes referred to as *compound F,* and most cortisone, *compound E,* are metabolized in the liver by reductases to tetrahydro forms and then conjugated to glucuronides. The glucuronides are more water soluble and are the major forms excreted into the urine.

The 24-hour urinary excretion of unmetabolized cortisol is in many ways the most accurate measure now available. Because only free cortisol is excreted into the urine, the total urinary free cortisol in normal people will be below 100 μg/day. However, if cortisol secretion rises and the binding capacity of transcortin is exceeded, at a level of plasma cortisol above 25–30 μg/dl, a progressively larger share will remain free and therefore available for filtration and excretion into the urine.

Additional metabolism of cortisol occurs through 5α-reductase activity in fat tissue, which may explain the higher levels of urinary cortisol in obese people. Despite increased turnover and excretion, plasma levels of cortisol remain normal, likely reflecting increased regeneration of cortisol from cortisone catalyzed by 11β-reductase in fat tissue.

Molecular Mechanisms of Action

As described in Chapter 3, adrenal steroids enter target cells by passive diffusion and are bound to a specific glucocorticoid receptor, a single-chain polypeptide (about 94,000 Da) that binds glucocorticoids with high affinity in a specific, saturable manner. The cytosolic steroid receptor is complexed with other proteins including a heat-shock protein. After the steroid is bound, the hormone–receptor complex translocates to the nucleus and binds to DNA (see Fig. 3-8). By interaction with specific regulatory DNA sequences, called *glucocorticoid response elements,* a change occurs in the transcriptional rate of specific genes, altering production of messenger RNA and changing the cell's synthesis of specific proteins.

Mineralocorticoids preferentially bind to receptors found primarily in their target tissues—kidney, colon, and salivary glands—that have a high affinity for aldo-

Fig. 14-8 Principal urinary metabolites of cortisol reflecting conversion to cortisone and the activity of reductase enzymes.

sterone. These are called *type I receptors,* where the glucocorticoid receptors in these tissues are called *type II.* The type I receptors have specificity for mineralocorticoids *in vivo* but not *in vitro,* where they bind glucocorticoids just as avidly as mineralocorticoids. *In vivo,* mineralocorticoid target tissues have an 11β-hydroxysteroid dehydrogenase enzyme that converts the natural glucocorticoid cortisol (which has a high affinity for the type I receptor) into cortisone, which has a low affinity (see Fig. 14-8). Therefore, despite the much higher concentration of cortisol in the glomerular filtrate, its conversion to cortisone prevents its binding to the type I receptors in the kidney and these receptors bind aldosterone passing through the tubule. A few patients lack the 11β-hydroxysteroid dehydrogenase enzyme, and the normal levels of cortisol are taken up by the type I receptors and exert a massive mineralocorticoid effect; this syndrome is called *apparent mineralocorticoid excess.* The glycyrrhizic acid present in licorice inhibits the 11β-hydroxysteroid dehydrogenase enzyme. People who consume large amounts of licorice, now added as a flavor to some chewing tobaccos, may manifest the same syndrome with all of the features of mineralocorticoid excess.

Functions
Cortisol, the primary glucocorticoid, is essential for life. Exactly why this is so is uncertain. In a simplistic way, cortisol is necessary to maintain critical processes at times of prolonged stress and to contain the reactions to inflammation. Most of its effects are *permissive,* or not directly responsible for the initiation of metabolic or circulatory processes but necessary for their full expression.

Intermediary Metabolism. Figure 14-9 demonstrates the balance between the anabolic and catabolic effects of cortisol, with a predominance of the catabolic. The major catabolic effect is to facilitate the conversion of protein in muscles and connective tissue into glucose and glycogen. Gluconeogenesis involves both the increased degradation of protein already formed and the decreased synthesis of new protein. Gluconeogenesis from amino acids is critical during prolonged fasting, as circulating glucose and stores of liver glycogen will be used up in less than 24 hours.

Carbohydrate Metabolism. Cortisol not only increases the supply of glucose through gluconeogenesis but also decreases the utilization of glucose by cells. The former likely reflects the activation of DNA transcription in liver cells to increase various enzymes involved in the conversion of amino acids into glucose and glycogen. The mechanism for the decreased utilization of glucose by cells involves direct inhibition of glucose transport into the cells.

As a result of these effects, a deficiency of cortisol increases the susceptibility to and decreases the recovery from hypoglycemia. An excess of cortisol raises the blood sugar and decreases the sensitivity to insulin.

Protein Metabolism. Cortisol reduces the utilization of amino acids for the formation of protein everywhere except in the liver. Extrahepatic protein stores are reduced and amino acid levels in the blood increase. Extrahepatic utilization is decreased because amino acids are not transported into muscle cells, thereby reducing protein synthesis. Breakdown of cellular proteins continues, so that plasma amino acids are further increased.

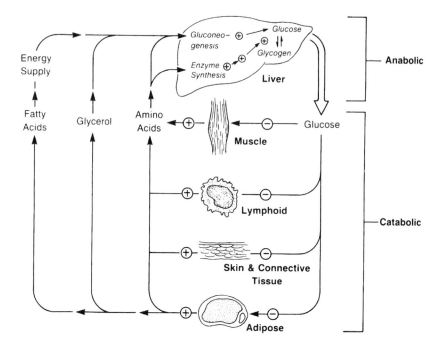

Fig. 14-9 Glucocorticoid influences on peripheral tissues. +, stimulation, and −, inhibition. (From Baxter JD, and Tyrrell JB: In: *Endocrinology and Metabolism,* 2nd ed., P Felig, JD Baxter, AE Broadus, and LA Frohman, eds., McGraw-Hill, New York, p. 545, 1987.)

In the liver, the higher levels of blood amino acids are transported more avidly into hepatic cells where they are utilized for gluconeogenesis, glycogen formation, and protein synthesis.

A deficiency of cortisol is not followed by any measurable increase in protein synthesis. An excess of cortisol, however, is associated with progressive loss of protein, atrophy and weakness of muscles, thinning of skin, and loss of bone matrix and mass. Bone formation is reduced, and less calcium is absorbed and more excreted into the urine.

Fat Metabolism. Cortisol also increases the mobilization of fatty acids and glycerol from adipose tissue, increasing their concentration in the blood and making more glycerol available for gluconeogenesis. Not only is fat broken down but less is formed, perhaps because less glucose is transported into fat cells.

The actions of cortisol on fat metabolism are not all lipolytic: it also stimulates appetite and the laying down of additional fat in the central or truncal areas. With an excess of cortisol, the extremities lose fat and muscle whereas the trunk and face become fatter. The mechanism for this redistribution of body fat is unknown.

These various effects of cortisol on intermediary metabolism contribute to the maintenance of blood glucose during food deprivation and the mobilization of extra glucose during stress. But these protective effects come at a cost of decreased protein and fat.

Circulatory. Cortisol is needed to maintain normal vascular integrity and responsiveness, and the volume of body fluids. In the absence of cortisol, abnormal vasodilation occurs, so that even without an external loss of fluid, the filling of the vascular bed is reduced and the blood pressure falls.

In addition, normal renal function requires cortisol. In its absence, glomerular filtration falls and water cannot be excreted as rapidly. Cortisol also has a mineralocorticoid effect that is responsible for part of normal sodium retention and potassium excretion. Although aldosterone is some 300–600 times more potent a mineralocorticoid than cortisol, under normal circumstances 200 times more cortisol than aldosterone is secreted. Therefore, a substantial part of overall mineralocorticoid activity is derived from cortisol. Of course, when blood pressure of body fluids are reduced, the renin–angiotensin mechanism (described in the next section) is activated to stimulate aldosterone, and not cortisol. Thus, when extra mineralocorticoids are needed, aldosterone and not cortisol serves that function.

Inflammatory and Immune Responses. Glucocorticoids suppress inflammation and immune reactions. As descried in Chapter 4, inflammation and immune reactions induce the synthesis of multiple cytokines, and the suppressive effects of glucocorticoids have logically been assumed to reflect their ability to inhibit the expression of multiple genes involved in proinflammatory cytokine synthesis. Recently, glucocorticoids have also been shown to increase the transcription of genes coding for anti-inflammatory proteins, including lipocortin-1, interleukin-10, and neutral endopeptidase. In addition, glucocorticoids upregulate the expression of various cytokine receptors and, when applied in combination, glucorticoids and cytokines may act synergistically.

These divergent effects may explain one of the clinical situations where administration of glucocorticoids has experimental support but clinical failure, namely the treatment of shock due to overwhelming sepsis. In animal experiments, glucocorticoids are usually given before the sepsis-inducing agent so that they inhibit the production of cytokines, which are involved in the manifestations of infection and are therefore protective. In clinical situations, glucocorticoids are given after septic shock has occurred and levels of proinflammatory cytokines are already high. Therefore, glucocorticoids cannot be protective and, because they induce cytokine receptors, they may worsen the situation.

Most of these anti-inflammatory effects are seen only with large amounts of cortisol. With large doses of cortisol derivatives, these glucocorticoid effects are widely utilized in clinical medicine in the treatment of many diseases in which the inflammatory reactions are harmful or there is a need to block immune responses. The treatment of rheumatoid arthritis is an example of the former and the prevention of rejection of transplanted organs is an example of the latter use of glucocorticoids.

Central Nervous System. In addition to the physiological negative feedback control of hypothalamic–pituitary release of ACTH, cortisol modulates perception and emotion. This is usually recognized only in disease: with cortisol deficiency, the senses of taste, hearing, and smell are accentuated; with cortisol excess, initial euphoria but subsequent depression is common and the threshold for seizure activity may be lowered.

Developmental Effects. Cortisol is important for the maturation of various fetal organs, again in a permissive manner. It is involved in the maturation of intestinal enzymes into various aspects of pulmonary function, including the synthesis of surfactant, a phospholipid needed for maintaining alveolar surface tension. In children, glucocorticoids inhibit linear skeletal growth by direct effects on bone and connective tissue.

Features of Cortisol Deficiency

The classic features of cortisol deficiency, as listed in Table 14-4, are seen with *primary* hypofunction of the adrenal glands (Addison's disease).This was once most commonly caused by destruction of the glands by tuberculosis, but now the process is usually of unknown cause or is related to antibodies against the person's own adrenal tissue—that is, to autoimmune disease.

Hypofunction of the adrenals can also be *secondary* to a loss of hypothalamic–pituitary function resulting in a deficiency of ACTH. The features of secondary adrenal insufficiency are usually intermingled with manifestations of deficiencies of other glands that are also under the control of the hypothalamic–pituitary system (Table 14-5). Although most instances of pituitary insufficiency involve all of its hormones, a few cases of isolated ACTH deficiency have been reported. The deficiency of ACTH, isolated or as part of panhypopituitarism, is rarely complete, so that cortisol deficiency is not usually as marked as in primary adrenal insufficiency. Moreover, the adrenal synthesis of the mineralocorticoid aldosterone, under the control of renin–angiotensin, is not affected by loss of ACTH, so that manifestations of mineralocorticoid deficiency usually do not arise.

The two forms of adrenal insufficiency, both quite rare, can be most easily diagnosed either by measurement of endogenous ACTH levels in the blood or by the response to exogenous ACTH. When the adrenal is destroyed, that is, as in primary hypofunction, and cortisol is deficient, the plasma level of ACTH increases markedly as the pituitary is no longer inhibited by the negative feedback control of circulating cortisol. Additional exogenous ACTH can do no more to stimulate damaged glands. Conversely, when the problem resides in the hypothalamus or pituitary and the adrenal becomes secondarily suppressed, plasma ACTH levels are low. The adrenals can respond to exogenous ACTH, although after prolonged suppression of their structure and function by the deficiency of ACTH their response may be sluggish.

Features of Cortisol Excess

Cortisol excess is usually exogenous, induced for management of various diseases. The multiple adverse effects of superphysiologic doses of glucocorticoids may be minimized by intermittent therapy with prednisone, one of the synthetic agents listed in Table 14-3 and one that remains in the circulation for about 36 hours. If given in even larger doses once every 48 hours, most of the beneficial effects will continue to be exerted in the areas of inflammation, but the hypothalamic–pituitary axis will not be suppressed and the noninflamed body tissues will not be exposed to high levels of steroid for the last 12 hours.

The much less common disorders causing endogenous cortisol excess may arise within the adrenal glands or, more commonly, from overproduction of ACTH either

Table 14-4 Major Functions of Cortisol and Their Clinical Expression

Effect	Clinical expression	
	Cortisol deficiency	Cortisol excess
Carbohydrate metabolism		
Increased gluconeogenesis, decreased glucose utilization	Hypoglycemia	Hyperglycemia
Decreased sensitivity to insulin	Insulin sensitivity	Insulin resistance
Protein metabolism		
Decreased extrahepatic amino acid utilization	Hypoglycemia	Decreased protein structure of bone, skin, muscle
Increased gluconeogenesis		Poor wound healing
Fat metabolism		
Increased lipolysis, decreased lipogenesis	Weight loss	Hyperlipemia
Distribution of fat		Redistribution of body fat, truncal obesity
Circulatory		
Maintain ECF volume	Vasodilation, hypotension	Hypertension
Maintain capillary integrity		
Mineralocorticoid		
Sodium retention	Hypovolemia	Hypervolemia
	Hyponatremia	Hypernatremia
Potassium excretion	Hyperkalemia	Hypokalemia
Inflammatory and immune responses		
Stabilize lysosomes	Propensity toward autoimmune disease	Decreased inflammatory response
Suppress synthesis of antibodies		Increased susceptibility to infection
Decrease capillary permeability		Decreased fibrous tissue formation
Decrease phagocytosis		
Hematopoietic		
Stimulate red cell production	Anemia	Erythrocytosis
Lympholysis	Lymphocytosis	Lymphopenia
Inhibit neutrophil accumulation at inflammatory sites		Leukocytosis
Central nervous system	Anorexia	Euphoria
	Fatigue	Depression
Hypothalamic–pituitary feedback control of ACTH	Increased ACTH secretion	Decreased ACTH secretion
		If excess is 2° to hypothalamic–pituitary drive, ACTH increased
	Pigmentation	

Table 14-5 Distinctions between Primary and Secondary Adrenal Insufficiency

	Primary	Secondary[a]
Site	Adrenal	Hypothalamic–pituitary
ACTH secretion	Increased	Decreased
Pigmentation	Increased	Decreased
Headaches, visual loss	Rare	Frequent
Body weight	Decreased	Variable
Other pituitary hormones		
Growth hormone	No change	Decreased
Gonadotropin	No change	Decreased
Adrenal hormones		
Aldosterone	Deficient	Normal
Androgens	Deficient	Variable
Cortisol	Markedly decreased	Moderately reduced
Response to exogenous ACTH	None	Sluggish

[a]Rare examples of isolated ACTH deficiency have been reported with normal levels of other pituitary hormones.

by the pituitary or by ectopic ACTH-producing tumors, with the adrenals secondarily stimulated (Table 14-6). The manifestations of cortisol excess (Cushing's syndrome), as delineated in Table 14-4, are similar in both conditions. They may be difficult to differentiate because their clinical features are almost exclusively related to the excess levels of circulating cortisol.

However, the maneuvers shown in Table 14-6 will usually differentiate the two, along with direct visualization of the sites by CT scans. If the problem arises primarily in the adrenal gland, usually from a tumor, pituitary ACTH secretion will be suppressed by the high levels of circulating cortisol. With hypersecretion from the pituitary or an ectopic tumor, levels of ACTH obviously should be elevated. Before measurements of plasma ACTH were easily obtained, the distinction was usually made by differential suppression of the pituitary and adrenals with exogenous glucocorticoids. This approach utilizes a number of principles of endocrine physiology, adapted to clinical circumstances. These principles are applied, first, to document cortisol excess and, second, to differentiate the source.

Table 14-6 Differential of Adrenal Hyperfunction

	Primary (30%)	Secondary (70%)	
Site	Adrenal	Hypothalamic–pituitary	Ectopic tumors
Adrenal pathology	Tumor	Bilateral hyperplasia	Bilateral hyperplasia
ACTH secretion	Decreased	Increased	Markedly increased
Suppression with exogenous glucocorticoid			
Low dose	None	Minimal	None
High dose	None	Marked	None

The suppression tests are based upon the ability of exogenous cortisol to exert negative feedback control on hypothalamic–pituitary release of ACTH. Those that are normal but are suspected of having cortisol excess because of suggestive features will be normally suppressed by amounts of glucocorticoid just beyond the normal, physiological level. Because exogenous cortisol would only take the place of endogenous cortisol, suppression as measured by levels of cortisol in the blood could not be demonstrated with cortisol itself. Recall, however, that potent glucocorticoid derivatives, with 20–30 times more suppressive activity per milligram than cortisol are available (Table 14-3). The one usually used is dexamethasone. A highly reliable screening test utilizes 1 mg of dexamethasone (equivalent to about 30 mg of cortisol) taken at bedtime to measure plasma cortisol the next morning. Normal suppression is to below 5 μg/dl; patients with adrenocorticol hyperfunction will not suppress to that level.

To elucidate further the nature of adrenal hyperfunction, more prolonged suppression tests can be done. One-half milligram of dexamethasone is given 4 times a day, for a total of 2 mg, which is equivalent to 60 mg of cortisol a day. That is enough to suppress completely the normal hypothalamic–pituitary axis, so that ACTH will not be released and the adrenal will make little cortisol. Cortisol measured in a urine or blood sample should be very low (Fig. 14-10). Those with cortisol excess, whatever the cause, will not be significantly suppressed.

The second differential suppression test builds on the same principles of pituitary–adrenal control. If the problem is caused by hyperfunction of the hypothalamic–pituitary axis with increased secretion of ACTH, near-normal amounts of cortisol will not go above the set point of negative feedback suppression, since by definition that set point has been raised to an abnormally high level in hyperfunctioning pituitary ACTH-secreting cells or in hypothalamic cells secreting excess CRF. However, the set point is suppressible if enough exogenous glucocorticoid is given. By trial and error, that dose was found to be 2.0 mg of dexamethasone 4 times a day for 2 days, a total of 8 mg of dexamethasone a day, which is equiva-

Fig. 14-10 Expected changes in plasma or urine cortisol values after 2 days of low (2 mg/day) and high (8 mg/day) dexamethasone in divided doses in normals and patients with Cushing's syndrome caused by hypothalamic–pituitary hyperfunction or an adrenal tumor.

lent to 240 mg of cortisol, or approximately 10 times the normal secretion. With that level, most hypothalamic–pituitary hyperfunctioning states will be suppressed, so that urine cortisol levels will fall by 40% or more.

In contrast, if the cortisol excess arises from an autonomous adrenal tumor or from an ectopic ACTH-producing tumor, no amount of exogenous glucocorticoid will usually stop the secretion of cortisol. The high levels of cortisol are suppressed slightly or not at all by the equivalent of 240 mg of cortisol.

Mineralocorticoids

Aldosterone is the primary mineralocorticoid. It arises from the outer zona glomerulosa and is under the control of angiotensin primarily, and of serum potassium and ACTH to a lesser degree. In its absence, fluid and electrolyte status is altered, although if enough cortisol is present, cortisol itself may exert a mineralocorticoid effect sufficient to prevent progressive depletion of body fluids.

Regulation of Mineralocorticoid Secretion

Because the major function of aldosterone is to control body fluid volume by increasing the reabsorption of sodium by the kidneys, it is appropriate that the major stimulus for aldosterone synthesis and secretion arises in the kidneys (Fig. 14-11). The juxtaglomerular apparatus consists of modified myoepithelial cells in the renal afferent arterioles, contiguous to the macula densa of the distal tubule. These cells synthesize and secrete the proteolytic enzyme renin, which splits off the 10-amino acid peptide, angiotensin I, from its protein substrate, angiotensinogen. Angiotensin I is inactive but is rapidly converted into the very active 8-amino acid, angiotensin II, by the action of a converting enzyme found throughout the body, arising from the plasma membrane of vascular endothelial cells.

Angiotensin II exerts two major actions, one as a direct arteriolar vasoconstrictor and the other as a stimulus to aldosterone secretion. These two actions, in concert, maintain the volume and pressure of the arterial circulation. They provide the major support to the circulation in times of fluid loss or falling blood pressure.

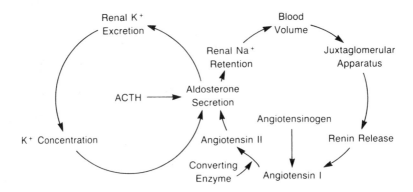

Fig. 14-11 Regulation of aldosterone secretion by the renin–angiotensin system, the potassium concentration, and corticotropin (ACTH). (From Griffin JE: *Manual of Clinical Endocrinology and Metabolism*, McGraw-Hill, New York, p. 78, 1982.)

Stimuli to Renin Release. The major stimulus to the release of renin is a decrease in the perfusion pressure of blood traversing the renal afferent arterioles, which is sensed by the juxtaglomerular apparatus functioning as a baroreceptor. When a decrease in either systemic blood volume or blood pressure leads to a fall in renal perfusion pressure, renin is secreted.

Other factors also stimulate renin secretion, including the concentration of sodium and chloride in the macula densa, the concentration of plasma electrolytes, and the concentration of circulating angiotensin II, a short feedback control loop. Some of these stimuli work through the stimulation of renal sympathetic nerves that innervate the juxtaglomerular apparatus.

Other Stimuli for Aldosterone. All of the actions of renin are mediated through its generation of angiotensin II, which serves as the primary stimulus to aldosterone synthesis. The stimulation occurs at various sites in the biosynthetic pathway. Plasma potassium concentration and ACTH also stimulate aldosterone. The potassium effect appears appropriate as the effects of aldosterone include a major increase in the renal excretion of potassium. If levels of plasma potassium are suddenly raised, as after a large meal of potassium-rich foods, the secretion of aldosterone is increased, acting on the kidney to excrete the excess potassium load. As described below, however, the effects of aldosterone to increase renal sodium retention and potassium excretion require an hour or more; thus, there must be more rapid ways to remove high levels of potassium entering the circulation, because such levels could lead to instant and serious trouble. The rapid transfer of potassium from extracellular fluid into cells is accomplished by a combination of insulin and epinephrine effects on potassium transport across cell membranes.

The effect of ACTH is powerful but short-lived. Although the physiological role of ACTH on aldosterone secretion is limited, when ACTH is deficient, the zona glomerulosa may atrophy and be less able to respond to other stimuli.

Secretion. Aldosterone is so powerful a mineralocorticoid that very little is needed for its primary effect. Only 0.05–0.20 mg (50–200 μg) is produced each day. Because there is no specific aldosterone carrier protein in the blood, very little circulating aldosterone is bound. Plasma concentrations are around 10 ng/dl. Secretion can be increased 2- to 6-fold by sodium depletion and even more so by persistent shrinkage of effective arterial blood volume as in cirrhosis of the liver with ascites and marked edema.

Metabolism. Aldosterone is metabolized mainly in the liver into a tetrahydroaldosterone derivative that is excreted in the urine as a glucuronide. Some is excreted as a glucuronide without being metabolized, and this acid-labile fraction, about 10% of total secretion, is what is usually measured. Therefore, a normal urine aldosterone level is 5–20 μg/day.

Functions
Aldosterone's primary action is to increase sodium reabsorption in the distal tubules. To do so, it is first bound to cytosolic receptors, then the hormone–receptor complex is transferred to the nucleus where it induces specific portions of DNA to form messenger RNA, which in turn increases the formation of enzymes involved in so-

dium transport across cell membranes. These processes take 30–60 minutes; thus, the effect of aldosterone is delayed by that length of time.

As aldosterone increases active sodium reabsorption, an electrochemical gradient is established that facilitates the passive transfer of potassium from tubular cells into the urine. Therefore, potassium is excreted, not as a direct exchange for sodium, but in a manner that depends directly upon the active reabsorption of sodium. If almost all sodium is reabsorbed more proximally, as in the presence of severe volume depletion, little will reach the distal reabsorptive site. Therefore, despite high levels of aldosterone, potassium excretion will be minimal in the absence of sodium delivery to the distal tubule. Conversely, a high sodium intake will increase potassium excretion. This is particularly true if the individual is receiving a diuretic that blocks part of the reabsorption of sodium higher in the tubule, causing even more sodium to reach the distal reabsorptive site.

Sodium Concentration. As sodium is reabsorbed in the kidney, an equivalent amount of water is also reabsorbed, thus preserving the normal concentration of sodium in the extracellular fluid. If not enough water is reabsorbed so that the concentration of sodium rises, the increase in osmotic pressure will activate the release of antidiuretic hormone, effectively increasing renal water reabsorption and increasing water intake via thirst.

Escape. Under usual circumstances of mild sodium depletion leading to increased aldosterone secretion, the extracellular fluid volume re-expands as more sodium is reabsorbed. The degree of expansion should be adequate to replenish the shrinkage that initiated the process so that it is then turned off. Under some circumstances, such as persistent leak of effective blood volume into the abdomen in a patient with cirrhosis of the liver and ascites, the stimulus to aldosterone never turns off. The extra sodium that is reabsorbed does not replenish the shrunken effective fluid volume because of the continuous leak. Therefore, very high levels of aldosterone, that is, secondary hyperaldosteronism, are seen in chronic edematous states.

When there is no continuous leak but aldosterone levels remain high, as with the administration of exogenous aldosterone or an aldosterone-secreting tumor, extracellular volume expands by a few liters but then the expansions stops. This *escape* phenomenon likely results from a confluence of effects: proximal reabsorption of sodium is decreased, probably because of a natriuretic factor that arises in the hypothalamus; glomerular filtration is increased, probably because of the actions of the atrial natriuretic factor (see Chapter 7); and renin–angiotensin levels are suppressed by the rise in systemic blood pressure, renal perfusion pressure, and sodium content in the macula densa.

Although sodium reabsorption escapes, potassium excretion continues because more sodium is delivered to the distal tubule.

Features of Primary Aldosterone Excess
Autonomous benign tumors of the adrenal gland that secrete large amounts of aldosterone have been recognized since 1954 as a rare but interesting form of curable hypertension. The clinical hallmarks are hypokalemia and hypertension. The blood pressure rises because plasma volume expands due to the aldosterone-mediated re-

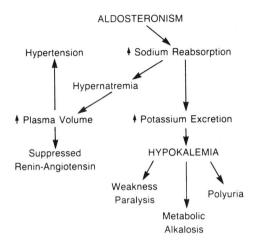

Fig. 14-12 The pathophysiology of primary aldosteronism. (From Kaplan NM: In: *Clinical Hypertension,* 5th ed., NM Kaplan, eds., Williams & Wilkins, Baltimore, 1990.)

absorption of sodium. Even though "escape" occurs, the extra few liters of body fluid volume are enough to keep the blood pressure high. Similarly, as noted above, the increase in potassium excretion continues so that hypokalemia, with its various manifestations, is typical (Fig. 14-12). The diagnosis is most easily made by finding high levels of aldosterone and low levels of renin in the blood.

Features of Secondary Aldosterone Excess

More common than aldosterone-secreting tumors are conditions in which effective arterial blood volume is shrunken, calling forth high levels of renin–angiotensin that continue to stimulate the adrenal synthesis of aldosterone, to the point that bilateral adrenal hyperplasia may develop (Table 14-7). These include chronic edematous diseases such as severe heart failure, cirrhosis of the liver with ascites, and the nephrotic syndrome. Despite the high levels of renin–angiotensin and the secondarily increased

Table 14-7 The Two Major Forms of Aldosterone Excess

	Primary	Secondary
Pathology	Adrenal tumor	Adrenal hyperplasia
Mechanism	Autonomous hypersecretion	Driven hypersecretion (renin–angiotensin)
Effective arterial blood volume	Expanded	Shrunken
Total body fluid volume	Slightly expanded	Markedly expanded (edema)
Renin–angiotensin	Suppressed	Activated
Clinical expression	Hypertension	Low-normal blood pressure
	Potassium wastage	Potassium wastage
		Edema

aldosterone excess, fluid volume remains shrunken and the blood pressure is low-normal.

It is possible to block aldosterone's effects in the kidney by use of spironolactone, a nonmineralocorticoid steroidal compound that competes directly with aldosterone for the mineralocorticoid receptors in the renal tubule. Because it is more weakly bound than aldosterone, amounts of 50–500 mg/day are needed to competitively block the 0.5–10 mg of aldosterone that may be secreted in secondary aldosteronism.

Extrarenal Effects

Aldosterone also increases the reabsorption of sodium in other places where sodium may be excreted—saliva, sweat, and stool. When physical activity is first begun in a hot climate, a great amount of sodium may be lost in the large volumes of sweat that are formed. The resulting shrinkage of fluid volume activates the renin–angiotensin–aldosterone mechanism that causes more and more sodium to be retained, which is the process of acclimatization to a hot environment. After a few days, sweat will be sodium-free. Thus, there is no need to increase sodium intake beyond the usual amounts obtained in the diet when undergoing continued exercise in hot climates. Water intake should be adequate to replenish the volume of sweat.

Androgens

Androgens, the third secretion of the adrenals, unlike the other two, are not critical for life, but in women they may contribute to sexual responsiveness. Libido, as well as axillary and pubic hair growth in both sexes, depends largely upon the androgens testosterone and dihydrotestosterone. In the male, these come almost entirely from the testes. In the female, the smaller amount of testosterone comes largely from peripheral conversion of androstenedione of ovarian and adrenal origin. In the postmenopausal women whose ovaries are no longer active, adrenal androgens also serve as the major source of estrogens, derived by peripheral conversion of adrenal androstenedione.

The clinical situations in which adrenal androgens are most prominent are the congenital adrenal hyperplasias that shuttle large amounts of precursors into the androgen pathway. As noted previously in this chapter and in Chapter 8, the presence and degree of androgen excess or deficiency depend upon the site of enzymatic defect.

Adrenal androgens are formed primarily in the zona reticularis and are largely under the control of ACTH and, perhaps, of prolactin.

ADRENAL MEDULLA

Catecholamines are the hormones secreted by the sympathetic nervous system. In the peripheral nerves, norepinephrine is the locally produced and secreted neurotransmitter; in the adrenal medulla, epinephrine is the major secretion. It is useful to regard norepinephrine as a local hormone that is involved in neurotransmission and that spills over into the general circulation only after rather intense activation of the sympathetic nervous system. In contrast, epinephrine is released from the adrenal medulla in response to stress and circulates throughout the body to prepare the organism for "flight-or-fight." The effects of adrenergic nervous activity are mediated via α- and β-receptors on effector tissues that often have antagonistic actions, such as α-vasoconstriction versus β-vasodilation.

Synthesis and Release of Epinephrine

The adrenal medulla is a modified sympathetic ganglion with postganglionic cells, but no axons, that is specialized to secrete catecholamines from chromaffin (take up chromium) cells. One preganglionic fiber from the splanchnic nerve innervates a number of medullary cells, so that a few impulses can cause a massive discharge of catecholamines.

Epinephrine is synthesized in the adrenal medulla (and probably in certain brain neurons) from norepinephrine by action of the enzyme phenylethanolamine-N-methyltransferase (PNMT) (Fig. 14-13). The synthesis of PNMT is induced by cortisol. As the adrenal medulla is cradled by the adrenal cortex, it is bathed with very high concentrations of cortisol, so that PNMT is available. About 80% of adrenal medullary catecholamine secretion is epinephrine; the other 20% is norepinephrine.

The synthesis of catecholamines is regulated by changes in the levels of the rate-limiting enzyme *tyrosine hydroxylase*. Acutely, when neural activity causes a

Fig. 14-13   Catecholamine biosynthesis.

release of cytoplasmic catecholamines, the enzyme is released from end-product inhibition. With chronic stimulation more of the enzyme is synthesized.

The release of catecholamines occurs by "stimulus–secretion coupling": preganglionic nerve impulses release acetylcholine, which increases membrane permeability, thus depolarizing the cell membrane, and increases calcium uptake. This induces reverse pinocytosis of the secretory granules or exocytosis.

Accurate assays for the very small quantities of catecholamines in the blood are now available. Increased levels under various clinical circumstances reflect the involvement of epinephrine in cardiovascular, metabolic, and other responses to stress. Repetitive sympathetic activation may eventuate in persistently high blood pressure and potentiate atherosclerosis.

Fate of Secreted Catecholamines

Catecholamines are rapidly removed from the synapses and circulation by a number of processes:

1. Reuptake by catechol-secreting cells for reuse or metabolism.
2. Uptake by receptors on effector cells.
3. Metabolism by inactivating mechanisms, mainly in the liver, involving the catecholamine-O-transferase and monamine oxidase enzymes. The products are mainly excreted through the kidney as metanephrines or vanilmandelic acid (VMA) (Fig. 14-14).

Fig. 14-14 Pathways of catecholamine metabolism.

Action of Epinephrine

Alpha- and β-receptors for epinephrine and norepinephrine are present in many tissues, and the responses are varied. Both epinephrine and norepinephrine can interact with both α- and β-adrenergic receptors, so that the response of a given system to adrenergic stimulation is largely determined by the type of receptors that populates that system (Table 14-8).

Because the adrenal medulla normally accounts for only about 10% of sympathetic nervous activation, we can live quite well without it. The major actions of epinephrine are as follows:

Arousal:

Alerting, pupillary dilation, piloerection, sweating, bronchial dilation, tachycardia, inhibition of smooth muscle in the gastrointestinal tract, constriction of sphincters, relaxation of uterine muscles.

Metabolic:

In keeping with the need for ready fuel, epinephrine's actions provide more glucose and free fatty acids. This occurs through the release of glucose from glycogen (glycogenolysis) by activation of phosphorylase in the liver and muscle via the Cori cycle (see Chapter 16). In muscle, without glucose-6-phosphatase the glucose is metabolized to lactate. Epinephrine also breaks down adipose cell lipids (lipolysis) by activating the lipase that converts triglycerides into free fatty acids and glycerol. As a result of these calorigenic effects, the metabolic rate increases by 20%–30%.

Cardiovascular:

In addition to direct stimulation of the heart rate and vasoconstriction, repeated bursts of epinephrine have been hypothesized to result in permanent hypertension via a number of possible effects.

Table 14-8 Adrenergic Receptors and Function

α-Receptor	β-Receptor
Vasoconstriction	Vasodilatation (β_2)
Iris dilatation	Cardioacceleration (β_1)
Intestinal relaxation	Increased myocardial strength (β_1)
Intestinal sphincter contraction	Intestinal relaxation (β_2)
	Uterus relaxation (β_2)
Pilomotor contraction	Bronchodilatation (β_2)
Bladder sphincter contraction	Calorigenesis (β_2)
	Glycogenolysis (β_2)
	Lipolysis (β_1)
	Bladder wall relaxation (β_2)

From Guyton AC: *Textbook of Medical Physiology,* Saunders, Philadelphia, p. 671, 1991.

Both agonists and antagonists of α- and β-adrenergic receptors are widely used in clinical medicine. Examples include β-agonists such as isoproterenol to dilate bronchi for the treatment of asthma and β-antagonists such as propranolol to decrease cardiac output for the treatment of hypertension. Epinephrine is also used for allergic reactions and norepinephrine is used as a pressor agent.

Features of Catecholamine Excess

Pheochromocytomas are usually benign tumors arising from the adrenal medulla, with clinical features that reflect the effects of epinephrine and norepinephrine (shown in Table 14-8) in excess. Thus, most patients have paroxysms of hypertension, tachycardia, sweating, tremor, palpitations, and nervousness. Most lose weight and are hyperglycemic. The diagnosis is made by measuring either plasma for free catecholamines or urine for metanephrine and by direct visualization of the typically large adrenal tumors, usually by computerized tomographic scan.

ASSESSMENT OF ADRENAL FUNCTION

The various forms of adrenal hypo- and hyperfunction are relatively rare, but many more patients than the few who turn out to have these diseases may be suspected of having them, in large part because of the multiple and diffuse effects of adrenal hormones. Thus, among the large number of women with obesity of predominantly truncal distribution and primary hypertension, some will be suspected of having cortisol excess (Cushing's syndrome), as truncal obesity and hypertension are typical features of the syndrome. Although only a few will have the syndrome, many may need an assessment to rule it out. Therefore, screening tests to assess adrenal function are rather frequently needed to exclude adrenal disorders. If they are positive, more definitive tests may be needed to establish the presence of the disorder and to determine its precise form (Table 14-9). In addition to these, anatomic localization and determination of the type of adrenal pathology may be obtained by various X-ray and isotopic scanning procedures—computerized tomography and magnetic resonance imaging.

As a general approach to screening for either hypofunction or hyperfunction, simple measurements of plasma or urine concentrations of adrenal hormones under basal conditions are usually not adequate in themselves, mainly because of the wide range of values seen in normal people. In screening for hypofunction, however, the presence of low levels of the adrenal hormone along with high levels of the physiological stimulating hormone, that is, ACTH for glucocorticoids and renin–angiotensin for mineralocorticoids, may be useful. Better results are obtained by measuring plasma levels after an appropriate stimulus, that is, ACTH for glucocorticoids and acute volume depletion by a diuretic for mineralocorticoids. For more definitive evidence, the responses of either plasma or urine levels of the hormones are measured after repeated administration of the appropriate stimulus.

To screen for hyperfunction, attempts at rapid suppression of the adrenal hormones are made. For glucocorticoid excess, the response of plasma cortisol to a single dose of the exogenous glucocorticoid dexamethasone is usually adequate. For

Table 14-9 Assessments of Adrenal Function

	Hypofunction		Hyperfunction	
	Screening	Definitive	Screening	Definitive
Cortical				
Glucocorticoid	Low cortisol, high ACTH Response to single ACTH injection	Response to repeated ACTH injections	High cortisol Response to single dose of glucocorticoid	Response to repeated doses of glucocorticoid
Mineralocorticoid	Low aldosterone, high renin Response to acute volume depletion	Response to chronic volume depletion	High aldosterone, low renin Response to acute volume expansion	Response to chronic volume expansion
Androgen	Low plasma levels	—	High plasma levels	—
Medullary	—	—	High catecholamines in single plasma or urine samples	Response to sympathetic nervous system suppressants

mineralocorticoid excess, the response of plasma aldosterone to acute volume expansion by a short infusion of normal saline is measured. For more definitive testing, the responses of either plasma or urine levels of the hormones after more prolonged attempts at suppression are used.

There are few indications to test for deficiencies of adrenal androgens and even fewer for catecholamine deficiency. Excesses of androgens are seen with congenital adrenal enzymatic defects. Catecholamine-secreting tumors (pheochromocytomas) are detected by measuring plasma and urine levels of the catecholamines or their metabolic products.

In summary, the assessment of adrenal function is similar to that of other endocrine disorders: hypofunction is best diagnosed by attempting to stimulate with the appropriate physiological trophic agent, and hyperfunction by suppressing with the appropriate physiological maneuver.

SUGGESTED READING

Andrew R, Phillips D IW, and Walker BR: Obesity and gender influence cortisol secretion and metabolism in man. J Clin Endocrinol Metab 83:1806–1809, 1998.

Barnes PJ: Anti-inflammatory actions of glucocorticoids; molecular mechanisms. Clin Sci 94:557–572, 1998.

Betito K, Mitchell JB, Bhatnagar S, Boksa P, and Meaney MJ: Regulation of the adrenomedullary catecholaminergic system after mild acute stress. Am J Physiol 267:R212–220, 1994.

Bornstein SR, and Vaudry H: Paracrine and neuroendocrine regulation of the adrenal gland—basic and clinical aspects. Horm Metab Res 30:292–296, 1998.

Boumpas DT, Chrousos GP, Wilder RL, Cupps TR, and Balow JE: Glucocorticoid therapy for immune-mediated diseases: basic and clinical correlates. Ann Intern Med 119:1198–1208, 1993.

Cooper M, and Stewart PM: The syndrome of apparent mineralocorticoid excess. Q J Med 91:453–455, 1998.

Ebeling P, and Koivisto VA: Physiological importance of dehydroepiandrosterone. Lancet 343:1479–1481, 1994.

Funder JW: Glucocorticoid and mineralocorticoid receptors: Biology and clinical relevance. Annu Rev Med 48:231–240, 1998.

Gomez MT, Magiakou MA, Mastorakos G, and Chrousos GP: The pituitary corticotroph is not the rate-limiting step in the postoperative recovery of the hypothalamic–pituitary–adrenal axis in patients with Cushing syndrome. J Clin Endocrinol Metab 77:173–177, 1993.

Griffin JE: *Manual of Clinical Endocrinology and Metabolism,* McGraw-Hill, New York, pp. 75–96, 1982.

Grinspoon SK, and Biller BMK: Laboratory assessment of adrenal insufficiency. J Clin Endocrinol Metab 79:923–931, 1994.

Guyton AC: The adrenocortical hormones. In: *Textbook of Medical Physiology,* 8th ed., AC Guyton, ed., Saunders, Philadelphia, pp. 667–678, 842–854, 1991.

Kallen CB, Arakane F, Christenson LK, Watari H, Devoto L, and Strauss JF: Unveiling the mechanism of action and regulation of the steroidogenic acute regulatory protein. Mol Cell Endocrinol 145:39–45, 1998.

Kaplan NM: Adrenal diseases: Pheochromocytoma; primary aldosteronism; Cushings syndrome and congenital adrenal hyperplasia. In: *Clinical Hypertension,* 7th ed., Williams & Wilkins, Baltimore, pp. 345–364, 365–382, 383–394, 1998.

Kater CE, and Biglieri EG: Disorders of steroid 17α-hydroxylase deficiency. Endocrinol Metab Clin North Am 23:341–357, 1994.

Mulatero P, Veglio F, Pilon C, Rabbia F, Zocchi C, Limone P, Boscaro M, Sonino N, and Fallo F: Diagnosis of glucocorticoid-remediable aldosteronism in primary aldosteronism: Aldosterone response to dexamethasone and long polymerase chain reaction for chimeric gene. J Clin Endocrinol Metab 83:2573–2575, 1998.

Newell-Price J, Trainer P, Besser M, and Grossman A: The diagnosis and differential diagnosis of Cushing's syndrome and pseudo-Cushing's states. Endocr Rev 19:647–672, 1998.

Rosmond R, Dallman MF, and Bjorntorp P: Stress-related cortisol secretion in men: Relationships with abdominal obesity and endocrine, metabolic and hemodynamic abnormalities. J Clin Endocrinol Metab 83:1853–1859, 1998.

White PC: Disorders of aldosterone biosynthesis and action. N Engl J Med 331:250–258, 1994.

White PC, and Speiser PW: Steroid 11β-hydroxylase deficiency and related disorders. Endocrinol Metab Clin North Am 23:325–339, 1994.

15

Calcium Homeostasis

NEIL A. BRESLAU

IMPORTANCE OF MAINTAINING CALCIUM HOMEOSTASIS

The physiological importance of calcium falls into two broad categories. The calcium salts in bone provide the structural integrity of the skeleton. The calcium ion in cellular and extracellular fluids is essential to the normal function of a number of biochemical processes including neuromuscular excitability, blood coagulation, hormonal secretion, and enzymatic regulation. The biochemical role of calcium requires that its extracellular and cellular concentrations be maintained within a very narrow range, and this is achieved by an elaborate system of controls.

The control of cellular calcium homeostasis is as carefully maintained as its concentration in extracellular fluids. The concentration of calcium ions in the cytoplasm is approximately one one-thousandth that in the extracellular fluids. Most of the intracellular calcium is contained in the mitochondria and microsomes. Three "pump–leak" transport systems located in the plasma, mitochondrial, and microsomal membranes control the concentration of calcium in the cytosol. Calcium leaks passively into the cytosol by diffusion across these three membranes, but each pump actively shifts calcium away from the cytosolic pool.

Several examples can serve to illustrate the importance of these three calcium transport systems in integrating cellular calcium metabolism. Calcium ion is the coupling factor linking excitation and contraction in skeletal and cardiac muscle. The sarcoplasmic reticulum, composed primarily of microsomes, is the main storehouse of intracellular calcium in muscle. Depolarization of the plasma membrane permits entry of a small amount of extracellular calcium into the muscle cell, which then triggers release of large quantities of stored calcium from the sarcoplasmic reticulum. The abrupt increase in cytosolic calcium interacts with troponin, a specific calcium-binding protein that undergoes conformational change culminating in the actin–myosin interaction that causes muscle contraction. Then the microsomes rapidly reaccumulate the cytosolic calcium, permitting relaxation.

Another important role of the intracellular calcium ion is in stimulus–secretion coupling. In secretory cells, it is frequently the mitochondria that act as the major intracellular storehouse of calcium. Once released from the mitochondria by an appropriate stimulus, cytosolic calcium links secretory vesicles to the plasma membrane, resulting in exocytosis of preformed cell products. Calcium has been implicated as an important coupling factor in neurotransmitter release, exocrine secretion (e.g., amylase), and endocrine secretion (e.g., insulin). In a number of these systems, cyclic adenosine monophosphate (cyclic AMP) operates as a second or intra-cellular messenger that modulates mitochondrial calcium transport, with the change in cytosolic calcium ion actually mediating cellular secretion.

Intracellular calcium ion is also important in the control of key enzymes regulating intermediary metabolism. In the kidney, increased intracellular calcium enhances gluconeogenesis by activating phosphoenolpyruvate carboxykinase and inhibiting pyruvate kinase. In mammalian skeletal muscle, which often works under hypoxic conditions and depends on glycogenolysis for its immediate energy needs, the major effect of calcium is upon the action of phosphorylase b kinase, a key enzyme in the glycogenolytic sequence. Thus, calcium, which is the coupling factor between excitation and contraction in muscle, may also play a role in providing the energy for contraction.

In humans, maintenance of extracellular calcium ion concentration within narrow limits is essential for a number of vital functions including mineralization, blood coagulation, and membrane function. Proper mineralization of bone requires maintenance of a normal calcium × phosphate ion product. The calcium ion serves as a co-factor for clotting factors VII, IX, and X. Ionic calcium also plays an important role in the permeability and excitability of plasma membranes. When the extracellular fluid concentration of calcium ion falls below normal, the nervous system becomes progressively more excitable because of increased permeability of the neuronal membrane to sodium. Nerve fibers become hyperexcitable, spontaneously depolarized, and initiate nerve impulses to peripheral skeletal muscles, thus eliciting tetanic contraction. This effect is the basis for the muscle spasms and marked hyperreflexia seen in hypocalcemic tetany. The traditional positive Chvostek sign— a twitching of the facial muscles in response to tapping over the facial nerve at the angle of the mandible—is one manifestation of hypocalcemic tetany. In severe hypocalcemia, increased central nervous system (CNS) irritability may lead to seizures. An increase in serum ionized calcium depresses central and peripheral neural excitability, resulting in mental sluggishness and hyporeflexia.

There are three definable fractions of calcium in serum: ionized calcium (50%), protein-bound calcium (40%), and calcium that is complexed to other constituents in serum, mostly citrate and phosphate forming soluble complexes (10%). Both complexed and ionized calcium are ultrafilterable, so that about 60% of the total calcium in serum crosses semipermeable membranes. Nearly 90% of the protein-bound calcium is bound to albumin and the remainder to globulins. The binding of calcium to albumin is pH dependent. Acute acidosis decreases binding and increases ionized calcium, whereas acute alkalosis increases binding with a consequent decrease in ionized calcium. Because it is the ionized fraction of calcium that is physiologically important, it is not surprising that patients who hyperventilate and develop an acute respiratory alkalosis may develop circumoral numbness, carpal spasm, and even seizures due to increased neural excitability.

REGULATION OF CALCIUM METABOLISM IN HUMAN BEINGS

Total serum calcium concentration in humans is maintained between 8.5 and 10.5 mg/dl by the flux of calcium between blood and three organs: bone, kidney, and intestine (Fig. 15-1). Calcium is constantly entering and leaving the blood by exchange

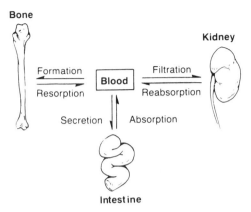

Fig. 15-1 Calcium homeostasis is regulated by the transfer of calcium between the blood and three major target organs.

through these organs. The movement of calcium in this system is controlled by three main hormones: parathyroid hormone (PTH), calcitonin, and the most important metabolite of vitamin D: 1,25-dihydroxyvitamin D [1,25-(OH)$_2$D]. PTH increases blood calcium concentration by increasing resorption of bone, by promoting reabsorption of calcium from the glomerular filtrate, and by increasing the rate of formation of 1,25-(OH)$_2$D in the kidney. This vitamin D metabolite accelerates the rate of absorption of calcium from the intestine. Moreover, it directly stimulates bone resorption and plays a permissive role in the action of PTH on bone. Calcitonin inhibits bone resorption but is not believed to play as important a role in the day-to-day regulation of calcium homeostasis as the previous two hormones.

The daily net changes in calcium transfer for an adult man in the steady state are approximately as follows. About 1000 mg of calcium is ingested per day, but only one-third of this amount is absorbed from the intestine (360 mg) and enters the extracellular fluid (ECF). Part of the calcium in the ECF is lost through enteric secretion (190 mg) back into the gut. The net absorption is thus 170 mg of calcium, approximately the same as that lost per day via urinary excretion. Bone is the principal reservoir of calcium in the body, containing 1000 g. Each day about 550 mg of calcium is exchanged between bone and body fluid. In the steady adult state, the transfer rates for calcium entering and leaving bone are the same. Obviously, in a growing child, calcium retention would occur in proportion to bone growth. The increased calcium entering bone would be balanced by greater intestinal absorption and less urinary excretion of calcium, thereby maintaining a constant serum calcium concentration.

BIOCHEMISTRY AND PHYSIOLOGY OF THE MAJOR CALCIUM-REGULATING HORMONES

Parathyroid Hormone (PTH)

Parathyroid hormone is produced in the parathyroid glands, of which there are generally two pairs situated behind the thyroid gland. Each parathyroid gland measures

6 × 4 × 2 mm and weighs 30–50 mg. Supernumerary parathyroids (up to eight glands) are present in 2%–5% of the population. The chief cell, the principal parenchymal parathyroid cell, is responsible for the synthesis and secretion of PTH.

PTH is a single-chain polypeptide composed of 84 amino acids with a molecular weight of 9500 Da. The structure of human PTH and its biosynthetic sequence are now known. The gene for PTH actually encodes a precursor termed *prepro-PTH*, which is a polypeptide of 115 amino acids with a molecular weight of 13,000 Da. This prehormone is short-lived, being rapidly cleaved to a smaller peptide, pro-PTH. Pro-PTH is composed of 90 amino acids and has a molecular weight of 10,200 Da. A second enzymatic cleavage of the 6-amino acid extension at the amino terminus of the molecule results in the final secretory product: 1–84 PTH. The function of the amino-terminal leader sequences in the precursor hormones may be to transport the polypeptide through the membrane channels of the endoplasmic reticulum. In the Golgi apparatus, PTH is packaged into secretory granules for storage and subsequent secretion. The precursor forms are not secreted and are biologically inactive.

The ability of the parathyroid cell to sense minute fluctuations in the extracellular ionized calcium concentration is essential for maintaining mineral ion homeostasis. Until recently, the mechanism(s) through which the parathyroid cell and other cells recognize and respond to changes in serum calcium has remained unclear. An extracellular calcium-sensing receptor has now been cloned and characterized. It is present in the cell membrane of parathyroid cells, renal tubule cells, and in the C cells of the thyroid gland. As shown in Figure 15-2, the protein is predicted to have three major structural domains. The first is a 613-amino acid, putatively extracellular amino-terminus that has several regions rich in acidic amino acids (glutamine and aspartic acids) that may potentially be involved in binding ionized calcium. The second comprises seven membrane-spanning segments that are characteristic of the superfamily of G protein–coupled receptors. The last structural domain is a 222-amino acid, presumably cytoplasmic carboxy-terminus. In response to an increase in extracellular ionized calcium, the receptor becomes activated and via a G protein–coupled mechanism, activates phospholipase C. This leads to the hydrolysis of polyphosphoinositides, accumulation of inositol triphosphate, and release of ionized calcium from intracellular stores. Moreover, the calcium-sensing receptor inhibits adenylyl cyclase via an inhibitory G protein, thereby reducing intracellular cyclic AMP. Both the increase in intracellular calcium and the decrease in cyclic AMP act to suppress PTH secretion. The calcium-sensing receptor also recognizes other divalent cations such as magnesium, and even trivalent cations such as gadolinium.

The major regulator of both the synthesis and secretion of PTH is the concentration of ionized calcium in the blood. There is an inverse relationship between PTH secretion and serum calcium. As serum calcium decreases acutely, PTH secretion may rise up to five times the normal secretion rate. If the hypocalcemia is chronic, gross parathyroid hyperplasia occurs and PTH secretion may approach 50 times the basal rate. A rising serum calcium will suppress PTH secretion, but there is a calcium-independent, nonsuppressible component of PTH secretion, which represents about 15% of the normal secretion rate. Within the physiological range, the effect of magnesium on PTH secretion is in the same direction as that of calcium, but much weaker. Severe hypomagnesemia is associated with an impairment in PTH

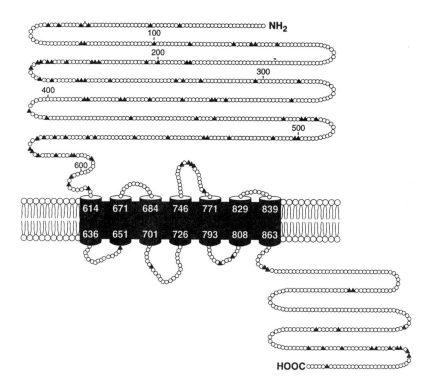

Fig. 15-2 Schematic diagram illustrating the principal structural features of the predicted parathyroid extracellular calcium-sensing receptor. Solid triangles indicate acidic amino acids. (Adapted from Brown EM, Pollak M, Hebert SC: Physiology and cell biology update: Sensing of extracellular Ca^{2+} by parathyroid and kidney cells: Cloning and characterization of an extracellular Ca^{2+}-sensing receptor. Am J Kidney Dis 25: 506–513, 1995).

secretion. β-adrenergic receptors have been identified in parathyroid cells, and isoproterenol and epinephrine have been shown to stimulate PTH secretion. The influence of catecholamines on PTH secretion may provide a partial explanation for the hypercalcemia noted in some patients with pheochromocytoma (see Chapter 14). There are receptors for 1,25-(OH)$_2$-D in the parathyroid glands, and this metabolite has been shown to suppress PTH secretion. There are also H$_2$ histamine receptors in the parathyroid glands, and under certain circumstances, the H$_2$ receptor blocker cimetidine has been shown to reduce PTH secretion. Glucocorticoids directly stimulate PTH secretion. Inorganic phosphorus has no direct influence on PTH secretion. Rather, it is the phosphorus-induced reduction in the concentration of serum ionized calcium that stimulates PTH secretion.

Intact, biologically active 1–84 PTH (molecular weight 9600 Da) is the major secretory product of the parathyroid glands. Its half-life is several minutes and it constitutes only about 10% of the circulating parathyroid fragments. However, it accurately reflects parathyroid function and its clearance is largely independent of kidney function. This peptide may be measured by a double antibody sandwich technique known as the *immunoradiometric assay* (IRMA) (see Chapter 5). Measurement of intact PTH by the IRMA technique has become the assay of choice for assessing parathyroid function. Intact PTH is metabolized by the kidney and liver to amino- and carboxy-terminal fragments. The amino-terminal 1–34 PTH (molecular weight 3000–4000 Da) possesses biological activity, but also has a short circulating half-life measured in minutes. It, too, constitutes 10% of circulating parathyroid fragments. Like intact PTH, the amino-terminal fragment is metabolized by its target tissues: kidney and bone. Carboxy-terminal fragments (molecular weight 6000–7000 Da), which are inactive, derive not only from hepatic and renal cleavage of the intact hormone, but also to some extent from the parathyroid glands themselves. The secretion of these inactive fragments is particularly evident at elevated ambient calcium concentrations. The carboxy-terminal peptides have a half-life measured in hours and constitute about 80% of the circulating PTH fragments. Carboxy-terminal fragments are not metabolized by target organs and are eliminated from the circulation solely by glomerular filtration. Therefore, patients with renal insufficiency may develop a very high concentration of these inactive fragments, which does not accurately reflect the parathyroid activity. In the presence of renal disease, the intact or amino-terminal PTH assays provide a more accurate assessment of parathyroid status.

By interacting with its three major target organs (bone, kidney, and intestine), PTH is primarily responsible for the regulation of calcium homeostasis in humans. In response to systemic needs, bone mineral is made available by the combined processes of osteocytic osteolysis and osteoclastic bone resorption. *Osteocytic osteolysis* refers to the rapid mobilization of bone mineral by lacunar osteocytes in haversian bone. This type of mineral mobilization may occur within minutes, involves activation of existing bone cells, and may proceed without actual resorption or destruction of bone. There is evidence that the rapid rise in serum calcium in response to PTH through this mechanism requires the presence of $1,25\text{-}(OH)_2D$. A more delayed (hours to days) response of bone to PTH is *osteoclastic resorption.* Following activation by PTH, precursor cells differentiate into multinucleated osteoclasts that resorb a localized area of mineralized bone. This process results in the destruction and removal of both bone mineral and bone matrix. Osteoclastic resorption is a delayed response occurring only after exposure of bone to prolonged stimulation by PTH. Over a period of many months or years, prolonged excess of PTH leads to increased bone resorption and development of large cavities filled with multinucleated osteoclasts (classic osteitis fibrosa cystica of severe hyperparathyroidism). If PTH is given intermittently, however, it increases osteoblastic activity and promotes bone growth through enhancement of bone remodeling in which a longer osteoblastic phase follows short-term induction of new osteoclasts.

In the kidney, PTH decreases proximal tubular phosphate reabsorption and increases calcium reabsorption in the distal nephron. Both effects are important in the minute-to-minute regulation of the serum concentrations of phosphorus and calcium. Another very important effect of PTH in the kidney is to stimulate $1,25\text{-}(OH)_2D$ synthesis, which exerts control over the intestinal absorption of calcium and phosphorus. In the proximal tubule, in addition to inhibiting phosphate reabsorption, PTH also inhibits reabsorption of sodium and bicarbonate. Thus, it has diuretic effects and may provoke a mild hyperchloremic acidosis. PTH decreases renal clearance of uric acid, and hyperparathyroidism may be associated with hyperuricemia and gout. Even though PTH stimulates distal tubular calcium reabsorption, the urinary calcium excretion is usually greater than normal in hyperparathyroidism because of the increase in filtered calcium load (owing to the bone and intestinal effects of PTH). Hypoparathyroid individuals with a normal serum calcium concentration of 9–10 mg/dl will excrete three times more calcium in the urine than will normal subjects because they lose the distal tubular effect of PTH.

Intact PTH binds to specific receptors on the surface of target cells in bone and kidney. This binding triggers the release of cytoplasmic "second messengers," which then mediate the multiple distant effects of PTH. Binding of PTH to its receptors requires only the first 34 residues at the amino-terminal of the PTH molecule.

The best-characterized mediator of PTH's action is *cyclic adenosine monophosphate* (cyclic AMP). Exposure of bone or kidney cells to PTH results in a rapid intracellular accumulation of cyclic AMP and an outpouring of cyclic AMP into the urine. Administration of analogs of cyclic AMP can mimic many of the effects of PTH. The rapid elevation of cyclic AMP in response to PTH and the actions of cyclic AMP strongly suggest that cyclic AMP mediates the effects of PTH. Binding of PTH to its receptor on the external surface of the cell triggers the release of guanosine diphosphate (GDP) from an intracellular protein called G_s and permits the binding of intracellular guanosine triphosphate (GTP) to G_s. The GTP-G_s then stimulates membrane-bound adenylate cyclase (see Chapter 3). The cyclic AMP produced by adenylate cyclase then activates protein kinase A, which then phosphorylates specific target proteins. The relevant target proteins and their precise modes of action remain uncharacterized, although proteins that activate genes responsive to cyclic AMP and ion channel proteins are strong candidates. The human disease *pseudohypoparathyroidism* (to be discussed later) provides evidence for the physiologic relevance of the above mechanism of PTH action.

In addition, PTH may stimulate cellular activity by another mechanism. PTH stimulates phosphotidylinositol turnover in cultured cell lines, causes a rapid rise in levels of free cytosolic calcium, and causes a shift of protein kinase C (to the cell membrane). These effects are different from the actions of cyclic AMP analogs, and they suggest that multiple second messengers may mediate some actions of PTH. The physiologic importance of metabolites of phosphotidylinositol and intracellular calcium as PTH-induced second messengers has not yet been established.

Calciferol (Vitamin D)

The biochemical activation of 7-dehydrocholesterol to the active metabolite 1,25-$(OH)_2D$ requires three separate organ systems (skin, liver, and kidney) plus interaction with the environment, so there are many potential loci for disease (Fig. 15-3). Vitamin D_3 (cholecalciferol) is produced in the skin from 7-dehydrocholesterol, an inert precursor whose availability in skin decreases with age. A "previtamin D_3" is synthesized photochemically in the high dermis and lower epidermis when the 7-dehydrocholesterol is exposed to photolytic wavelengths of 250–310 nm (mid-ultraviolet). Melanin absorbs the same wavelengths and interferes with calciferol synthesis. Overproduction is also prevented by a photochemical equilibrium that favors synthesis of lumisterol and tachysterol (inert metabolites) during prolonged sun exposure. Intensity and duration of solar 286–310 nm radiation is strongly depen-

Fig. 15-3 Chemical structure and site of formation of the major vitamin D metabolites.

dent on the angle of the sun (time of day, season of year), clouds, air pollution, and habitat (window glass and most electrical fixtures absorb all radiation less than 315–350 nm). Clothing and social customs further modify mid-ultraviolet exposure. Calciferol deficiency was common in temperate latitudes before diets were fortified, and it still occurs in elderly or housebound individuals.

Over a period of several days, the previtamin D_3 formed in the skin undergoes a temperature-dependent isomerization to vitamin D_3. The vitamin D–binding protein in blood has a 1000-fold higher affinity for vitamin D_3 than previtamin D_3, so that vitamin D_3 is preferentially transported from the skin into the circulation. The vitamin D_3 removed into the circulation is replaced by slow thermal conversion of previtamin D_3 to vitamin D_3. This series of steps appears to constitute an important mechanism whereby relatively brief exposure to ultraviolet radiation may lead to a continuous supply of vitamin D for days to weeks.

The terms *parent vitamin D* and *calciferol* are synonyms that actually refer to two sterols. Cholecalciferol (vitamin D_3) is the form of the vitamin found in animal tissues, fish liver oils, and irradiated milk. Ergocalciferol (vitamin D_2) is the form of vitamin D found in plants and irradiated yeast and bread. Most foodstuffs, from either plant or animal sources, contain only inactive vitamin D precursors and require ultraviolet irradiation for the conversion of these precursors to the calciferols. In addition to the photochemical synthesis of vitamin D_3 in the skin, humans may supplement their vitamin D stores by dietary intake of vitamin D_2 or D_3. In humans, the storage, transport, metabolism, and potency of vitamin D_2 and vitamin D_3 are identical, and the net biological activity of vitamin D *in vivo* results from the combined effects of the hydroxylated derivatives of vitamin D_2 and vitamin D_3. The adult requirement for calciferol is considered to be 400 USP units daily (1 mg of calciferol is equivalent to 40,000 USP or international units). In the United States, vitamin D additives are present in a number of foods including milk, milk products, and cereals.

Cholecalciferol, a biologically inactive prohormone, is transported to the liver bound to vitamin D-binding protein. There it is hydroxylated at C-25 to form 25-$(OH)D$, a partially active product (Fig. 15-3). The 25-$(OH)D$ constitutes the major circulating form of vitamin D in humans and is a good index of the vitamin D status of the individual. The typical concentration of 25-$(OH)D$ in serum is 7–42 ng/ml with a circulating half-life of 15 days. The circulating pool of this metabolite is in equilibrium with a storage pool of 25-$(OH)D$ in muscle and fat. 25-Hydroxylation of vitamin D takes place in the hepatic microsomes. Clinical studies have shown that 25-hydroxylation of vitamin D is inhibited by vitamin D and 1,25-$(OH)_2D$. Whether 25-$(OH)D$ plays a physiologic role in regulating its own synthesis has not been established. Inhibition of 25-hydroxylation by vitamin D seems to be a relatively ineffective control mechanism in view of the fact that marked increases in circulating 25-$(OH)D$ are responsible for the abnormal mineral metabolism in vitamin D intoxication. In contrast, feedback regulation of 25-$(OH)D$ production by 1,25-$(OH)_2D$ appears to be effective. Also, 1,25-$(OH)_2D$ completely inhibits the increase in serum 25-$(OH)D$ produced by vitamin D challenge in normal subjects. The mechanism by which hepatic production of 25-$(OH)D$ is modulated by 1,25-$(OH)_2D$ is not known. Systemic calcium and phosphorus status do not influence hepatic 25-hydroxylase activity, and the importance of this enzyme as a biological control site is questionable. Anticonvulsants induce hepatic microsomal mixed oxidase enzymes that convert vitamin D metabolites to more polar hydroxylated, biologically inactive products, which are excreted in the bile. This mechanism may partially explain the reduced circulating 25-$(OH)D$ levels and/or clinical osteomalacia (impaired mineralization of bone) in patients receiving prolonged high-dose anticonvulsant therapy.

The 25-$(OH)D$ is transported to the kidney, where it is hydroxylated either at C-1 to produce 1,25-$(OH)_2D$, the most potent vitamin D metabolite, or at C-24 to produce 24,25-$(OH)_2D$, a less active compound of unclear biological significance. Although there is evidence of regulation of both cholecalciferol production in the skin and the initial hydroxylation of vitamin D in the liver, the hydroxylase reactions in the kidney are the key points of biological regulation of the metabolic activation of vitamin D. The principal regulator of the renal synthesis of 1,25-(OH)$_2$D is PTH. Serum 1,25-(OH)$_2$D is increased in primary hyperparathyroidism and is reduced in hypoparathyroidism. Circulating 1,25-(OH)$_2$D is increased when parathyroid extract is given to normal subjects and to patients with hypoparathyroidism. In normal adults, the renal production of 1,25-(OH)$_2$D is tightly regulated, and serum 1,25-(OH)$_2$D changes very little in response to vitamin D challenge. This occurs because an increase in circulating 1,25-(OH)$_2$D raises intestinal calcium absorption and hence the serum-ionized calcium concentration. The rise in serum-ionized calcium concentration suppresses PTH secretion and thereby inhibits the renal production of 1,25-(OH)$_2$D. Moreover, as already noted, receptors for this vitamin D metabolite have been demonstrated in parathyroid cells, and there is considerable evidence for a direct feedback inhibition of PTH synthesis and secretion by 1,25-(OH)$_2$D.

In addition, PTH may control 1-hydroxylation by promoting urinary phosphate excretion, which in turn lowers the serum phosphate level. In animals and humans it has been shown that 1-hydroxylation can be stimulated even in the absence of the parathyroid glands by decreasing serum phosphate concentration. The action of PTH on the renal tubular cell, which is mediated by cyclic AMP, probably also involves decreased intracellular phosphate concentrations owing to inhibition of phosphate reabsorption. The importance of these biochemical stimuli is underscored by the observation that urinary cyclic AMP and phosphate excretion change very little, and serum 1,25-(OH)$_2$D remains low in response to parathyroid extract in patients with a PTH-resistant state known as *pseudohypoparathyroidism.* These same patients have a brisk rise in serum 1,25-(OH)$_2$D associated with a marked phosphaturia in response to dibutyryl-cyclic AMP infusions.

Another major regulator of the renal production of 1,25-(OH)$_2$D is the vitamin D status of an individual. In the absence of PTH, as in hypoparathyroidism, serum 1,25-(OH)$_2$D varies with the concentration of serum 25-(OH)D, suggesting that there is substrate dependency. There is also evidence that 1,25-(OH)$_2$D itself and an elevated serum calcium level inhibit synthesis of 1,25-(OH)$_2$D. Moreover, 1,25-(OH)$_2$D induces renal 25-hydroxyvitamin D 24-hydroxylase activity. Thus, in the vitamin D–replete state, the production of the relatively inactive metabolite 24,25-(OH)$_2$D is enhanced.

The normal serum level of 1,25-(OH)$_2$D is 20–50 pg/ml and its circulating half-life is about 3 hours. As noted, the renal production of this potent vitamin D metabolite is carefully regulated. However, under certain circumstances, extrarenal production of 1,25-(OH)$_2$D may occur without appropriate regulation, resulting in disturbances in calcium metabolism. A classic example is a granulomatous disorder known as *sarcoidosis,* in which sarcoid lymph node tissue produces 1,25-(OH)$_2$D. Patients with this disorder may have elevated calcium levels in the blood and urine, sometimes resulting in kidney stones. Defective regulation of circulating 1,25-(OH)$_2$D in sarcoid can be shown by the lack of change in serum 1,25-(OH)$_2$D in response to increased calcium intake as compared with the reduction of circulating 1,25-(OH)$_2$D that occurs in normal subjects. Other granulomatous conditions in which hypercalcemia associated with abnormal elevation of 1,25-(OH)$_2$D has been reported include tuberculosis, disseminated candidiasis, silicon-induced granuloma, and lymphoma. The human placenta has also been demonstrated to produce 1,25-(OH)$_2$D, which may be important in meeting the increased calcium demands of pregnancy.

Both 1,25-$(OH)_2$D and 24,25-$(OH)_2$D may undergo an additional hydroxylation to form 1,24,25-trihydroxyvitamin D [1,24,25-$(OH)_3$D]. *In vivo*, the synthesis of 1,24,25-$(OH)_3$D from 1,25-$(OH)_2$D is probably the more important pathway as 1,25-$(OH)_2$D induces the 24-hydroxylase that can use 1,25-$(OH)_2$D as substrate. Moreover, 1,24,25-$(OH)_3$D has only one-third the activity of 1,25-$(OH)_2$D in the intestine and it is only marginally active in bone resorption. Many investigators favor the view that the hydroxylation of the vitamin D nucleus at C-24 represents a step in the direction of inactivation of the hormone. Because 24-hydroxylase activity has been detected in the intestine and bone as well as in the kidney, it is conceivable that this may represent an initial inactivation step when 1,25-$(OH)_2$D reaches its target organs. Upon oxidative cleavage of its side chain, 1,25-$(OH)_2$D forms a C-23 carboxylic acid, calcitroic acid, which is biologically inactive. Production of calcitroic acid in target tissues might be another important mechanism for inactivation of the biologically potent 1,25-$(OH)_2$D. Side-chain oxidation appears to proceed more rapidly in the presence of hydroxyl groups at C-24 and C-25, a finding compatible with the view that 24-hydroxylation may represent an initial inactivation step. In addition, vitamin D metabolites undergo an enterohepatic circulation in which they are concentrated in bile, secreted into the intestine, and then reabsorbed. Consequently, certain gastrointestinal disorders may result in vitamin D deficiency despite adequate synthesis of cholecalciferol in the skin.

The major target tissues for vitamin D action are the intestine, bone, and kidney. There is general agreement that 1,25-$(OH)_2$D is the main metabolite of vitamin D regulating intestinal absorption and bone resorption. Whether other hydroxylated metabolites of vitamin D have physiologically important actions on any of the target organs remains unclear.

In the intestine, 1,25-$(OH)_2$D promotes calcium absorption by a mechanism that conforms generally to the steroid hormone model. Initially, the hormone is bound to a cytosolic receptor. The 1,25-$(OH)_2$D receptor complex becomes tightly associated with the cell nucleus and stimulates transcription of DNA to synthesize messenger RNA and translation of proteins to carry out the biological action of the hormone. Not all of the proteins that are synthesized in response to 1,25-$(OH)_2$D have been identified, but one of them is *calcium-binding protein* (CaBP), which cannot be detected in the intestines of vitamin D–deficient animals. The role of CaBP in intestinal calcium absorption is still controversial, but it probably facilitates calcium uptake by the intestinal cell. Vitamin D also stimulates phosphate and magnesium absorption by the intestine. A recently described human disorder known as *vitamin D–dependent rickets type II* points to the importance of the 1,25-$(OH)_2$D receptor in mediating the biological effects of vitamin D. This disorder is characterized by impaired intestinal calcium absorption resulting in rickets or osteomalacia, despite marked increases in circulating 1,25-$(OH)_2$D. It is caused by abnormalities in the receptor for 1,25-$(OH)_2$D.

Although 1,25-$(OH)_2$D produces bone resorption [100 to several thousand times more potent than 25-(OH)D], the mechanism by which this occurs is not known. Autoradiographic studies show uptake of labeled 1,25-$(OH)_2$D by osteoprogenitor cells and osteoblasts but not by osteoclasts. If bone resorption produced by 1,25-$(OH)_2$D is mediated by osteoclasts, it is unlikely to be a direct effect in view of the absence of a receptor for the hormone. Evidence indicates that osteoclasts may be derived from circulating peripheral monocytes that do have receptors for 1,25-

(OH)$_2$D. Under the influence of 1,25-(OH)$_2$D, circulating monocytes may fuse into multinucleated macrophage-like cells that produce bone resorption and at least resemble osteoclasts. High-dose 1,25-(OH)$_2$D activated both osteoclasts and peripheral monocytes to produce bone resorption in a patient with malignant osteopetrosis, a disease characterized by impaired osteoclast function. Thus, 1,25-(OH)$_2$D may be important in regulating cellular differentiation in osseous tissue. Both PTH and 1,25-(OH)$_2$D clearly potentiate each other in bone resorption, and a maximum rate of resorption is observed only in response to the combined effects of both hormones. Present evidence indicates that the mechanism of action of 1,25-(OH)$_2$D in bone is identical to its mechanism of action in the intestinal mucosal cell, although the specific target cells in bone and the protein translation products induced by 1,25-(OH)$_2$D remain largely unknown.

Although the main defect in vitamin D deficiency is a failure of normal mineralization (e.g., rickets or osteomalacia), the exact role of vitamin D metabolites in bone formation remains uncertain. One view is that 1,25-(OH)$_2$D participates with PTH in regulating bone resorption but that bone mineralization is a passive process that proceeds normally given an adequate calcium $\times$ phosphate product in the extracellular fluid. Indeed, the infusion of calcium and phosphate into vitamin D–deficient humans sufficient to normalize the mineral ion product is associated with remineralization of bone. However, the mineralization that occurs is patchy and disordered, in contrast to the orderly mineralization process following vitamin D repletion. Perhaps a vitamin D metabolite controls the bone-forming cells responsible for mineralization (osteoid osteocytes). In addition to impaired mineralization, vitamin D–deficient states are characterized by retarded bone formation. The osteoblasts responsible for laying down the protein matrix of bone are flattened and inactive during vitamin D depletion. Following vitamin D treatment, the osteoblasts become cuboidal and active, and there is histologic evidence of increased bone formation. In human bone cells with many of the features of osteoblasts, 1,25-(OH)$_2$D stimulates production of alkaline phosphatase and osteocalcin, both of which may play a role in mineralization of newly formed bone matrix. In some human studies of vitamin D deficiency and end-stage renal disease, osteomalacic changes in bone could be completely cured only by administering 25-(OH)D, whereas 1,25-(OH)$_2$D produced only a partial reversal of the abnormalities. Thus, although most investigators regard 1,25-(OH)$_2$D as the vitamin D metabolite that mediates bone resorption, considerable evidence shows that one or more additional metabolites of vitamin D might directly or indirectly influence the processes of bone formation and mineralization.

In the kidney, both 25-(OH)D and 1,25-(OH)$_2$D have been reported to increase renal tubular reabsorption of both calcium and phosphate. The physiological relevance of these effects has been questioned. The potential effects of vitamin D on other tissues remain largely speculative and require additional investigation. Muscle weakness is a dominant symptom of vitamin D deficiency and responds rapidly to vitamin D repletion. This weakness is usually attributed to coincident hypophosphatemia, but may represent a more fundamental effect of vitamin D in muscle. The finding of receptors for 1,25-(OH)$_2$D in a number of cells and tissues other than those of established target organs indicates that the hormone might have a number of biological effects in addition to those related to mineral metabolism. A recently investigated role for this vitamin D metabolite may be in the regulation of cell growth and differentiation, particularly for those cells derived from bone marrow. The 1,25-

(OH)$_2$D receptors were demonstrated in promyelocytic leukemia cells (HL-60), and 1,25-(OH)$_2$D inhibited growth and induced differentiation of these cells into multi-nucleated macrophage-like cells that resorbed bone. Also, 1,25-(OH)$_2$D and two fluorinated analogs induced macrophage differentiation of normal human and leukemic stem cells and prolonged survival of nude mice inoculated with leukemia cells. Moreover, 1,25-(OH)$_2$D has been shown to promote differentiation of human skin cells. This property has been utilized to reduce the abnormal turnover of skin cells in psoriasis. These observations have stirred excitement over the possible use of 1,25-(OH)$_2$D in the treatment of certain human leukemias and psoriasis.

Calcitonin

Calcitonin is a 32-amino acid peptide derived from a larger precursor called *procalcitonin*. Calcitonin's primary action is to inhibit bone resorption by inhibiting osteoclasts. It is synthesized by the parafollicular or "C cells" of the thyroid gland. The C cells are actually neuroendocrine cells that originate in the neural crest. They are included in the amine precursor uptake and decarboxylation (APUD) cell family, which may explain the association of medullary carcinoma of the thyroid (C-cell adenocarinoma) with another tumor of the APUD series, that is, pheochromocytoma in a polyglandular endocrine syndrome termed *multiple endocrine neoplasia type II* (Sipple's syndrome).

Several different products of the calcitonin gene have been recognized, each with different properties. The calcitonin gene generates multiple RNAs as a consequence of alternative processing events. One encodes the precursor of the 32-amino acid hormone, calcitonin, which also contains a flanking carboxy-terminal peptide, katacalcin, with hypocalcemic properties. The others encode precursors of two 37-amino acid peptides, α- and β-calcitonin gene-related peptide (CGRP). The β-CGRP differs from α-CGRP at only three positions in the amino acid sequence, and both are equally effective in causing arterial vasodilation. CGRP is widely distributed in the central and peripheral nervous systems and in many organs, including the heart, lungs, thyroid, and gastrointestinal tract. It is found in association with the smooth muscles of blood vessels and perivascular nerves. It is believed that CGRP functions as a neurotransmitter and in the regulation of peripheral vascular tone.

Circulating calcitonin consists of heterogeneous forms owing to peripheral metabolism, as well as the secretion of multiple peptide fragments. However, detailed studies have revealed that the entire 32-amino acid sequence of calcitonin is required for biological activity and that even single amino acid deletions at either end of the molecule result in virtually complete loss of biological activity. According to most well-established radioimmunoassays, calcitonin normally fluctuates between 5 and 50 pg/ml in human serum. The half-life of human calcitonin is approximately 5 minutes. Salmon calcitonin, derived from the ultimobrachial body (an embryologic analog of human C cells), is ten times more potent than human calcitonin in its hypocalcemic effect. The increased potency of salmon calcitonin appears to result both from a prolonged circulating half-time and from an increased affinity for and/or an increased duration of binding to calcitonin receptors in the hormone's target tissues.

The main stimuli for the secretion of calcitonin are (*1*) an elevated serum calcium and (*2*) certain gastrointestinal hormones, particularly gastrin. The rate of calcitonin secretion is a direct function of the level of serum calcium above 9 mg/dl.

Calcitonin secretion appears to proceed at a low basal rate within the normal range of serum calcium and is reduced to undetectable levels during hypocalcemia. Although the level of ionized calcium is the principal regulator of calcitonin secretion, evidence shows that gastrin also plays a role. For example, one study showed that calcitonin secretion could be elicited by oral calcium without a demonstrable change in circulating ionized calcium concentration, but with a rise in serum gastrin. An interpretation of this experiment is that the gastrin-secreting stomach cell senses calcium in the food contents and alerts the calcitonin-secreting parafollicular cell to its imminent absorption. The incoming calcium is met by a hormone that protects against alimentary hypercalcemia. The main organs responsible for the clearance and destruction of calcitonin are the kidney, liver, and possibly bone.

Acute administration of calcitonin causes hypocalcemia and hypophosphatemia. Both effects are due largely to the influence of the hormone on bone, although in pharmacological doses calcitonin also affects the renal handling of calcium and phosphate. The most important effect of calcitonin is the inhibition of bone resorption. There is little evidence for any direct effect of calcitonin on bone formation. Osteoclasts, the multinucleated bone-resorbing cells, contain membrane receptors for calcitonin. Within a few minutes after the administration of this hormone, the osteoclasts lose their ruffled borders (indicators of phagocytic activity), and there is a reduction in serum calcium and hydroxyproline excretion, indicating inhibition of both mineral and matrix resorption. In patients with Paget's disease, in whom both bone resorption and bone formation are excessive, calcitonin has a prolonged and marked inhibitory effect on osteoclasts. It is therefore very effective in the treatment of this disease. Because bone formation is "coupled" to bone resorption, chronic exposure to calcitonin leads ultimately to a decrease in all aspects of bone turnover, including osteoblast number and function. Calcitonin's ability to inhibit bone resorption acutely has also been utilized in the treatment of hypercalcemia associated with malignant disease. Within days, however, the inhibitory influence of calcitonin may be lost because of down-regulation of calcitonin receptors in bone ("escape phenomenon"). The reduction in serum phosphate produced by calcitonin appears to result from an inhibition of phosphorus mobilization from bone and from the renal phosphaturic effect.

There are calcitonin receptors in the kidney, and, infused in sufficient dosage, calcitonin leads to a transient increase in the excretion of calcium, phosphate, sodium, potassium, and magnesium. The calciuric and phosphaturic effects of calcitonin augment the hypocalcemia and hypophosphatemia that result from the actions of the hormone on bone. Some evidence shows that calcitonin may increase the synthesis of $1,25\text{-}(OH)_2D$ by the kidney, even in parathyroidectomized animals. Cyclic AMP serves as the intracellular mediator of calcitonin's effects in both bone and kidney, although the exact mechanism by which the stimulation of cyclic AMP in these cells mediates calcitonin's effect on ion transport remains unknown. Calcitonin and PTH interact with different target cells in the renal tubule. Moreover, the two hormones differ in their effects on cyclic AMP excretion in the urine. Urinary cyclic AMP excretion provides a sensitive reflection of the effects of circulating, active PTH, whereas large doses of calcitonin have no influence on urinary cyclic AMP excretion (presumably because the target cells of calcitonin are less permeable to cyclic AMP).

The physiological significance of calcitonin in humans has been questioned because there are no known metabolic consequences of calcitonin deficiency or excess. Serum calcium is well regulated within normal limits after total thyroidectomy. When calcitonin is present in inappropriately high concentrations (as in medullary carcinoma of the thyroid), it appears to have little effect on mineral homeostasis or bone density. Clinically, calcitonin measurements have been useful in detecting the presence of medullary carcinoma of the thyroid, particularly after provocative tests involving infusion of calcium or pentagastrin. Measurements of basal and stimulated levels of serum calcitonin are also valuable as indices of the success or failure of treatment of these C-cell tumors. Salmon calcitonin injections have been utilized in the long-term treatment of Paget's disease, to prevent further bone loss in osteoporosis, and in the short-term treatment of hypercalcemia of malignancy. Salmon calcitonin is also available as a nasal spray.

Overall Control of Calcium Ion Concentration

The maintenance of a steady serum calcium concentration by the major calcium-regulating hormones is diagrammed in Figure 15-4.

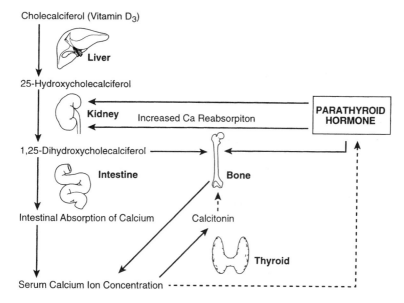

Fig. 15-4   Regulation of serum calcium homeostasis by the major calcium-regulating hormones. The solid arrows indicate activation; the dashed arrows indicate inhibition. When serum calcium concentration rises, for example, after a calcium-containing meal, parathyroid (PTH) secretion is inhibited. The normal actions of PTH to stimulate 1,25-$(OH)_2D$ production, increase renal calcium reabsorption, and promote bone resorption become suppressed. The reduction of 1,25-$(OH)_2D$ production lowers intestinal calcium absorption and bone resorption. Calcitonin release is stimulated by the rise in serum calcium concentration and inhibits bone resorption. These effects return the serum calcium level back to normal.

OTHER HORMONES THAT AFFECT BONE
AND CALCIUM METABOLISM

Although PTH, vitamin D, and, to a lesser extent, calcitonin are the major calcium-regulating hormones, a number of other hormones are known to have an important influence on bone and mineral metabolism. These include estrogens and androgens, glucocorticoids, thyroid hormones, and growth hormone.

Estrogens and Androgens

Gonadal steroids are involved in the pubertal growth spurt and in closure of the epiphyses. In childhood and puberty, the steroids of both sexes favor bone formation over resorption. In the adult female, estrogen inhibits PTH-mediated bone resorption by mechanisms that are incompletely understood. Estrogen receptors have been detected in osteoblasts, and conceivably these cells may release factors (e.g., transforming growth factor [TGF]-β) that inhibit osteoclastic resorption. Estrogens have also been demonstrated to reduce the amount of bone-resorbing cytokines such as interleukin (IL)-1 and IL-6 in bone and to reduce prostaglandin E_2 levels. Thus, estrogens protect the skeleton from the development of osteoporosis or decreased bone mass. Following oophorectomy or menopause, there is an increased rate of bone resorption that in many women causes osteoporosis, which can lead to vertebral compression fractures and hip fractures. Estrogen replacement therapy, although not without side effects, has been shown to slow or arrest the progress of postmenopausal osteoporosis. Interestingly, despite blocking the resorptive action of PTH on bone, estrogen appears to facilitate PTH action at the kidney. An increase in serum PTH concentration also occurs, owing to the hypocalcemic effect of the inhibition of bone resorption. Consequently, estrogen treatment results in greater urinary cyclic AMP and phosphate excretion and greater production of 1,25-$(OH)_2D$. The higher levels of this metabolite lead to greater intestinal calcium absorption and more positive calcium balance. These changes brought about by estrogen administration are beneficial for women at risk of developing osteoporosis and also for those with primary hyperparathyroidism who are unable to have surgical parathyroidectomy. Testosterone protects men from the development of osteoporosis, as evidenced by the occurrence of excessive bone loss in hypogonadal conditions such as Klinefelter's syndrome (see Chapter 8).

Glucocorticoids

At physiological levels, glucocorticoids are necessary for skeletal growth. When chronically present in excess, however, as in naturally occurring or iatrogenic Cushing's syndrome, these hormones have deleterious effects on nearly every target organ involved in calcium homeostasis. Glucocorticoids acutely decrease renal tubular calcium reabsorption, leading to hypercalciuria. More chronically, they interfere with intestinal calcium absorption, although it is not yet clear whether any alteration in vitamin D metabolism occurs. Because of the urinary calcium losses and reduced intestinal absorption of calcium, secondary hyperparathyroidism develops. Glucocorticoids also directly stimulate PTH secretion. Consequently, bone resorption is stimulated, but normal coupling does not occur because a major effect of glu-cocorticoids is to inhibit osteoblastic bone formation. Furthermore, glucocorti-coids suppress gonadal estrogen and testosterone production. This combination of events explains the rapidly progressive and severe nature of glucocorticoid-induced osteoporosis.

Thyroid Hormones

The thyroid hormones are extremely important for the development and growth of the skeleton in infancy and childhood. A major feature of hypothyroidism is retarded bone age, as indicated by delayed ossification of the cartilaginous bone growth cen-ters. In hyperthyroidism, both thyroxine and triiodothyronine in excess cause in-creased bone resorption. As excessive calcium enters the circulation from bone, PTH is suppressed and hypercalciuria results. Because serum PTH is suppressed and serum phosphate may be increased, levels of $1,25\text{-}(OH)_2D$ and intestinal calcium absorption are reduced. The enhanced bone resorption is of sufficient magnitude that 10%–20% of patients with thyrotoxicosis have increased serum calcium levels, although usually not to a degree sufficient to cause symptoms. Negative calcium balance induced by excessive thyroid hormone levels, either due to thyrotoxicosis or overreplacement with thyroid hormone, may cause osteoporosis.

Growth Hormone

Growth hormone (GH) affects a number of target organs involved in mineral home-ostasis. It has striking effects on bone growth by way of somatomedin C (or insulin-like growth factor [IGF]-I), a growth hormone-dependent peptide produced in the liver and bone that is mitogenic for chondrocytes and osteoblasts. Somatomedin C generation is required for normal skeletal growth in children. Laron dwarfs are re-sistant to GH (see Chapter 12) and are unable to produce sufficient somatomedin C levels. In adults, excess GH produces striking bony deformities (acromegaly), which are associated with accelerated bone formation and resorption, the former process predominating. In GH-deficient children, administration of GH not only stimulates bone growth via somatomedin C but also increases intestinal calcium absorption by a vitamin D–independent mechanism, and increases renal tubular phosphate reab-sorption. The latter effect appears to explain the high values for serum phosphorus noted in growing children and adults with active acromegaly.

LOCAL REGULATORS OF BONE REMODELING—EMERGING INSIGHTS INTO THE PATHOPHYSIOLOGY OF OSTEOPOROSIS

Bone is remodeled continuously during adulthood through the resorption of old bone by osteoclasts and the subsequent formation of new bone by osteoblasts. These two closely coupled events are responsible for renewing the skeleton while maintaining its anatomical and structural integrity. Under normal conditions, bone remodeling proceeds in cycles in which osteoclasts adhere to bone and subsequently remove it by acidification and proteolytic digestion. Shortly after the osteoclasts have left the resorption site, osteoblasts invade the area and begin the process of forming new bone by secreting osteoid (a matrix of collagen and other proteins), which is eventually mineralized. After bone formation has ceased, the surface of the bone is covered by lining cells, a distinct type of terminally differentiated osteoblasts. In adults, approximately 25% of trabecular bone is resorbed and replaced every year, as compared with only 3% of cortical bone, indicating that the rate of remodeling is controlled primarily by local factors.

In recent years, important advances have occurred in our understanding of the origin of osteoclasts and osteoblasts, the interplay between them, and the systemic and local factors that regulate their development. The process of remodeling and its intimate relationship to the bone marrow (the source of the stem cells for osteoclasts and osteoblasts) is shown in Figure 15-5. Osteoblasts originate from pluripotent mesenchymal stem cells of the bone marrow. Stromal cells with the potential to become osteoblasts, or to become fibroblasts, chondrocytes, adipocytes, or muscle cells as well, can be identified in marrow cell cultures as adherent colonies. The common progenitors that give rise to these colonies are termed *fibroblast colony-forming units* (CFU). Osteoclasts are derived from the hematopoietic granulocyte-macrophage CFU, which also give rise to monocytes and macrophages. Osteoclast progenitors

Fig. 15-5 The bone remodeling process and its relationship to bone marrow stem cells. Remodeling is accomplished by cycles involving the resorption of old bone by osteoclasts and the subsequent formation of new bone by osteoblasts. The osteoclasts and osteoblasts are replenished from their respective hematopoietic progenitors (granulocyte–macrophage colony-forming units [CFU-GM]) and mesenchymal progenitors (fibroblast colony-forming units [CFU-F]) in the bone marrow. (Adapted with permission from Manolagas SC and Jilka RL: Bone marrow, cytokines and bone remodeling: Emerging insights into the pathophysiology of osteoporosis. N Engl J Med 332:305–311, 1995. Copyright Massachusetts Medical Society. All rights reserved.)

move from bone marrow to bone either through the circulation or by direct migration from the marrow.

The effects of bone systemic hormones and locally produced factors that stimulate the development of osteoclasts are mediated by cells of the stromal–osteoblastic lineage. Figure 15-6 shows the pathways of differentiation of osteoclasts and osteoblasts, with the development of osteoclasts dependent on cells of the stromal–osteoblastic lineage. Interleukins (IL) are autocrine or paracrine mediators produced by hematopoietic and bone cells that permit communication between cells. IL-6, which stimulates the early stages of osteoclastogenesis, is produced by both stromal cells and osteoblastic cells in response to stimulation by systemic hormones such as PTH, PTH-related peptide, and 1,25-(OH)$_2$D, and also in response to bone-resorbing cytokines such as IL-1 and tumor necrosis factor (TNF). IL-6 has a pathogenetic role in the abnormal bone resorption associated with multiple myeloma, Paget's disease, rheumatoid arthritis, and Gorham-Stout disease (also known as van-

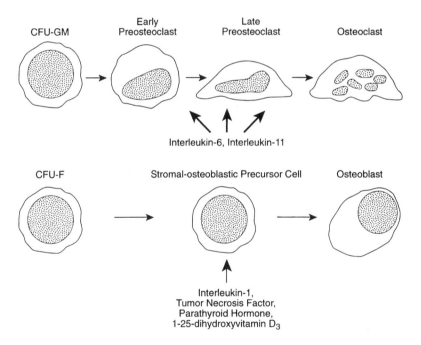

Fig. 15-6 Pathways of differentiation of osteoclasts and osteoblasts. Osteoclasts arise from granulocyte–macrophage CFU (CFU-GM), and osteoblasts from fibroblast CFU (CFU-F). The development of osteoclasts is controlled by stromal-osteoblastic cells that produce factors, including interleukin-6 and interleukin-11, that regulate the differentiation pathway of osteoclasts. Systemic hormones, such as parathyroid hormone and 1,25-dihydroxyvitamin D$_3$, and local factors, such as interleukin-1 and tumor necrosis factor, promote the development of osteoclasts through their ability to stimulate the production of cytokines such as interleukin-6 and interleukin-11. (Adapted with permission from Manolagas SC and Jilka RL: Bone marrow, cytokines and bone remodeling: Emerging insights into the pathophysiology of osteoporosis. N Engl J Med 332:305–311, 1995. Copyright Massachusetts Medical Society. All rights reserved).

ishing- or disappearing-bone disease)—four conditions characterized by excessive osteoclast development and focal osteolytic lesions.

Bone Remodeling and Osteoporosis

The hallmark of osteoporosis is a reduction in skeletal mass caused by an imbalance between bone resorption and bone formation. Loss of gonadal function and aging are the two most important factors contributing to the development of this condition. Starting around the fourth or fifth decade of life, both women and men lose bone at a rate of 0.13%–0.5% per year. For about 5 years after menopause (or after castration in men), the rate of bone loss increases as much as 10-fold. In humans, the loss of bone mass that follows the loss of ovarian function is associated with an increase in the rates of bone resorption and bone formation, with the former exceeding the latter, and an increase in the number of osteoclasts in trabecular bone.

Role of IL-6 in Stimulating Osteoclastic Bone Resorption in Gonadal Deficiency

Evidence has accumulated that IL-6 plays a role in osteopenia associated with loss of gonadal function. The production of IL-6 by cultured bone marrow stromal and osteoblastic cell lines is inhibited by estrogens or androgens. These sex steroids act through a specific receptor in the promoter region of the IL-6 gene and inhibit transcription. The loss of gonadal function in mice stimulates osteoclastogenesis *in vivo* through increased production of IL-6 in the marrow. Administration of estrogen or an IL-6-neutralizing antibody prevents the osteoclastogenesis in ovariectomized mice. Similarly, the secretion of IL-6 is increased in human bone marrow cells after menopause or the discontinuation of estrogen replacement therapy.

Although IL-6 is an essential mediator of bone loss associated with loss of gonadal function, it does not seem to play a role in the development of osteoclast precursors in the marrow or to influence the number of osteoclasts in trabecular bone in animals with sufficient sex steroids. Under physiologic conditions (i.e., the estrogen-replete state), it appears that the production of IL-6 is below a critical threshold of sensitivity for osteoclastogenesis. Therefore, it seems that other cytokines are responsible for the development of osteoclasts in the estrogen-replete state. For example, the osteoclastogenic effects of IL-11 are independent of estrogen status.

In addition, IL-1 may contribute to bone loss associated with the loss of ovarian function. The production of IL-1 is increased in bone marrow mononuclear cells from ovariectomized rats. Administering IL-1 receptor antagonist to these animals prevents the late but not the early stages of bone loss induced by the loss of ovarian function. Estrogens do not seem to regulate the IL-1 gene directly.

Senescence and Osteoblast Development in Marrow

Bone loss associated with aging has characteristics that are different from those of bone loss associated with the early years of gonadal deficiency. The amount of bone formed during each remodeling cycle decreases with age in both sexes, most likely because the supply of osteoblasts is reduced in proportion to the demand for them. The cause of the impaired ability of the marrow to produce osteoblasts with aging remains uncertain, but one possibility is a deficiency of bone growth factors that normally stimulate osteoblast formation.

Several growth factors have now been identified in either extracts of bone matrix or conditioned mediums of cultured bone and bone cells. Among these bone-derived growth factors, insulin-like growth factor (IGF-I) seems particularly likely to be an important physiologic regulator. The IGF-I present in the skeletal matrix may be derived from the systemic circulation (hepatic production under the influence of growth hormone) or it may be synthesized by a variety of cells present in bone, including osteoblasts (stimulated by growth hormone or parathyroid hormone). IGF-I has been shown to promote replication and differentiation of osteoblasts associated with increased production of osteocalcin and type I collagen (matrix proteins). It is now recognized that circulating concentrations of growth hormone decline with advancing age, and that this is accompanied by reduced levels of IGF-I in bone. Indeed, there is a 60% loss of human skeletal IGF-I between 20 and 60 years of age. Decreased IGF-I content in bone could have important relevance to the diminished osteoblast availability of aging and hence ↔o the pathogenesis of senile osteoporosis. Small clinical trials involving treatment with recombinant human growth hormone or IGF-I have been disappointing, but treatment with intermittent PTH injections has shown some promise.

Another important local regulator of bone formation that declines with age is *transforming growth factor-β* (TGF-β). TFG-β is synthesized by many tissues, but bone and platelets are the major sources of this polypeptide; TGF-β induces cartilage formation but also stimulates replication and differentiation of osteoblast progenitors. TGF-β inhibited osteoclast formation in marrow cultures. When bone is resorbed, TGF-β is released from the bone matrix, and may act as the critical "coupling factor" in turning off further osteoclastic resorption and switching on osteoblastic bone formation. It is noteworthy that estrogen and fluoride, two agents proven highly effective in the treatment of osteoporosis, have been shown to stimulate TGF-β production or to increase TGF-β receptors in osteoblast-like cells.

EFFECT OF DIET AND ACTIVITY ON BONE AND MINERAL METABOLISM

Diet

In addition to all of the factors delineated above, bone and mineral metabolism is importantly influenced by nutrition and activity. Important dietary factors include calcium, sodium, animal protein, and simple carbohydrates. Because of reduced renal production of $1,25\text{-}(OH)_2D$ and a deficiency of intestinal receptors for this metabolite, elderly women suffer from low calcium absorption and are subject to negative calcium balance, especially at low calcium intakes. The amount of calcium intake required to achieve zero calcium balance increases by approximately 500 mg/day to a total of 1500 mg/day with the onset of menopause, yet the estimated calcium intake of postmenopausal American women is only about 500 mg daily. Conflicting reports have appeared concerning the relationship between calcium intake and bone mass or occurrence of skeletal fractures, but in a widely quoted Yugoslavian study, the incidence of hip fracture was significantly higher in the region with low calcium intake than in a region with high calcium intake. Thus, prolonged adherence to a diet deficient in calcium may lead to secondary hyperparathyroidism and cortical bone loss.

An excessive intake of sodium may cause renal hypercalciuria by impairing renal calcium reabsorption, resulting in a compensatory increase of PTH secretion (Fig. 15-7). In young individuals and premenopausal women in whom the capacity for 1,25-(OH)$_2$D production is intact, stimulation of intestinal calcium absorption ensues from the sodium load consequent to PTH-dependent augmentation of 1,25-(OH)$_2$D synthesis. Thus, calcium balance is maintained. However, in postmenopausal women, the compensatory rise in intestinal calcium absorption does not develop following sodium-induced calciuria because of impaired 1,25-(OH)$_2$D synthesis (related to aging kidney or estrogen deficiency) and reduced intestinal vitamin D receptors. Therefore, postmenopausal women are at least theoretically at risk for bone loss from habitual high sodium intake.

Administration of animal proteins increases urinary calcium and causes negative calcium balance, without altering intestinal calcium absorption. These effects

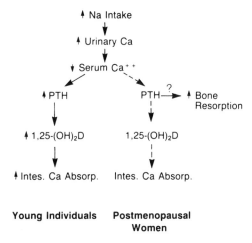

Fig. 15-7 Relationship of excessive dietary sodium intake to calcium homeostasis. In young individuals, there is an adaptive response to sodium-induced calciuresis. Stimulation of the parathyroid–vitamin D (PTH–1,25-(OH)$_2$D) axis from transient decrements in serum ionized calcium raises intestinal calcium absorption, thereby sustaining serum calcium concentration while permitting continued excessive urinary calcium excretion. Thus, in young individuals, the skeleton is protected but chronic hypercalciuria may pose a risk for nephrolithiasis. In elderly postmenopausal women, a sluggish response of the parathyroid–vitamin D axis prevents sufficient intestinal adaptation. Consequently, negative calcium balance and increased bone resorption would likely ensue in an effort to maintain normal serum ionized calcium concentration.

are probably attributable to the acid load from the sulfur-containing amino acids that would stimulate bone dissolution. An excessive ingestion of readily metabolizable refined sugar has been shown to acutely increase urinary calcium excretion by altering renal tubular calcium reabsorption. It is not known whether the calciuric response to carbohydrate ingestion elicits the same hormonal and metabolic changes that have been described for sodium-induced hypercalciuria.

Activity

The importance of activity is indicated by the fact that normal people at total bed rest show a preponderance of bone resorption over bone formation and quickly go into negative calcium balance. In individuals with increased bone turnover such as growing children or patients with Paget's disease, sudden immobilization from injury may cause hypercalciuria and even hypercalcemia, often within weeks of the accident. Apparently, normal bone cell function requires the pressures generated in bone by movement against gravity. During immobilization or the weightlessness of spaceflight, increased osteoclastic bone resorption is stimulated by an unknown mechanism. Moreover, there is reduced osteoblastic activity and less calcium enters bone from the circulation. Meticulous studies of patients paralyzed after spinal cord injury have shown that this abnormal bone turnover pattern leads to suppression of the PTH–vitamin D axis with an accompanying reduction in intestinal calcium absorption. Bone loss rapidly progresses and there is a further risk of kidney stone formation due to the ensuing hypercalciuria. In astronauts, calcium balance studies during Skylab flights demonstrated combined urinary and fecal calcium losses at a rate of 2.5% of total body calcium per month. Bone mineral loss and hypercalciuria are currently major impediments to long-term space travel.

In contrast, several studies have shown that regular weight-bearing exercise may have beneficial effects on the skeletal leading to increased bone density. A regular exercise program has been recommended for women hoping to prevent postmenopausal osteoporosis. However, if female joggers or ballet dancers exercise excessively to the point at which gonadotropin suppression and amenorrhea occur, bone density diminishes because of the overriding effect of estrogen deficiency. The relationship of immobilization and exercise to bone and calcium homeostasis is summarized in Figure 15-8.

INTEGRATED CONTROL OF CALCIUM HOMEOSTASIS

Under normal circumstances, the circulating concentration of ionized calcium is maintained within a narrow range by various homeostatic mechanisms. This integrated control is so precise that, in a normal individual, ionized serum calcium probably fluctuates by no more than 0.1 mg/dl in either direction from its normal set point throughout the day. Three types of homeostatic control mechanisms are involved in maintaining the serum calcium level: hormonal, physiological, and physicochemical.

Fig. 15-8 (*A*) Relationship of immobilization and exercise to calcium homeostasis. The scheme of "resorptive hypercalciuria" that occurs during immobilization has been well validated. Enhanced urinary calcium excretion following parathyroid (PTH) suppression, and the accompanying reduction in 1,25-(OH)₂D and intestinal calcium absorption are protective against development of hypercalcemia. At times, the amount of calcium entering the circulation is so great that these adaptive mechanisms are overwhelmed and hypercalcemia occurs. (*B*) The depiction of the sequence of events during exercise has also been largely confirmed. This scheme may account for the increased mineralization of bone that occurs during an exercise program.

Hormonal Regulation

The parathyroid glands are exquisitely sensitive to minor changes in serum ionized calcium. A decline in serum calcium stimulates secretion of PTH. The integrated actions of PTH on bone resorption, distal renal tubular calcium reabsorption, and 1,25-(OH)₂D-mediated intestinal calcium absorption are chiefly responsible for the precise regulation of serum ionized calcium in humans. The rapid mobilization of calcium from bone, requiring both PTH and 1,25-(OH)₂D, and the stimulation of distal tubular calcium reabsorption are the major control points in minute-to-minute serum calcium homeostasis. Adjustments in the rate of intestinal calcium absorption via the calcium–PTH–1,25-(OH)₂D axis require several days to be maximal. Another role of the increased PTH secretion in response to hypocalcemia is to decrease tubular phosphate reabsorption so that the increased amount of phosphate mobilized from bone and absorbed from the intestine along with calcium will be excreted into the urine. A decline in serum calcium also inhibits secretion of calcitonin and 24,25-(OH)₂D, which conceivably could help to restore serum calcium, although the physiological importance of the latter two metabolites in humans remains unclear. It is of interest that during a prolonged hypocalcemic challenge, the initial requirement for calcium mobilization from the skeleton is largely replaced by a more efficient absorption of calcium from the intestine. However, when severe intestinal malabsorption of calcium and vitamin D (e.g., steatorrhea) precludes intestinal adaptation, a marked secondary hyperparathyroidism develops to defend the serum calcium level at the expense of the skeleton.

A rise in serum calcium suppresses secretion of PTH and synthesis of 1,25-(OH)₂D, thereby returning serum calcium to normal as outlined in Figure 15-4. This system functions quite well in meeting routine mild hypercalcemic challenges such as the absorption of calcium following a dairy meal. A small rise in the serum ionized calcium (<0.1 mg/dl) is capable of suppressing parathyroid function by 30% or more. The main result of this suppression is a decrease in distal tubular calcium reabsorption, so that the postprandial increase in the filtered load of calcium is "spilled" into the urine. In more severe hypercalcemic challenges such as enhanced bone resorption due to osteolytic metastases, despite suppression of the PTH–1,25-$(OH)_2D$ axis, the quantity of mobilized calcium may overwhelm the renal capacity for calcium excretion (800 mg calcium/day) and result in hypercalcemia.

Physiological Regulation

As already noted, the kidney plays an important role in calcium homeostasis. This regulation is partly hormone independent because the renal excretion of calcium is a function of the filtered load of calcium, that is, increased serum calcium → increased filtered load → increased urinary calcium. Moreover, there is a calcium-sensing receptor in the renal tubule cells such that hypercalcemia leads to a reduced renal tubular reabsorption of calcium. It is this calcium sensor that is impaired in the inherited condition, *familial hypocalciuric hypercalcemia* (FHH), resulting in a sustained high renal calcium reabsorption despite the presence of hypercalcemia. (PTH levels are also inappropriately elevated in FHH because of a defective parathyroid calcium-sensing receptor).

Compensatory changes in intestinal calcium absorption occur in response to alterations in dietary calcium. Intestinal calcium absorption is most efficient at low calcium loads. As increasing amounts of calcium are ingested, the percentage of calcium absorbed declines. One may examine the amount of calcium appearing in the urine after an oral calcium load as an indirect measure of intestinal calcium absorption. A progressive increase occurs in urinary calcium excretion as oral calcium loads are increased incrementally from 100 to 500 mg, but beyond 500 mg, there is little further change in urinary calcium excretion. It is thus more advantageous to provide calcium supplements as 500 mg four times daily than to provide 2000 mg of calcium all at once. In addition to the intrinsic ability of the intestine to absorb calcium less efficiently at higher calcium loads, a sustained higher calcium intake would also suppress the PTH-1,25-$(OH)_2D$ axis and thereby reduce calcium absorption.

Physicochemical Regulation

It has been hypothesized that serum concentrations of ionized calcium and phosphate reflect the solubility of the bone mineral. This assumes that circulating concentrations of ionized calcium and phosphate are maintained at a constant product, representing saturation with respect to a particular phase of calcium phosphate in bone. This hypothesis could explain the decline in serum calcium that accompanies a rise in serum phosphate. Unfortunately, various physiocochemical studies have failed to identify the particular phase of calcium phosphate with which serum calcium and phosphate might be in steady state. Nevertheless, when the Ca × P product exceeds 60 (in mg/dl), soft tissue deposition of calcium salts is likely to occur.

LOSS OF CALCIUM HOMEOSTATIC CONTROL: HYPERCALCEMIA

Hypercalcemia may occur when there is a loss of calcium homeostatic control. For it to develop, there must first be a sufficient, unabated input of calcium into the circulation, as might occur from a continued excessive rate of bone resorption or of intestinal calcium absorption. Second, the extent of the influx of calcium into the circulation must exceed the capacity of the kidneys to remove the calcium load. These conditions are met in two fairly common disorders: primary hyperparathyroidism and hypercalcemia of malignancy. Together, these two disorders account for over 90% of the hypercalcemia that is clinically encountered.

PRIMARY HYPERPARATHYROIDISM

In primary hyperparathyroidism, calcium homeostatic control is lost as a result of excessive PTH secretion. Thus, PTH is secreted by adenomatous or hyperplastic parathyroid tissue in amounts that are inappropriately high for the level of circulating calcium. Hypercalcemia develops from the combined effects of PTH-induced stimulation of bone resorption, intestinal calcium absorption, and renal tubular reabsorption of calcium. Hypercalciuria also often occurs because even though PTH augments renal tubular reabsorption of calcium, this action of the hormone is usually insufficient to overcome the increased renal filtered load of calcium.

The major symptoms of primary hyperparathyroidism may be ascribed to the PTH-induced resorption of bone, hypercalciuria, and hypercalcemia. These abnormalities are in turn pathophysiologically related to the bihormonal defect, that is, an excessive production of both PTH and 1,25-$(OH)_2$D.

The classical bone disease of hyperparathyroidism is *osteitis fibrosa cystica.* This disorder is characterized by bone pain, pathological fractures of long bones, and compression fractures of the spine. Radiologically, the bones appear demineralized and may reveal a frayed erosion of the outer and inner cortical surfaces. These cortical erosions are referred to as *subperiosteal resorption* and are best demonstrated on the radial aspect of the middle phalanges and in the distal clavicles. Locally, destructive lesions known as *brown tumors* may appear as well-demarcated lucent areas. These brown tumors or bone cysts are composed largely of osteoclasts, intermixed with poorly mineralized woven bone. Histologically, extensive fibrosis replaces normal marrow and bone cell elements. The pathogenesis of osteitis fibrosa cystica is believed to be related to overstimulation of osteoclastic bone resorption by very high PTH levels. Increased 1,25-$(OH)_2$D levels may also activate bone remodeling. Osteitis fibrosa cystica appears to be a complication of severe and rapidly progressive hyperparathyroidism associated with large parathyroid adenomas or carcinomas. Following successful parathyroidectomy, the subperiosteal resorption, brown tumors, and marrow fibrosis all resolve. Hyperparathyroidism tends to affect the cortical bone more than trabecular bone. In mild, asymptomatic primary hyperparathyroidism, the spine is often spared.

Up to one-third of patients present with nephrolithiasis. They may form pure calcium phosphate stones, calcium oxalate stones, or mixed calcium stones. Hypercalciuria is an important factor in the pathogenesis of renal stone disease.

Hypercalciuria probably contributes to stone formation by rendering urine supersaturated with respect to calcium phosphate and calcium oxalate. Patients with hyperparathyroidism who form kidney stones frequently have a pronounced hypercalciuria, but only a modestly elevated serum calcium level. Some investigators have found that the hyperparathyroid patients with marked elevations in serum 1,25-$(OH)_2D$, intestinal hyperabsorption of calcium, and resulting hypercalciuria are the most prone to stone disease. The greater intestinal absorption of calcium with associated parathyroid suppression could explain the tendency for smaller parathyroid glands and disproportionate hypercalciuria in these patients. It remains unclear why certain patients with hyperparathyroidism have near-normal circulating levels of 1,25-$(OH)_2D$, whereas in others the concentration of this active metabolite is markedly elevated. Moreover, hypercalciuria is not the only factor in stone formation; some patients do not form stones despite hypercalciuria and supersaturation of the urine with respect to calcium salts. Perhaps the stone formers have an excess of as yet unidentified promoters or a deficiency of inhibitors of stone formation. In any case, nephrolithiasis generally ceases following successful parathyroidectomy.

Hypercalcemia may account for many of the other symptoms of primary hyperparathyroidism. Hypercalcemia is known to cause CNS depression, mental aberrations, fatiguability and weakness, as well as constipation and anorexia. Hypercalcemia may also play a role in the development of peptic ulceration in hyperparathyroidism as it is associated with hypersecretion of gastrin and hydrochloric acid. Moreover, hypercalcemia may cause polyuria by impairing vasopressin-mediated renal concentrating ability. The fact that an increased calcium concentration inhibits the renal tubule's ability to conserve water may lead to a vicious spiral of dehydration, prerenal azotemia, and worsening hypercalcemia.

Bone disease, nephrolithiasis, and peptic ulcer disease constitute a clinical triad that should alert the physician to the possibility of primary hyperparathyroidism. When one or more of the triad is present in patients with hypercalcemia, a vigorous search for evidence supporting this diagnosis should be conducted. The hypercalcemia may be asymptomatic, or associated with mental aberrations, anorexia, constipation, or polyuria. A dramatic change in the usual clinical presentation of hyperparathyroidism has occurred since the introduction of automated clinical chemistry techniques to measure serum calcium. Over half the patients now present with asymptomatic hypercalcemia, perhaps reflecting an earlier or milder form of the disease. Biochemically, the diagnosis may be made from determinations of serum calcium, phosphate and PTH.

Hypercalcemia of Malignancy

The underlying cause of hypercalcemia is generally excessive bone resorption. Three major pathogenetic mechanisms have been recognized: (1) local osteolytic hypercalcemia, (2) humoral hypercalcemia of malignancy (HHM), and (3) 1,25-$(OH)_2D$ synthesis by lymphomas. Each of these mechanisms will be briefly discussed.

Typically, patients with local osteolytic hypercalcemia (LOH) have extensive skeletal involvement with either breast cancer, multiple myeloma, or lymphoma. LOH accounts for about 20% of all hypercalcemia of malignancy. Hypercalcemia results largely from osteoclastic bone resorption, which is mediated by osteoclast-activating factors (IL-I, TNF) secreted by malignant cells. The mediator in breast cancer is not clear, but it may be one of the above cytokines, prostaglandin E_2, or other unknown factors. There is also evidence for direct resorption of the skeleton by mononuclear cells and by breast cancer cells. Biochemically, patients with LOH display reductions in circulating PTH and urinary cyclic AMP levels. Urinary calcium excretion is usually markedly increased, reflecting the increased filtered load of calcium together with parathyroid suppression. The serum 1,25-$(OH)_2D$ concentration and, therefore, intestinal calcium absorption are also reduced as a consequence of parathyroid suppression.

The term *humoral hypercalcemia of malignancy* (HHM) can be used generically to describe malignancy-associated hypercalcemia that occurs in the absence of skeletal metastases and results from the secretion by the neoplasm of a circulating, bone-resorbing, calcemic factor. Typical tumors where this occurs would include squamous cell carcinoma of the lung and renal carcinoma. A few cases have been reported of true native PTH production by ovarian carcinoma or small cell carcinoma of the lung. However, HHM generally refers to patients in whom hypercalcemia results from the overexpression of a novel class of peptide hormones, PTH-related protein (PTHrP). Explosive growth has occurred in the understanding of the pathogenesis of this syndrome in recent years.

The existence of PTHrP was first suspected clinically because cancer patients were evaluated and found to have hypercalcemia, hypophosphatemia, and elevated urinary cyclic AMP excretion, in the absence of immunologically detectable PTH. Moreover, the tumors causing the hypercalcemia did not contain mRNA encoding PTH. The patients with HHM also differed from patients with primary hyperparathyroidism in that they had reduced serum 1,25-$(OH)_2D$ concentration and uncoupling between exaggerated osteoclastic bone resorption and reduced osteoblastic bone formation.

Meanwhile, in the laboratory, the PTHrP obtained from tumor extracts was isolated and purified based on its ability to stimulate cyclic AMP production in canine renal cortical cells or rat osteosarcoma cells. The next step was the partial sequencing of the purified peptide from carcinomas of the lung, breast, and kidney, which provided uniform results. This permitted the synthesis of oligonucleotide probes for use in screening HHM tumor-derived complementary DNA libraries. Full-length PTHrP complementary DNAs were isolated and found to encode products that were approximately twice the size of native PTH (Fig. 15-9). Actually, three forms of PTHrP were detected, one of 139, one of 141, and one of 173 amino acids in length (compared to PTH which has 84 amino acids). One of the most striking features was that each of these tumor-derived peptides displayed marked homology with PTH through the first 13 amino acids (8 of the first 13 amino acid residues were identical). This structural homology to PTH allowed the PTHrP to attach to and activate the PTH receptor. However, beyond amino acid 13, the sequences of the two classes of peptides were completely different.

The availability of the complete PTHrP sequence from the complementary DNAs permitted the chemical synthesis and recombinant expression of a variety of PTHrPs for use in biologic and immunologic studies. Studies using these peptides have shown that they reproduce the full spectrum of PTH-like bioactivities, including the stimulation of adenylyl cyclase in renal membranes and bone cells, the stim-

Fig. 15-9 Comparison of the structures of native human parathyroid hormone (PTH) with that of PTH-related protein (1 to 141), the first of the PTH-related protein complementary DNAs to be identified. The heavy portions of the two lines indicate the binding domain of parathyroid hormone (amino acids 25 to 27) and the putative receptor-binding domain of PTH-related protein at amino acids 19 to 21. Note the homology between PTH and PTH-related protein in the −2 to +13 region. Positions −1 and −2 are identical in both peptides and represent the proteolytic cleavage site between the N-terminal of the mature peptide and their "*pro*" sequences. Homology in the −2 to +13 region is equally striking at the nucleotide level. (Reproduced with permission from Stewart AF, and Broadus AE: In: *Advances in Endocrinology and Metabolism,* Vol. 1, EL Mazzaferri, RS Bar, and RA Kreisberg, eds., Mosby, St. Louis, pp. 1–21, 1990.)

ulation of bone resorption *in vitro* and the production of hypercalcemia *in vivo*, the stimulation of renal 1α-hydroxylase activity, and the stimulation of renal tubular calcium reabsorption.

The evidence that PTHrPs are indeed the factors responsible for the clinical and biochemical manifestation of HHM is compelling. The peptides are present only in HHM-associated tumors and not in control tumors. In one elegant study, immunodeficient mice implanted subcutaneously with human HHM-associated tumors developed localized neoplasms associated with hypercalcemia, hypophosphatemia, and elevated urinary cyclic AMP excretion. Infusion of the mice with PTHrP antisera, but not control serum, reversed the hypercalcemia as well as the other manifestations of the HHM syndrome. Radioimmunoassays for PTHrP have been developed, and elevated circulating PTHrP concentrations have been found in the vast majority of patients with HHM. This mechanism is believed to account for at least 80% of the hypercalcemia of malignancy.

Another mechanism for hypercalcemia of malignancy that has been validated is 1,25-$(OH)_2$D synthesis by certain lymphomas. Whereas some lymphomas produce hypercalcemia through the local osteolytic mechanism described above, hypercalcemia has been reported in at least a dozen patients with a variety of histologic types of lymphoma in whom skeletal involvement was either absent or negligible. In these patients, circulating 1,25-$(OH)_2$D concentrations were markedly elevated, but were normalized with either glucocorticoid therapy, surgical tumor resection, or chemotherapy, suggesting that the lymphomas were the source of the 1,25-$(OH)_2D$. The overproduction of 1,25-$(OH)_2D$ in these patients is analogous to the overproduction of 1,25-$(OH)_2D$ that occurs in patients with granulomatous disorders (e.g., sarcoidosis and tuberculosis). It is believed to represent dysregulated production of 1,25-$(OH)_2D$ by macrophages or lymphocytes within the lymphomatous tissue. Hypercalemia in these patients results from 1,25-$(OH)_2D$-induced intestinal hyperabsorption of calcium in addition to accelerated bone resorption. Biochemically, patients are characterized by hypercalcemia together with suppression of circulating PTH and urinary cyclic AMP levels. Circulating 1,25-$(OH)_2D$ values are elevated.

Other Causes of Hypercalcemia

Although primary hyperparathyroidism and hypercalcemia of malignancy are the most commonly encountered forms of hypercalcemia, the clinician must keep in mind other potential causes of hypercalcemia. A detailed discussion of these disorders is beyond the scope of this chapter, but a useful classification scheme is presented in Table 15-1. It is helpful to divide the various causes of hypercalcemia into those related primarily to increased calcium *input into* the circulation and those related to decreased calcium *removal from* the circulation.

Table 15-1 Classification Scheme for Hypercalcemias

Increased calcium input into circulation
  High bone resorption
    Primary hyperparathyroidism
    Neoplasms
    Thyrotoxicosis
    Vitamin D toxicity
    Sarcoidosis and other granulomatous disorders
    Immobilization

  High intestinal calcium absorption
    Primary hyperparathyroidism
    Vitamin D toxicity
    Sarcoidosis and other granulomatous disorders
    Milk-alkali syndrome
    Phosphorus depletion syndrome

Reduced calcium removal from circulation
  Reduced renal calcium excretion
    Primary hyperparathyroidism
    Familial hypocalciuric hypercalcemia
    Extracellular volume depletion
    Thiazide therapy
    Milk-alkali syndrome

  Reduced bone formation
    Immobilization
    Phosphorus depletion syndrome

LOSS OF CALCIUM HOMEOSTATIC CONTROL: HYPOCALCEMIA

Hypocalcemia occurs when there is an inadequate response of the parathyroid–vitamin D axis to a hypocalcemic stimulus, when there is target organ resistance to the major calcium-regulating hormones, or when excessive phosphate accumulates in the circulation. Various disorders may cause hypocalcemia (Table 15-2). In narrowing down the possibilities, a useful initial step is to consider whether the serum phosphate is increased or decreased.

The cause of hypocalcemia is often multifactorial. In renal failure, for example, hypocalcemia occurs because of phosphate retention and inadequate production of 1,25-$(OH)_2D$ by the damaged kidney. The low 1,25-$(OH)_2D$ level reduces intestinal calcium absorption and impairs the mobilization of calcium from bone. In another condition, severe hypomagnesemia, there is reduced PTH secretion as well as resistance of bone and kidney to the actions of PTH. In endocrinology, the classic cause of hypocalcemia is hypoparathyroidism.

HYPOPARATHYROIDISM

The diagnosis of hypoparathyroidism must be considered when hypocalcemia and hyperphosphatemia occur in the presence of normal serum creatinine and magnesium concentrations, and in the absence of a source of massive phosphate leakage into the circulation. Hypoparathyroidism is a bihormonal disease in which the abnormalities in serum chemistry are the sequelae of reduced PTH action and 1,25-$(OH)_2D$ deficiency. Hypocalcemia is invariably found in hypoparathyroidism; it is the result of (1) reduced PTH-dependent osteoclastic resorption, (2) decreased osteocytic calcium transfer (rapid bone calcium mobilization) consequent to 1,25-$(OH)_2D$ deficiency and reduced PTH action, (3) low renal tubular reabsorption of calcium from reduced PTH action, and (4) impaired intestinal calcium absorption from 1,25-$(OH)_2D$ deficiency. Hyperphosphatemia results primarily from the impaired renal phosphate clearance consequent to reduced PTH action. The retained

Table 15-2 Classification of Causes of Hypocalcemia Based on Serum Phosphate Level

Low calcium, high phosphate
Renal insufficiency
Hypomagnesemia
Excessive phosphate intake
Massive cell destruction (e.g., chemotherapy rhabdomyolysis)
Hypoparathyroidism
Low calcium, low phosphate
Vitamin D deficiency
Abnormal vitamin D metabolism
Vitamin D resistance
Acute pancreatitis

buildup of phosphate in the serum lowers the serum calcium by physicochemical means and by further reducing synthesis of 1,25-(OH)$_2$D.

Most of the symptoms of hypoparathyroidism may be ascribed to the abnormal levels of calcium and phosphate in the blood. Hypocalcemia is responsible for the increased neuromuscular irritability that may produce carpopedal spasm, prickling sensations in the lips, fingers, and toes, and occasionally muscle cramps. If the serum calcium decreases to very low levels, laryngospasm or seizures may occur. Latent tetany may be revealed by Chvostek's or Trousseau's sign (carpal spasm developing within 3 minutes of inflating the blood pressure cuff above the systolic level). The hyperphosphatemia may result in soft tissue calcifications. Basal ganglia calcification is not uncommon in hypoparathyroidism, and, if extensive, may lead to disturbances of the extrapyramidal motor system such as Parkinsonism or chorea. Other disorders that may accompany chronic hypocalcemia include cataracts, congestive heart failure, and mental impairment.

Within recent years, the development of assays for PTH, 1,25-(OH)$_2$D, urinary cyclic AMP, and components of the adenylyl cyclase enzyme system has permitted the separation of hypoparathyroidism into several distinct types. Table 15-3 represents a current classification scheme for the various forms of hypoparathyroidism. Each type has a unique pathogenetic basis, a discussion of which should nicely illustrate the variety of ways the calcium homeostatic system may be deranged.

PTH-Deficient Hypoparathyroidism

This condition is characterized by a reduced or absent synthesis of PTH; the target tissues are responsive to the action of PTH. Thus, the serum concentration of PTH is low or undetectable and the basal urinary cyclic AMP level is low. When challenged by exogenous PTH, PTH-dependent adenylyl cyclase in bone and kidney is stimulated, as shown by a marked increase in the renal excretion of cyclic AMP and phosphate. The circulating concentration of 1,25-(OH)$_2$D is low, accounting for the subnormal intestinal calcium absorption. During exogenous PTH challenge, there is a rapid rise in serum calcium ("calcemic response") attributed to the combined action of PTH and newly synthesized 1,25-(OH)$_2$D.

The most common cause of PTH-deficient hypoparathyroidism is the inadvertent removal of excessive parathyroid tissue during thyroid or parathyroid surgery. A rarer condition is idiopathic hypoparathyroidism, which results from absence, fatty

Table 15-3 Classification of Hypoparathyroidism

PTH-deficient hypoparathyroidism
Postoperative
Idiopathic
PTH ineffective hypoparathyroidism
PTH-resistant (pseudo)hypoparathyroidism
Type Ia
Type Ib
Type Ic
Type II

replacement, or atrophy of the parathyroid glands. This condition may be inherited in families, or it may occur sporadically. In either case, it may occur in combination with pernicious anemia, Addison's disease (see Chapter 14), Hashimoto's thyroiditis (see Chapter 13), gonadal failure, and mucocutaneous candidiasis. The finding of circulating antibodies against parathyroid, thyroid, and other tissues has strengthened the suspicion that idiopathic hypoparathyroidism may be an autoimmune disease. Recently, a familial form of hypoparathyroidism has been attributed to an activating mutation in the calcium-sensing receptor gene. In affected patients, serum PTH levels are suppressed by lower than normal serum calcium levels.

PTH-Ineffective Hypoparathyroidism

This very rare condition is characterized by synthesis of PTH that is biologically inactive; the target tissues are responsive to the action of exogenous PTH. Typically, a patient presents with hypocalcemia, hyperphosphatemia, and normal renal function, but increased serum PTH. Infusion of exogenous PTH elicits normal cyclic AMP and phosphaturic responses.

PTH-Resistant Hypoparathyroidism (Pseudohypoparathyroidism)

Pseudohypoparathyroidism was first described by Albright as a disease characterized by the biochemical signs of hypoparathyroidism, hypocalcemia, and hyperphosphatemia, resulting from PTH resistance rather than PTH deficiency. Indeed, these patients have large parathyroid glands and very high circulating levels of PTH. In almost all patients, urinary cyclic AMP excretion after PTH infusion is significantly reduced, implicating a defect in the hormone receptor–adenylyl cyclase complex (pseudohypoparathyroidism, type I). As a consequence of the inability to generate cyclic AMP in the renal tubule, phosphate excretion and the production of $1,25\text{-}(OH)_2D$ are impaired. Therefore, intestinal calcium absorption is reduced and the rapid mobilization of calcium from bone in response to administered PTH is subnormal. Osteoclastic bone resorption responds to the high circulating PTH levels, however. Thus, in contrast to PTH-deficient hypoparathyroidism, bone density is usually diminished and hydroxyproline excretion is increased. Some patients with pseudohypoparathyroidism actually develop frank osteitis fibrosa cystica.

It is now known that peptide hormone receptors are coupled to adenylyl cyclase by guanine nucleotide-binding proteins (G proteins; see Fig. 15-10 and Chapter 3). Patients with pseudohypoparathyroidism type Ia have reduced activity of the stimulatory G protein (G_s) associated with adenylyl cyclase. As a consequence of this generalized G_s deficiency, patients are resistant not only to PTH, but also to many other peptide hormones including TSH, glucagon, and gonadotropins. Clinical hypothyroidism and gonadal dysfunction are quite common in these patients. Deficient G_s activity is presumed to limit cyclic AMP production and thereby cause resistance to multiple hormones in pseudohypoparathyroidism type Ia. Patients also tend to have a characteristic physical appearance that has come to be known as *Albright's hereditary osteodystrophy.* It consists of a short, stocky stature, round face, short neck, and short fingers and toes, most often affecting the fourth digits due to short fourth metacarpals and metatarsals.

Fig. 15-10 The adenylyl cyclase–cyclic AMP system. H_s and H_i, stimulatory and inhibitory agents, respectively; R_s and R_i, stimulatory and inhibitory receptors; G_s and G_i, stimulatory and inhibitory guanine nucleotide-binding proteins; C, the catalytic unit of adenylyl cyclase; PDE, phosphodiesterase; cAMP, cyclic AMP. Hormones act by facilitating exchange of guanine nucleotides at a binding site on the regulatory G protein. Formation of a ternary complex consisting of hormone, receptor, and G protein allows GTP to exchange for GDP. The GTP-bound G protein in turn interacts with the catalytic unit of adenylyl cyclase. Most peptide hormones including PTH stimulate G_s resulting in cyclic AMP generation. The cyclic AMP acts as the second messenger to carry out the physiological effect of the hormone. The message is ended when cyclic AMP is broken down by phosphodiesterase. (Modified from Spiegel AM, Gierschik P, Levine MA, and Downs RW Jr: N Engl J Med 312:26–33, 1985.)

In contrast, subjects with pseudohypoparathyroidism type Ib have a normal appearance, normal G_s activity, and, in most instances, resistance to PTH alone. The pathogenesis of pseudohypoparathyroidism Ib is unknown, but as resistance is limited to PTH, it has been suggested that a defect in the PTH receptor could be involved. This concept has been supported by the observation that skin fibroblasts from many, but not all, subjects with pseudohypoparathyroidism Ib have selective resistance to PTH in terms of cyclic AMP response. Recently, pseudohypoparathyroidism type Ic has been recognized. These patients have Albright's hereditary osteodystrophy and multiple hormone resistance, but unlike pseudohypoparathyroidism type Ia, they have normal G_s levels. The defect appears to reside in an abnormal adenylyl cyclase catalytic subunit.

The type II form of pseudohypoparathyroidism is extremely rare. This type of patient presents with hypocalcemia, hyperphosphatemia, and increased serum PTH concentration. Exogenous PTH causes a marked rise in urinary cyclic AMP without provoking a phosphaturic response. In type II pseudohypoparathyroidism, the defect is thought to be distal to cyclic AMP generation, perhaps at the level of the protein kinase. It is also possible that a defect exist in a more distal site, for example, a substrate for the protein kinase, such as a phosphate transport protein in the renal tubular luminal brush border.

SUGGESTED READING

Bell NH: Vitamin D–endocrine system. J Clin Invest 76:1–6, 1985.

Breslau NA, McGuire J, Zerwekh JE, Frenkel E, and Pak CYC: Hypercalcemia associated with increased serum 1,25-dihydroxyvitamin D in three patients with lymphoma. Ann Intern Med 100:1–7, 1984.

Breslau NA: Pseudohypoparathyroidism: Current concepts. Am J Med Sci 298:130–140, 1989.

Breslau NA: Calcium, estrogen and progestin in the treatment of osteoporosis. In: *Rheumatic Disease Clinics of North America,* N Lane, eds., Saunders, Philadelphia, pp. 691–716, 1994.

Breslau NA, and Zerwekh JE: Pharmacology of vitamin D preparations. In: *Vitamin D,* D Feldman, F Glorieux, and W Pike, eds., Academic Press, San Diego, pp. 607–618, 1997.

Brown EM, Pollak M, and Hebert SC: Physiology and cell biology update: Sensing of extracellular Ca^{2+} by parathyroid and kidney cells: Cloning and characterization of an extracellular Ca^{2+}-sensing receptor. Am J Kidney Dis 25:506–513, 1995.

Heller HJ, and Breslau NA: Clinical evaluation of parathyroid tumors. In: *Comprehensive Management of Head and Neck Tumors,* 2nd ed., SE Thawley, WR Panje, JG Batsakis, and RD Lindberg, eds., Saunders, Philadelphia, pp. 1752–1774, 1999.

Kronenberg HM: Parathyroid hormone: Mechanism of action. In: *Primer on the Metabolic Bone Diseases and Disorders of Mineral Metabolism,* 3rd ed., MJ Favus, ed., Lippincott-Raven, Philadelphia, pp. 68–70, 1996.

Manolagas SC, and Jilka RL: Bone marrow, cytokines and bone remodeling: Emerging insights into the pathophysiology of osteoporosis. N Engl J Med 332:305–311, 1995.

Naveh-Many T, and Silver J: Regulation of parathyroid hormone gene expression by hypocalcemia, hypercalcemia and vitamin D in the rat. J Clin Invest 86:1313–1319, 1990.

Nicolas V, Prewett A, Bettica P, Mohan S, Finkelman RD, Baylink DJ, and Farley JR: Age-related decreases in IGF-I and TGF-β in femoral cortical bone from both men and women: Implications for bone loss with aging. J Clin Endocrinol Metab 78:1011–1016, 1994.

Pollak M, Brown EM, Chou Y-HC, Herbert SC, Marx SJ, Steinman B, Levi T, Seidman CE, and Seidman JG: Mutations in the human Ca^{2+}-sensing receptor gene cause familial hypocalciuric hypercalcemia and neonatal severe hyperparathyroidism. Cell 75:1297–1303, 1993.

Pollak MR, Brown EM, Estep HL, McLaine PN, Kilfor U, Park J, Hebert SC, Seidman CE, and Seidman JG: Autosomal dominant hypocalcemia caused by a Ca^{2+}-sensing receptor gene mutation. Nat Genet 8:303–307, 1994.

Silverberg SJ, Gartenberg F, Jacobs TP, Shane E, Siris E, Staron RB, and Bilezikian JP: Longitudinal measurements of bone density and biochemical indices in untreated primary hyperparathyroidism. J Clin Endocrinol Metab 80:723–728, 1995.

Silverberg SJ, Gartenberg F, Jacobs TP, Shane E, Siris E, Staron RB, McMahon DJ, and Bilezikian JP: Increased bone mineral density after parathyroidectomy in primary hyperparathyroidism. J Clin Endocrinol Metab 80:729–734, 1995.

Spiegel AM, Gierschik P, Levine MA, and Downs RW Jr: Clinical implications of guanine nucleotide-binding proteins as receptor-effector couplers. N Engl J Med 312:26–33, 1985.

Stewart AF, Adler M, Byers CM, Segre GV, and Broadus AE: Calcium homeostasis in im-
    mobilization: An example of resorptive hypercalcuria. N Engl J Med 306:1136–1140,
    1982.
Stewart AF, and Broadus AE: Humoral hypercalcemia of malignancy. In: *Advances in En-
    docrinology and Metabolism,* Vol. 1, EL Mazzaferri, RS Bar, and RA Kreisberg, eds.,
    Mosby, St. Louis, MO, pp. 1–21, 1990.

16

Glucose, Lipid, and Protein Metabolism

DANIEL W. FOSTER
J. DENIS McGARRY

The maintenance of life requires a constant supply of fuels for body tissues. These fuels are used to generate energy and preserve organ structure. The process is in principle quite simple. Energy is derived when ingested food is oxidized to carbon dioxide and water in the presence of oxygen, generating adenosine triphosphate (ATP). A portion of the ingested foodstuff is also utilized, either directly or after transformation into other substrates, to replace cell membranes and organelles that turn over naturally during the process of living. The remainder is stored as potential energy in the form of glycogen or fat. Under normal circumstances, each individual remains in a near steady state with weight and appearance stable over prolonged periods. Despite the outward evidence of stability, however, fuel metabolism changes dramatically several times a day, particularly during the overnight fast. Two distinct phases, anabolic and catabolic, alternate one with the other. The *anabolic* phase begins with food ingestion and lasts for several hours. It is in this period, when caloric intake ordinarily exceeds caloric demands, that energy storage occurs. The *catabolic* phase usually begins 4–6 hours after the last food intake and lasts until the person eats once again. During this phase the body shifts from exogenous to endogenous fuels, a change heralded by the mobilization of substrate from storage sites in liver, muscle and adipose tissue. This endogenous substrate sustains the organism between meals.

Both anabolic and catabolic phases exhibit characteristic biochemical processes (Fig. 16-1). In the anabolic phase glycogen synthesis occurs in liver and muscle. Fatty acid synthesis and triglyceride formation are stimulated in hepatocytes and adipose tissue, and protein synthesis is initiated. Flux of substrate is from intestine through the liver to storage and utilization sites. After a mixed meal, glucose, triglyceride, and amino acid concentrations increase in plasma, whereas free fatty acids, ketones (acetoacetic and β-hydroxybutyric acids), and glycerol decrease. In the catabolic phase the biochemical activities are reversed. Glycogen breaks down, glycolysis is impaired, gluconeogenesis is activated (first in liver and then in kidney), lipogenesis and triglyceride formation cease, and lipolysis in the adipocyte increases manyfold. Free fatty acid oxidation is enhanced in most tissues, and ketone body formation is initiated in the liver. Finally, proteolysis is activated in muscle to sup-

State	Hormones	Fuel Source	Process
Anabolism	↑ Insulin ↓ Glucagon	Diet	Glycogen Synthesis Triglyceride Synthesis Protein Synthesis
Catabolism	↓ Insulin ↑ Glucagon	Storage Depots	Glycogenolysis Lipolysis Proteolysis Ketogenesis

Fig. 16-1 Fuel metabolism in anabolic and catabolic phases.

ply amino acids as substrate for gluconeogenesis. Flux of fuel is from storage depots to liver and other utilization sites. Glucose and triglyceride levels in plasma decrease, whereas certain amino acids, long-chain fatty acids, acetoacetate, and β-hydroxybutyrate increase.

When food is readily available (and the diet is not nutritionally unbalanced), the only risk of the anabolic phase in the normal individual is that it may be entered too frequently or maintained too long so that obesity results. Ingestion of food in certain inborn errors of metabolism such as fructose intolerance or intestinal lactase deficiency can cause symptoms, but these anabolic-phase diseases are rare. In contrast, the absence of food is potentially dangerous, for without major adaptations death or permanent brain injury may occur fairly rapidly because of a fall in plasma glucose concentrations to levels too low to sustain function in the central nervous system. Indeed, it can be stated that the primary aim of the acute metabolic changes accompanying the catabolic state is the prevention of hypoglycemia. Two changes are required to maintain plasma glucose within the normal range in the absence of food (Fig. 16-2).

First, the liver must be converted to an organ of glucose production. This is accomplished initially by glycogen breakdown, but subsequently new glucose production occurs via gluconeogenesis, a process in which amino acids, lactate, pyruvate, and glycerol are converted to glucose by a linked series of enzymatic reactions. The second major change is the conversion of tissues other than the central nervous system to a lipid economy. Most organs utilize long-chain free fatty acids (FFA) directly (adipose tissue → FFA → utilization sites), but a one-fourth to one-third of the total fatty acids are taken up by the liver for conversion to ketone bodies (adipose tissue → FFA → liver → ketones → utilization sites). In contrast to long-chain fatty acids, the ketones can be efficiently oxidized by the central nervous system and, thus, can be considered a backup substrate to glucose; that is, in the presence of ketone bodies at concentrations usually found after several days of fasting, the brain can function normally despite levels of glucose low enough to cause loss of consciousness or convulsions in the absence of ketones. Because ketogenesis is not activated immediately by the absence of food, this protective mechanism is not available in the first few hours of a fast. Acetoacetic and β-hydroxybutyric acids are also readily utilizable by all other nonhepatic tissues. The liver, by contrast, has only a minimal capacity to oxidize ketones. The shift to lipid metabolism is critical to survival in a prolonged fast because the liver, even at maximal glucose production, can-

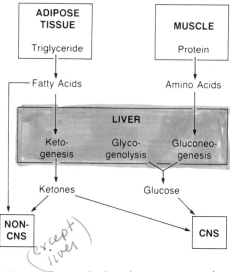

Fig. 16-2 The catabolic sequence. The liver becomes a net glucose producer first via glycogen breakdown and subsequently by gluconeogenesis. Glucose is preserved for use by the central nervous system (CNS) because other tissues (non-CNS) preferentially utilize long-chain fatty acids and their derivative products, the ketone bodies. Ketones can also be used by the brain. Glycerol (released by triglyceride breakdown) and pyruvate–lactate (from muscle glycogen) are additional substrates for gluconeogenesis (not shown in the figure). See text for details.

not provide adequate carbohydrate to sustain all tissues in the body simultaneously. If fat oxidation is impaired for any reason, hypoglycemia supervenes.

When the adaptive mechanisms are functioning properly, human beings can survive for long periods of time in the total absence of food, provided water is available. For example, most normal-sized (nonobese) adults have 100,000–150,000 kcal stored as fat that, at a utilization rate of 2000 kcal/day, would assure survival for 50–75 days.

REGULATION OF GLUCAGON AND INSULIN SECRETION

The primary regulatory organ for fuel metabolism is the endocrine pancreas, and the two key hormones are insulin and glucagon. Insulin is the primary mediator of anabolism, whereas glucagon is the preeminent inducer of catabolism. There is no backup hormone for insulin, but four other hormones exhibit catabolic functions similar to those of glucagon. They are epinephrine, norepinephrine, cortisol, and growth hormone. Most norepinephrine reaches target sites via release from sympathetic nerve endings rather than through the bloodstream. Glucagon and the other four hormones are often designated *counterregulatory,* indicating that they oppose the actions of insulin and protect the body against hypoglycemia.

Insulin and glucagon release normally are smoothly coordinated, so that substrate flow in the alternating anabolic–catabolic phases maintains the plasma glucose levels in the normal range, avoiding both hypo- and hyperglycemia. Concentrations of the two hormones ordinarily vary reciprocally: when insulin concentrations in plasma rise, glucagon levels fall, and vice versa. Each hormone influences release of the other within the pancreatic islet. Insulin inhibits glucagon secretion directly. The venous drainage from the centrally located β- (insulin-producing) cells appears to pass directly to the peripherally situated α- (glucagon-producing) cells. There insulin binds to the insulin receptor and induces an inhibitory signal (nature unknown) that impairs glucagon release. Glucagon stimulates insulin secretion both directly and indirectly. The former mechanism involves binding of the α-cell hormone to its receptor on the β-cell with subsequent enhancement of insulin release, possibly mediated by cyclic AMP. The indirect effect stems from the ability of glucagon to cause a transient rise in the plasma glucose concentration (through its stimulatory action on hepatic glycogenolysis), which, in turn, promotes insulin release from the β-cell. Hypoglycemia inhibits insulin release and stimulates glucagon secretion. Hyperglycemia has an inhibitory effect on glucagon secretion that is independent of insulin, but the mechanism is poorly understood.

Hypoglycemia is such a powerful stimulus to glucagon secretion that it can override, at least acutely, the inhibitory effect of insulin on the α-cell. Thus, when plasma glucose is significantly lowered by the injection of exogenous insulin, glucagon levels rise to protect against that hypoglycemia despite high concentrations of insulin in plasma. Although it is presumed that the primary stimulus to the α-cell is hypoglycemia per se, acting through some form of a glucose sensor, hypoglycemia-induced catecholamine release doubtless also plays a role. The catecholamine initiation of glucagon secretion is independent of the glucose-sensing mechanism.

Overall it seems safe to say that the primary regulatory signal to both α- and β-cells is the plasma glucose concentration, although glucose-induced changes in glucagon and insulin modulate islet cell response. Stimulatory and inhibitory levels of glucose vary, depending on interactions with other nutrients and hormones, but in general, insulin release becomes negligible or absent when the plasma glucose concentration declines to the 80–85 mg/dl range. Above this level, insulin secretion increases in near linear fashion as the plasma glucose rises. Glucagon release begins to occur at a plasma glucose concentration of approximately 50 mg/dl. Maximal suppression of the α-cell hormone occurs when the plasma glucose reaches 150 mg/dl.

The mechanisms controlling insulin release have also been slow to emerge. Well established is the fact that glucose enters the β-cell by a specific glucose transport molecule called *GLUT-2* (which also transports glucose into the hepatocyte). The sugar is then phosphorylated and subsequently metabolized with the generation of ATP. The ATP closes an ion channel, the (ATP)-sensitive K^+ channel, which depolarizes the β-cell membrane. This depolarization activates a voltage-dependent calcium channel that increases intracellular calcium and stimulates insulin release. Sulfonylureas, drugs that stimulate insulin release, interact with a receptor that appears to act through the (ATP)-sensitive K^+ channel. What has only recently come to light is that in the fasted state, the elevated level of circulating fatty acids, and to a lesser extent the ketone bodies (see below), play a key role in pancreatic β-cell function: first, they synergize with glucose to maintain a low, but critically important output of insulin (see below); second, they are essential for the robust secretion of insulin following termination of the fast.

While glucose appears to be the preeminent regulatory signal coordinating islet hormone traffic in the basal state, other fuels and hormones may play a role under certain conditions. For example, a high-protein, carbohydrate-free meal stimulates both glucagon and insulin release, in contrast to carbohydrate-containing meals after which insulin increases and glucagon decreases as just described. The teleologic interpretation is that the protein-induced insulin release would cause hypoglycemia in the absence of carbohydrate were it not for the protective effect of glucagon that induces breakdown of hepatic glycogen to "cover" the insulin. This is the only physiological circumstance in which insulin and glucagon rise simultaneously.

Meals of all kinds induce hormonal and autonomic nervous system signals that enhance insulin secretion. These include the hormones cholecystokinin, secretin, gastrin, gastric inhibitory peptide, glucagon-like polypeptide 1, and acetylcholine. Acetylcholine is released in the pancreas from parasympathetic nerve endings. These regulatory molecules, controlled from the gastrointestinal tract, are thought to function in anticipatory fashion, readying the β-cell to release insulin promptly as the products of digestion enter the bloodstream. They also account for the fact that insulin response to oral glucose is greater than that seen when the same amount of glucose is given intravenously.

In stress and exercise, insulin–glucagon interrelationships are altered by adrenergic mechanisms. Epinephrine released from the adrenal medulla and norepinephrine reaching the islets from sympathetic nerve endings block insulin release and stimulate glucagon secretion so that hepatic glucose production rises as much as 4- to 5-fold over the rate seen after an overnight fast (approximately 10 g/hour overnight fast → 40–50 g/hour extreme exercise). Epinephrine and norepinephrine act via α_2-adrenergic receptors in the β-cell, inhibiting insulin release (mechanism unclear), whereas in the α-cell their action is mediated by β-adrenergic receptors that causes a rise in cyclic AMP with stimulation of glucagon secretion. Were it not for the marked increase in the [glucagon]:[insulin] ratio induced by the catecholamines, hepatic glucose output would not be sufficient to protect against hypoglycemia during strenuous exercise; that is, if muscle were using 40 g glucose/hour, whereas the liver was producing only 10 g/hour (the normal response to the hormonal signals operative in fasting), hypoglycemia would rapidly supervene.

The role of somatostatin in regulating insulin and glucagon release from the islets is problematic. Produced by the pancreatic δ-cell, somatostatin conceivably could act in a paracrine fashion (direct cell-to-cell interaction) within the islet, but in fact this probably does not occur. Somatostatin is a powerful inhibitor of both insulin and glucagon secretion. Its concentration in pancreatic venous effluent is so high that essentially no glucagon or insulin would be released if the α- and β-cells were exposed to similar levels. For this reason it is thought that somatostatin acts as a true hormone, released into the systemic circulation for action at distal sites. One interpretation is that its central role is to slow intestinal absorption of fat. In animals, blockade of somatostatin action by the infusion of antisomatostatin antibodies results in the accelerated appearance of chylomicrons after a fat meal, suggesting enhanced absorption of triglycerides.

It seems probable that cortisol, growth hormone, and thyroid hormone modulate metabolism primarily through extrapancreatic effects, although all exert permissive regulatory actions in the islets. Cortisol, in particular, increases the gluconeogenic capacity of the liver, probably by stimulating synthesis of key enzymes.

MECHANISM OF ACTION OF INSULIN AND GLUCAGON

Despite intensive study over many years, the mechanism(s) by which insulin acts is still not fully understood. As with other peptide hormones, the initial step involves binding to a specific receptor localized in the plasma membrane. The receptor itself is now well characterized, its gene having been localized to the nineteenth chromosome in humans. Cloning has made it possible to define its primary structure, which has two α-subunits (M_r 135,000) and two β-subunits (M_r 95,000). The hormone-binding site is on the α-subunit. The β-subunit expresses a specific enzyme, tyrosine kinase, that phosphorylates proteins on tyrosine molecules rather than the serines and threonines that are phosphorylated by the more common cyclic AMP-dependent protein kinase. Once insulin is bound, it stimulates autophosphorylation of the receptor and phosphorylation of other proteins by the tyrosine kinase. An early substrate is insulin receptor substrate-1 (IRS-1), which acts as a signaling molecule for a host of subsequent events.

For example, in certain tissues, such as muscle and fat (the predominant extrahepatic insulin-sensitive tissues), tyrosine phosphorylation of IRS-1 causes activation of phosphatidylinositol-3'-kinase (PI-3-kinase), which in turn appears to be involved in translocation of a member of the glucose transporter family (GLUT-4) from intracellular storage sites to the cell surface, thus allowing more rapid entry of glucose into the cell. Another role for phosphorylated IRS-1 is its interaction with the regulatory proteins Grb2 and SoS to activate the proto-oncogene RAS by exchanging GTP for GDP (GTP is the "on" signal). RAS in turn activates a related protein, RAF-1, which then activates a kinase sequence, mitogen-activated protein kinase kinase (MAPK-K) and mitogen-activated protein kinase (MAP-K), which then carry out subsequent phosphorylations leading to gene activation and other effects, including movement of GLUT-1 to the cell surface, and stimulation of mitogenesis and protein synthesis. Thus, insulin acts through a complicated series of protein kinases to exert its actions. The kinase pathways are influenced by phosphatases; for example, a vanadate-activated tyrosine phosphatase may reverse early tyrosine phosphorylations by the insulin receptor.

In hormone interactions, agonists often regulate other agonists, frequently by dominant negative action. By way of illustration, the stimulatory effects of cyclic AMP and glucocorticoids on the gluconeogenic enzyme phosphoenolpyruvate carboxykinase can be inhibited by insulin, whereas insulin stimulation of the enzymes of glycogen synthesis and glycolysis can be overridden by glucagon.

It is of interest that in vitro acute actions of insulin on the liver are readily demonstrable only against a background of prior glucagon activation. Thus, in the hepatocyte, insulin can be considered primarily a counterregulatory agent for glucagon. Conversely, in nonhepatic tissues, direct effects of insulin may predominate; that is, insulin is regulatory rather than counterregulatory.

The actions of glucagon are better understood than those of insulin. Its primary effect is to raise intracellular levels of cyclic AMP rapidly. The hormone binds to the glucagon receptor and stimulates adenylate cyclase through a coupling mechanism with a guanine nucleotide-binding protein usually called G_s (s = stimulatory). An inhibitory guanine nucleotide-binding protein, G_i (i = inhibitory), also interacts with the system, and balance between stimulatory and inhibitory subunits determines net activity of the cyclase. Their interactions are very complex and need not be reviewed here (see Chapter 3). Cyclic AMP levels in liver rise very rapidly after exposure to glucagon. The cyclic nucleotide binds to inactive protein kinase, thereby dissociating the catalytic subunit that then initiates the phosphorylation of multiple proteins. Some of the effects of glucagon may be mediated by cyclic AMP-independent events involving changes in intrahepatic calcium stores. In either case, the net result is phosphorylation of key enzymes, an event that may either activate or inhibit them. For example, hepatic glycogen synthase is *inactivated*, whereas glycogen phosphorylase is *activated*, accounting for the fact that glucagon inhibits glycogen synthesis and stimulates glycogen breakdown.

ANABOLIC PATHWAYS

The absorptive process that follows food intake requires intraluminal and brush-border enzymes in the intestine that break down complex carbohydrates, lipids, and proteins to constituent sugars, fatty acids, and amino acids. In a normal mixed diet all three components are present (together with vitamins and minerals); their absorption occurs in parallel but at different rates.

Carbohydrate

Starch, sucrose, and lactose are the important carbohydrates in the normal diet. In Western societies about 60% of the daily carbohydrate intake is in the form of starch, 30% is sucrose, and 10% is lactose. About 20% of the starch is made up of amylose, which consists of straight chains of glucose molecules in $\alpha 1 \rightarrow 4$ linkage. The remainder is amylopectin, which has branching chains that occur about every 25 molecules, the branch point representing an $\alpha 1 \rightarrow 6$ linkage. Digestion of starch begins in the oral cavity with salivary amylase and is continued by the pancreatic version of that enzyme in the intestine. The initial products from the amylose chains are maltotriose and maltose, whereas branched oligosaccharides averaging 8 glucose units (called α-limit *dextrins*) are produced from amylopectin. The products of starch digestion, together with dietary lactose and sucrose, are hydrolyzed to single sugars by oligosaccharidases localized in the brush border of the intestinal mucosa. Glucose and galactose are transported across the intestinal membrane by an energy-requiring process after being bound to "carrier" protein molecules (distinct from the glucose carriers mentioned earlier that mediate insulin's action on glucose transport). The reaction depends on active pumping of sodium ions out of the cell. Fructose is absorbed by the carrier as well, but this process, called *facilitated diffusion,* is energy and sodium independent.

As noted above, the ingestion of a meal is followed by anticipatory priming of the pancreas that makes insulin available to control the metabolism of glucose ab-

sorbed directly and of glucose produced by interconversion from fructose and galactose. Some dietary glucose is oxidized in the postprandial (after ingestion of a meal)
period for energy production. The remainder is converted to glycogen and fat. In
muscle the glucose molecule is phosphorylated and incorporated directly into glycogen via the sequence glucose → glucose-6-phosphate → glucose-1-phosphate →
UDPglucose → glycogen. The same reaction sequence occurs in the liver, but in this
organ glycogen is also formed by an "indirect pathway" (Fig. 16-3), in which glucose is first metabolized to lactate and the lactate is then converted into glucose 6-
phosphate and subsequently into glycogen via gluconeogenesis. Precisely where the
glucose → lactate conversion takes place is unclear. It is likely that nonhepatic tissues (e.g., muscle, intestine, red blood cells, skin) are partly responsible, but some
of the lactate could arise in the liver itself, particularly if the hepatic parenchyma is
architecturally divided into zones of predominant glycolysis and predominant gluconeogenesis, as some have postulated. With refeeding after an overnight fast, the
direct and indirect pathways contribute about equally to hepatic glycogen repletion.

Because release of glucose from the liver rapidly stops after a carbohydrate
meal with concomitant insulin release, glucose-6-phosphatase is probably inhibited,
thereby favoring conversion of glucose 6-phosphate to glycogen. A second factor
assuring efficient glycogen synthesis is glucose-induced inactivation of glycogen
phosphorylase, which slows or stops glycogen breakdown. The conversion of phosphorylase *a*, the active form, to phosphorylase *b*, the inactive form, has another
effect. Phosphorylase *a* inhibits the specific phosphatase that dephosphorylates

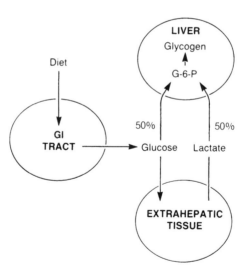

Fig. 16-3   The formation of glycogen in the liver. Glucose absorbed from the diet enters hepatic glycogen by two pathways. About 50% enters directly without degradation. The remainder enters indirectly after conversion to lactate in extrahepatic tissues.
The precise site of this conversion is not known, although muscle, intestine, and red
blood cells have all been postulated. Lactate then returns to the liver and is converted
to glucose-6-phosphate (G-6-P) via gluconeogenesis. Essentially all muscle glycogen is
formed by the direct pathway.

glycogen synthase and converts it from an inactive to active form. Thus, a glucose-induced fall in glycogen phosphorylase a allows conversion of inactive glycogen synthase b to active glycogen synthase a with the result that glucose 6-phosphate is "pulled" into glycogen. The combined effect of inhibition of glucose-6-phosphatase and activation of glycogen synthase accounts for the rapid glycogen repletion that characterizes the postprandial state.

Substantial evidence now supports the view just articulated that at physiological concentrations of plasma glucose, such as those seen after a normal meal, a significant fraction of hepatic glycogen is formed by the indirect pathway. For many years it was believed that the gluconeogenic sequence (required by the indirect pathway) was shut down almost immediately after meal ingestion. This turns out not to be true, for it has been shown both in experimental animals and in humans, using isotopic techniques, that gluconeogenesis continues unimpaired for several hours after a meal. Indeed, it is likely that some basal rate of gluconeogenesis operates at all times. In humans, gluconeogenic flux has been found to increase earlier in the postprandial state than was once believed. The control of gluconeogenesis is ordinarily thought to be vested in the regulatory glycolytic intermediate fructose-2,6-bisphosphate (F-2,6-P_2); high levels of F-2,6-P_2 normally inhibit gluconeogenesis (see Fig. 16-6 and discussion of gluconeogenesis below). In isolated hepatocytes, F-2,6-P_2 concentrations rapidly rise after exposure to glucose, but in intact animals its concentration in the liver does not increase until glycogen stores are repleted. This late rise readily explains continued gluconeogenesis. In contrast, when fructose or sucrose is ingested, F-2,6-P_2 levels rise promptly to levels that should be inhibitory to gluconeogenesis, yet the process continues. This paradox remains to be explained (see below).

As noted, dietary carbohydrate not utilized for energy production is converted to glycogen first and then to fat. Triglyceride synthesis from carbohydrate takes place primarily in the liver with lesser *in situ* synthesis occurring in adipose tissue. Thus, most glucose-derived fat is made in the liver and transported via lipoproteins to the adipocyte rather than being formed *de novo* in adipose tissue. The biochemical pathways are well understood. The primary substrate is lactate (pyruvate) derived from glucose. Pyruvate, which is formed in the cytosol, then enters the mitochondria and is decarboxylated to acetyl-coenzyme A (CoA) by the pyruvate dehydrogenase complex. Acetyl-CoA condenses with oxaloacetate to form citrate under the influence of citrate synthase. Citrate may proceed through the reactions of the tricarboxylic acid cycle, but a portion exits the mitochondria and is reconverted to acetyl-CoA and oxaloacetate in the cytosol by citrate cleavage enzyme. Acetyl-CoA is converted to malonyl-CoA under the influence of acetyl-CoA carboxylase, and the sequential addition of malonyl-CoA to an anchoring acetyl-CoA, carried out by fatty acid synthase, leads to the formation of palmitic acid. The latter (after conversion to its CoA ester) can then undergo changes such as elongation and desaturation. The sequence, in summary, is glucose → lactate/pyruvate → citrate → acetyl-CoA → malonyl-CoA → palmitate → other fatty acids. Once formed, the long-chain fatty acids are esterified to glycerol-3-phosphate, and the newly synthesized triglyceride is incorporated into a very-low-density lipoprotein (VLDL) molecule. Fatty acids are transferred from VLDL into adipocytes after hydrolysis of VLDL-borne triglycerides by endothelial-bound lipoprotein lipase. Adipose tissue also has the capacity to synthesize long-chain fatty acids *de novo* by the mechanism just described.

Fat

Fat absorption is mediated by pancreatic lipase. Enzymatic activity is manifest only after the lipase is bound to triglyceride in complex formation with colipase, a small protein molecule that is formed from its precursor, procolipase, by the action of trypsin. Complexing of lipase with colipase prevents the former's inactivation by intraluminal bile salts whose concentration increases after a meal. Pancreatic lipase splits off long-chain fatty acids from triglyceride, leaving a monoglyceride with the fatty acid in position 2. In the presence of bile salts, fatty acids and the 2-mono-glyceride form a soluble complex called a *micelle,* which is then able to pass the diffusion barriers of the intestinal mucosa. Micelle formation, required because fatty acids and monoglycerides are poorly soluble in water, provides an efficient mechanism for delivery of these components to the absorptive surface of the intestinal epithelial cell. Inside the cell triglycerides are re-formed and packaged into large, round lipoprotein particles called *chylomicrons,* which are rapidly secreted into the lymph. Medium- and short-chain fatty acids are not reesterified to triglycerides, nor are they transported out of the intestinal cell in chylomicrons; rather, they pass directly into the portal vein for transport to the liver as free fatty acids.

Chylomicrons are the largest lipoprotein particles found in the blood; about 90% of their bulk is made up of triglyceride. Clinically they can be separated from VLDLs, the endogenous fat transport molecules formed in the liver, by allowing plasma to stand overnight in the cold. Chylomicrons then separate out as a cream layer at the top of the tube with clear plasma underneath, whereas VLDL remains distributed throughout the plasma volume, giving the appearance of dilute skim milk. Chylomicrons contain a variety of apolipoproteins including AI, AII, and AIV. They also have a characteristic apolipoprotein B that is designated *apo-B48.* Apo-B48 is clearly distinguishable from apolipoprotein B100, which is synthesized in liver and is the counterpart protein of VLDL. Once in the plasma, the chylomicron's apolipoprotein composition changes rapidly; most of the A proteins are lost, and apolipoproteins CI, CII, CIII, and apolipoprotein E are added (Fig. 16-4). Apolipoprotein CII appears to play a critical role in activating lipoprotein lipase, thereby assuring rapid clearance of dietary fat from the plasma. Individuals with a congenital absence of apolipoprotein CII characteristically have major hypertriglyceridemia when eating fat because of difficulty in clearing chylomicrons. Lipoprotein lipase, which is located on the luminal surface of capillary endothelial cells, acts in a fashion similar to pancreatic lipase described above, removing the long-chain fatty acids from positions 1 and 3 and leaving a 2-monoglyceride, which is then hydrolyzed intracellularly.

In adipose tissue, most of the long-chain fatty acids are reesterified to glycerol derived from glucose (the original glycerol released from the chylomicron passes via plasma to the liver), but in muscle, heart, and other tissues a significant portion of the fatty acid is oxidized for energy production. Most of the triglyceride in chylomicrons is removed in a single pass through tissues, only 10%–15% of the original mass remaining in the "remnant" particle (Fig. 16-4). The small amounts of

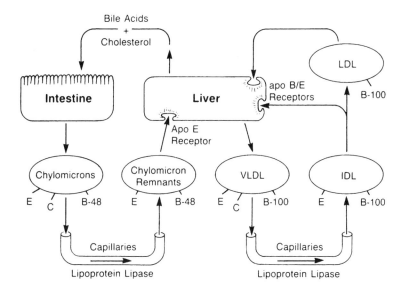

Fig. 16-4 The transport of dietary and endogenous fat. Capital letters stand for apolipoproteins. B-48 and B-100 refer to apolipoprotein B arising in intestine and liver, respectively. Dietary fat is transported to peripheral tissues as chylomicrons that pass to the liver after being stripped of triglyceride through the action of lipoprotein lipase. Uptake in the liver is mediated by a specific receptor designated the "apo E" receptor. Very-low-density lipoprotein (VLDL) carrying endogenously synthesized fat follows a similar sequence except that the "remnant" particle is designated intermediate-density lipoprotein (IDL). IDL can be taken up directly by the liver but is also the precursor for low-density lipoprotein (LDL). Both IDL and LDL are taken up by the LDL receptor designated here as the "apo B/E" receptor. (Redrawn with permission from Goldstein JL, Kita T, and Brown MS: Defective lipoprotein receptors and atherosclerosis: Lessons from an animal counterpart of familial hypercholesterolemia. N Engl J Med 309:288–296, 1983.)

cholesterol and cholesteryl esters present are not deleted. The primary apolipoproteins left in the remnant are apo-B48 and apo-E. The remnant particle then passes to the hepatocyte where it is cleared from the plasma by a specialized receptor called the *apo-E receptor*. The apo-E receptor has now been renamed the *LDL receptor-related protein* (LRP). It is also sometimes called the *chylomicron remnant receptor*.

The pathway of fat metabolism just described is often designated the *exogenous* or *dietary pathway*. A similar series of events occurs in the *endogenous* or *hepatic pathway* in which free fatty acids derived from diet, adipose tissue triglyceride stores, or synthesis in the liver are reesterified to form triglycerides and packaged as VLDL, as mentioned previously. Lipoprotein lipase (activated by VLDL-bound apolipoprotein CII) acts on VLDL in a manner similar to that described for chylomicrons except that not all the triglyceride is removed in a single pass. Lipoprotein transformations in the endogenous pathway are complicated. The remnant particle of VLDL, called *intermediate-density lipoprotein* (IDL), exchanges apolipoproteins with high-density lipoprotein (HDL) and is finally converted to low-density lipoprotein (LDL), the major cholesterol-carrying transport protein in the blood. Both IDL and LDL are then cleared from the plasma via a receptor on hepatocytes called the *apo-B/E* or *LDL receptor*. Identical receptors are present on other tissues of the body, and binding of LDL to these receptors allows entry of cholesterol into cells for membrane synthesis and hormone formation. Partial or complete absence of the LDL receptor leads to the disease *familial hypercholesterolemia.*

HDL molecules are not directly involved in fat transport but play a key role in reverse cholesterol transport out of tissues. LDL itself is innocent in atherogenesis but becomes atherogenic after oxidation to minimally modified LDL; the latter binds to a receptor distinct from the LDL receptor. The oxidized LDL receptor is known as the *acetyl LDL* or *scavenger receptor*. HDL functions as an antioxidant opposing the oxidation of LDL. Hence, it protects against atherosclerosis by two mechanisms: by removing cholesterol from blood vessels and by preventing the formation of oxidized LDL.

Cholesterol Metabolism

Although cholesterol is not a fuel, a brief discussion of its metabolism is included here because it is intimately involved in triglyceride metabolism, and because elevation of plasma cholesterol is a major risk factor in the development of atherosclerosis. Cholesterol in the body arises from two sources: diet and endogenous synthesis. The latter takes place via a linked series of enzymatic reactions starting from acetyl-CoA. An overview of the sequence is acetyl-CoA → acetoacetyl-CoA → hydroxymethylglutaryl-CoA (HMG-CoA) → mevalonic acid → isopentenylpyrophosphate → squalene → lanosterol → desmosterol → cholesterol. The rate-limiting step is the conversion of HMG-CoA to mevalonic acid, a reaction catalyzed by the enzyme HMG-CoA reductase. The general rule is that dietary and synthetic sources of cholesterol are reciprocally related: when dietary cholesterol intake is high, cholesterol synthesis is low and vice versa. Inhibitors of HMG-CoA reductase are the primary means of treating clinically significant hypercholesterolemia.

The average daily intake of cholesterol in Western diets is 500–1000 mg. This is mostly esterified because of a high intake of eggs, dairy products, and meat. Esterified cholesterol is hydrolyzed before absorption by a pancreatic cholesteryl esterase that acts in the presence of bile acids. It is presumed that cholesterol is absorbed in the form of mixed micelles made up of bile salts, fatty acids, and phospholipid. The process has limited efficiency; absorption ranges from one-third to two-thirds of the ingested load. By means that are not well understood, cholesterol is transferred from the absorptive micelles to lipoproteins, the two major carriers being chylomicrons and HDL. The former predominates, particularly if the meal contains fat. As discussed earlier, absorbed cholesterol reaches the liver via the production of chylomicron remnants (Fig. 16-4). Cholesterol taken up by the liver has several functions and fates. It may be excreted into the bile directly or may be converted to bile acids. It also causes inhibition of HMG-CoA reductase, thus slowing endogenous cholesterol synthesis in the hepatocyte. Simultaneously, cholesteryl ester formation is stimulated through activation of acyl-CoA:cholesterol acyltransferase (ACAT).

Finally, the lipoprotein-borne cholesterol suppresses synthesis of LDL receptors, thereby controlling entry of LDL into the cell. Dietary cholesterol, like newly synthesized cholesterol, can be repackaged into VLDL molecules, which lead to the production of LDL molecules, as described in the previous section. LDL is the principal means by which cholesterol reaches extrahepatic tissues for membrane synthesis and, in the endocrine glands, for steroid hormone formation.

Elucidation of the LDL receptor pathway has provided insight into a general mechanism whereby a variety of larger molecules pass from the plasma into cells. The system is called *receptor-mediated endocytosis*. Specificity is determined by the various receptors involved (i.e., insulin enters cells after binding to the insulin receptor, epidermal growth factor [EGF] by binding to the EGF receptor, and so forth). The LDL binds to its receptors in specialized areas of the plasma membrane called "coated pits" (the "coat" is a distinctive protein called *clathrin*). The receptor, bearing its LDL, is then pinched off to form a coated vesicle. The vesicle next merges with lysosomes, and lysosomal enzymes rapidly degrade LDL to constituent amino acids with release of cholesteryl esters. The latter are hydrolyzed to free cholesterol. Empty LDL receptors cycle back to the cell surface. The speed of the process is quite remarkable, each receptor making the trip from coated pit to lysosome and back to the plasma membrane in 10 minutes. Normally about 60%–70% of cholesterol traffic enters the cell via the LDL receptor, but about one-third traverses a nonspecific uptake pathway. Disturbances in the LDL receptor cycle ordinarily cause difficulty because cholesterol concentrations in plasma rise, leading to atherosclerosis via conversion of LDL to oxidized LDL. Interestingly, even the complete absence of the LDL receptor system is not accompanied by clinical hormonal deficiency states, presumably because the combination of endogenous cholesterol synthesis and entry of cholesterol by receptor-independent pathways satisfies cellular needs.

Protein

The absorption of protein is more complicated than the absorption of fat and carbohydrate. The process appears to start in the stomach through the action of pepsin in the presence of an acid environment. Pepsin is not necessary for protein absorption, however. Most of the absorptive process takes place in the small intestine with pancreatic proteases doing the bulk of the work. The major endopeptidases (trypsin, chymotrypsin, and elastase) act on peptide bonds to produce free amino acids and oligopeptides. Exopeptidases (aminopeptidase and carboxypeptidase) act after the initial formation of longer peptides by trypsin, chymotrypsin, and elastase to produce the final luminal products. Ordinarily the combined activities yield about 30% free amino acids and 70% oligopeptides, with a chain length ranging from 2 to 6 amino acids. The fate of the oligopeptides is complicated, some being broken down by brush border enzymes and others being transported into the cell where cytoplasmic peptidases complete the degradative process. The high specific activity amino-oligopeptidase of the brush border has its action blocked by the presence of a proline in the penultimate position of the oligopeptide chain. This regulatory proline thus appears to determine whether intraluminal/brush-border digestion is complete or whether intracellular digestion is required. Surprisingly, the transport of free amino acids from the lumen into the cell is a slower process than the transport of oligopeptides. Absorbed amino acids pass to the liver via the portal vien.

The rise in amino acid concentrations in arterial blood that follows a protein

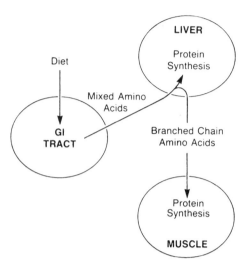

Fig. 16-5 Amino acid transport following a meal. Mixed amino acids reach the liver via the portal vein. Branched-chain amino acids preferentially pass through the hepatic circulation and account for 60% of the rise in amino acid concentrations in the general circulation. They appear to be utilized for protein synthesis under the influence of insulin.

meal does not reflect the makeup of the ingested protein. That is, all amino acids are not metabolized or transported in identical fashion. Although branched-chain amino acids make up no more than one-fifth of the total residues in meat, about 60% of the increase in amino acids following the protein meal is made up of leucine, valine, and isoleucine. Presumably they escape uptake by the liver and are transported to muscle where they serve as the major substrate for protein synthesis (Fig. 16-5). Insulin has the capacity to stimulate the process of protein synthesis in general and the utilization of branched-chain amino acids in particular. The mechanism is not completely understood, but at least one action of insulin is to stimulate the formation of "initiation complexes" that start the series of reactions leading to peptide formation. Some investigators believe that phosphorylation–dephosphorylation reactions may be important, as mentioned earlier in the discussion of insulin actions. Leucine may be a special stimulatory signal for protein synthesis, but again, the mechanism is not clear. Net buildup of muscle following a meal is also a consequence of insulin-induced diminution in proteolysis; that is, insulin has the capacity to simultaneously stimulate protein synthesis and block protein breakdown.

CATABOLIC PATHWAYS

To review briefly, the catabolic phase of metabolism is a series of metabolic adaptations designed to ensure adequate fuels for body tissues in the absence of exogenous substrate. The preeminent concern is to maintain the plasma glucose at safe levels for the central nervous system until ketone concentrations rise into the protective range. If acetoacetic and β-hydroxybutyric acids are not present in sufficient concentrations, the brain is vitally dependent on glucose, and absence of glucose is as devastating as the absence of oxygen. As noted earlier, the protective processes required are glycogen breakdown, gluconeogenesis, lipolysis, and ketogenesis.

Glycogenolysis and Gluconeogenesis

In the early postabsorptive state and the initial phases of fasting, maintenance of the plasma glucose depends almost entirely on glycogen stores. Although glycogenolysis can be induced by catecholamines acting as β-agonists (and, in humans, to a small extent via a-receptors), it is generally accepted that the bulk of glycogen breakdown occurs through a glucagon-mediated rise in cyclic AMP. Activation of cyclic AMP-dependent protein kinase phosphorylates phosphorylase b, converting it to the active a form. Simultaneously, phosphorylation of glycogen synthase a converts it to the inactive b form. In consequence, glycogen formation ceases, avoiding a futile cycle of coexistent glycogen breakdown and formation. It is likely that glucose-6-phosphatase activity also increases in the catabolic phase, assuring that glucose 6-phosphate (G-6-P) formed from glycogen will pass immediately into the plasma as free glucose. This would be a mirror image of the inhibition postulated to occur after feeding. The nature of regulation at the G-6-P reaction, if any exists, is not known. If the enzyme is not regulated, flux is probably substrate controlled; that is, a rise in G-6-P concentrations secondary to glycogen breakdown and impaired glycogen synthesis would drive the reaction.

The mechanisms by which carbon flow between G-6-P and pyruvate is controlled are now reasonably well understood. As noted earlier, in the catabolic phase, glycolysis (G-6-P → pyruvate) is blocked and gluconeogenesis (pyruvate → G-6-P) is enhanced. The key regulatory site appears to be the interconversion of fructose-6-phosphate (F-6-P) and fructose-1,6-bisphosphate (F-1,6-P$_2$) (see Fig.16-6). Although most of the reactions of the glycolytic–gluconeogenic pathway are reversible,

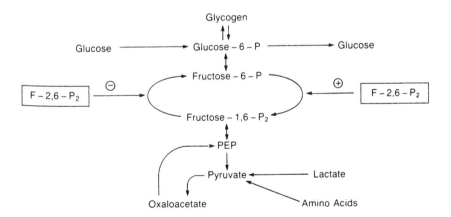

Fig. 16-6 The regulation of glycolysis and gluconeogenesis. Fructose-2,6-bisphosphate (F-2,6-P$_2$) stimulates glycolysis by activating phosphofructokinase, which converts fructose-6-phosphate to fructose-1,6-bisphosphate and inhibits gluconeogenesis by deactivating fructose-1,6-bisphosphatase, which converts fructose-1,6-bisphosphate to fructose-6-phosphate.

separate enzymes operate at this site. In the glycolytic pathway, F-6-P is converted to F-1,6-P_2 via the enzyme 6-phosphofructo-1-kinase, whereas the reverse reaction, the major regulatory step in gluconeogenesis, is mediated by fructose-1,6-bisphosphatase. Glucagon control of the opposing reactions is effected by changing the concentrations of a regulatory intermediate, fructose-2,6-bisphosphate, which is itself not a direct participant in glycolysis. Fructose-2,6-bisphosphate is formed from F-6-P by a bifunctional enzyme called 6-phosphofructo-2-kinase/fructose-2, 6-bisphosphatase (PFK_2/$FBPase_2$). This remarkable enzyme shifts from a kinase to a phosphatase when phosphorylated. When insulin levels are high and glucagon levels are low, the enzyme is dephosphorylated and functions as a kinase, which leads to the synthesis of fructose-2,6-bisphosphate. When insulin levels fall and glucagon concentrations increase, the enzyme is phosphorylated, kinase activity is lost, and phosphatase activity appears. This causes, simultaneously, decreased synthesis and increased hydrolysis of fructose-2,6-bisphosphate with the result that its concentration in the hepatocyte rapidly falls. When fructose-2,6-bisphosphate levels are high, phosphofructokinase activity is stimulated and glycolysis is active, whereas fructose bisphosphatase is inhibited, blocking gluconeogenesis. The catabolic sequence can be summarized as follows: increased glucagon → increased cAMP → increased cAMP-dependent kinase → increased phosphorylation of PFK_2/$FBPase_2$ → decreased F-2,6-P_2 → decreased glycolysis + increased gluconeogenesis. Activation of gluconeogenesis assures sustained hepatic glucose production after preformed glycogen is depleted while the block in glycolysis indirectly allows the liver to become a ketogenic organ, as described below.

In quantitative terms, hepatic glucose production averages about 2 mg/kg body weight/minute after an overnight fast. About 70%–80% of the output is derived from glycogen and about 20% from gluconeogenesis under these conditions. If fasting is combined with exercise, glycogen stores are depleted much more rapidly and the percentage contribution from gluconeogenesis increases. The gluconeogenic substrates are lactate, glycerol, and amino acids. Lactate derives from two sources. The first is from glucose incompletely oxidized in peripheral tissues. That is, during the initiation of the catabolic state, glucose passes from the liver to peripheral tissues where it is metabolized to pyruvate-lactate. A portion of the pyruvate undergoes terminal oxidation to CO_2 and water with energy production, but the remainder of the pyruvate-lactate returns to the liver. Lactate concentrations in plasma are ten times higher than those of pyruvate so that it is the principal member of the couple. The glucose → lactate → glucose sequence is known as the *Cori cycle*. Note that the Cori cycle does not result in net glucose synthesis in the body as the lactate was originally derived from preformed glucose. Net glucose synthesis from lactate requires its production from glucose derived from muscle glycogen.

Glycerol, which is a relatively minor contributor to gluconeogenesis, is released from triglycerides hydrolyzed in adipose tissue (see lipolysis below). The major substrate for gluconeogenesis is amino acids, which flows from muscle. As is the case in the anabolic phase, where the rise in amino acid concentrations in arterial blood does not reflect the amino acid makeup of ingested proteins, the output of amino acids from muscle is also asymmetrical. Thus, alanine and glutamine account for over 50% of the amino acids released, although alanine represents only about 7% of the total amino acid residues in muscle (Fig. 16-7). Glutamine is primarily taken

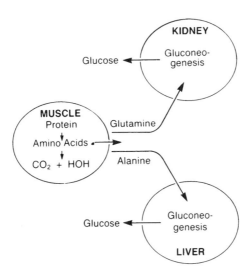

Fig. 16-7 Release of amino acids from muscle and their use in gluconeogenesis. Glutamine and alanine are the primary amino acids delivered to the liver and kidney for conversion to glucose. See text for details.

up by extrahepatic splanchnic tissues and is also utilized for gluconeogenesis in the kidney after prolonged fasting. Studies in humans suggest that it may be a more significant substrate for hepatic gluconeogenesis than previously thought. Alanine is the primary amino acid utilized for glucose production by the liver. Its fractional extraction and total uptake are increased in the fasting state.

The explanation for the excess release of alanine from muscle is thought to be a transamination reaction wherein branched-chain amino acids (leucine, isoleucine, valine) donate their amino groups to pyruvate derived from muscle glycogen. A teleological explanation might be that alanine is the best precursor for hepatic gluconeogenesis, entering the gluconeogenic sequence after reversed transamination to pyruvate. The a-keto analogues of branched-chain amino acids remaining after amino group donation can be oxidized in muscle for energy purposes, although some are released into the general circulation.

The signals for proteolysis in muscle are not completely understood. It is likely that both insulin deficiency and the presence of counterregulatory hormones play a role. For example, small physiological increments in plasma cortisol concentrations clearly stimulate proteolysis. Catecholamines (and perhaps glucagon) probably have similar effects. Protein breakdown occurs by both lysosomal and nonlysosomal pathways. At least a portion of the latter is calcium dependent.

The amino acids utilized in gluconeogenesis do not come from nonfunctional storage pools but from working muscle. It is assumed, therefore, that enzymes, transport molecules, and membrane proteins may be broken down. Their loss puts cellular integrity at risk. Indeed, in most cases death from starvation is due to protein wastage, often from cardiac arrhythmias. It thus becomes crucial that proteolysis be limited when fasting is prolonged. This in fact occurs. A great part of the physiological adaptation is the previously mentioned shift to a lipid economy in which most tissues of the body are sustained by the oxidation of fat, either as free fatty acids or ketone bodies. This markedly reduces the demand for glucose and, as a result, the requirements for gluconeogenic substrate diminish. This is reflected in a lessening of the negative nitrogen balance that is so characteristic of starvation. How the muscle is notified to diminish proteolysis is not clear. The thesis, once widely held, that ketone bodies represent the off signal is no longer tenable. One possibility is that rising free fatty acid and ketone body concentrations stimulate insulin release from the β-cell and that it is insulin that is the antiproteolytic signal.

However, refeeding studies with fructose indicate that this sugar alone, in the absence of an increase in plasma insulin levels, also reverses all manifestations of starvation, including protein breakdown, suggesting that insulin is not an obligatory mediator for cessation of proteolysis. Conceivably the message is carried through amino acid concentrations in plasma. A diminished need for glucose either because of refeeding or because of fat oxidation might slow the uptake of alanine and other amino acids by the liver, leading to a transient rise in plasma and subsequently in muscle amino acid concentrations. This might somehow activate a negative feedback sequence that would blunt protein breakdown. Although it is clear that proteolysis slows with prolonged fasting, the mechanisms must be considered speculative at this time.

When the catabolic state induced by fasting is reversed by feeding there is a complete reversal of the metabolic changes just described. The triggering event is almost certainly a rise in the [insulin]:[glucagon] ratio. One interesting characteristic of the reversal in carbohydrate metabolism has been commented on earlier—namely that gluconeogenesis continues for several hours after feeding, allowing hepatic glycogen repletion to take place in large measure via an "indirect" rather than a "direct" pathway. Continued gluconeogenesis is not difficult to explain after glucose feeding as fructose-2,6-bisphosphate levels do not rise for several hours, as noted earlier. Conversely, with sucrose refeeding, F-2,6-P$_2$ levels rise early on and yet gluconeogenesis is not impaired. Two possible explanations suggest themselves. First, there might be a regulatory intermediate substance (not yet identified) that can override normal F-2,6-P$_2$ inhibition of gluconeogenesis. Second, the measured rise in F-2,6-P$_2$ might not be uniform in all hepatocytes; that is, some zones of the liver would contain cells that do not manifest an early rise in F-2,6-P$_2$ and thus continue gluconeogenesis.

Lipolysis and Ketogenesis

The switch to a lipid economy in the catabolic phase of metabolism requires changes in both adipose tissue and liver. The hydrolysis of triglycerides in the adipocyte delivers long-chain fatty acids, together with glycerol, into the circulation. Two-thirds to three-fourths of the mobilized fatty acids are utilized directly, whereas the remainder are taken up by the liver for conversion to ketone bodies. Under normal anabolic conditions the liver produces only tiny amounts of acetoacetic and β-hydroxybutyric acids. Dietary fatty acids entering the hepatocyte are simply esterified to triglycerides and transported into the circulation as VLDL. After a few hours of fasting, or under the influence of counterregulatory hormones induced by stress, fatty acid oxidative capacity is activated and significant ketone body production becomes possible, provided long-chain fatty acids are available. Conceptually, adipose tissue can be viewed as the substrate supply depot and the liver as the factory for ketone production. Full-blown ketosis requires both an adequate delivery of FFA to the liver and activation of the enzyme system that converts these substrates to acetoacetic and β-hydroxybutyric acids. Failure of either substrate delivery or enzyme activation causes ketogenesis to fail. Once the liver is activated, rates of ketone body production are simply the consequence of the rate of delivery of long-chain fatty acids; that is, the higher the concentration of long-chain fatty acids in plasma, the greater the production rate of ketones by the liver until V_{max} rates are obtained. Qualitatively, there is no difference in the metabolic adaptations in adipose tissue and liver that accompany the very mild ketosis of a brief fast and the raging ketoacidosis of uncontrolled diabetes mellitus. The differentiating determinant is that FFA concentrations are very much higher in the latter state.

The hydrolysis of triglycerides in adipocytes is due to activation of an intracellular lipase generally designated *hormone-sensitive lipase* to distinguish it from the extracellular lipoprotein lipase responsible for hydrolysis of triglyceride in plasma lipoproteins. The hormone-sensitive lipase is inhibited by insulin and adenosine and activated by counterregulatory hormones (Fig. 16-8). In humans, catecholamines appear to play the primary role in activation, whereas glucagon, growth hormone, cortisol, and corticotropin (ACTH) have much lesser effects. Epinephrine and norepinephrine act through cyclic AMP-stimulated protein kinase in classic fashion. Removal of the insulin inhibitory effect, expected from a fall in plasma insulin accompanying the catabolic phase, also plays a role. The quantitative contribution of the removal of insulin inhibition in relation to the positive activating effects of catecholamines has not been completely worked out. Experimentally, the hormone-sensitive lipase can also be inhibited by adenosine and ketone bodies. Some evidence suggests that the effects of adenosine may be physiologically important.

The fatty acid-oxidizing system of the body is quite complicated and involves multiple enzymes. It can be divided into two components: a transport system re-

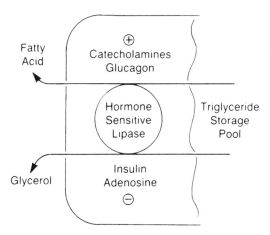

Fig. 16-8 Hormone-sensitive lipase in adipocytes and its regulation. +, activation; −, inhibition. Although not shown, ketone bodies may also inhibit the lipase.

quired to get long-chain fatty acids into the mitochondria and the intramitochon-drial oxidizing system (β-oxidation) that cleaves the long-chain fatty acid to acetyl-CoA. In most tissues, the fatty acid-derived acetyl-CoA undergoes terminal oxidation to CO_2 and water in the tricarboxylic acid cycle for the generation of energy. In the liver, however, the bulk of the acetyl-CoA in the catabolic phase (about 95%) is con-verted to acetoacetic and β-hydroxybutyric acids via the hydroxymethylglutaryl-CoA cycle. The transport step appears to be rate limiting under most circumstances so that any fatty acids traversing the inner mitochondrial membrane are rapidly ox-idized. When long-chain fatty acids are taken up in liver or other tissues, they are converted to CoA derivatives, with ATP as an energy source (Fig. 16-9). The long-chain fatty acyl-CoA cannot penetrate the inner mitochondrial membrane, however; it requires a transesterification step in which CoA is exchanged for carnitine, a car-rier molecule in lipid transport. The transesterification is carried out by an enzyme located on the outer mitochondrial membrane called *carnitine palmitoyltransferase I* (CPT I). Fatty acylcarnitine is then transported across the inner mitochondrial mem-brane by a translocase enzyme and reconverted to the CoA derivative under the in-fluence of carnitine palmitoyltransferase II (CPT II). The newly reformed fatty acyl-CoA appears to be committed to oxidation in the β-oxidative sequence. The

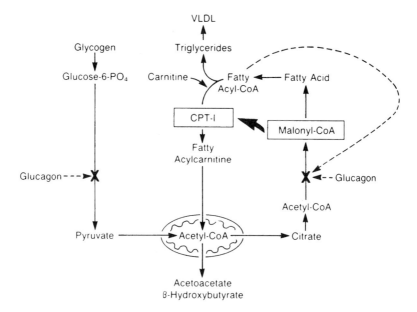

Fig. 16-9. The regulation of ketogenesis. In the transition from anabolic to catabolic phases glucagon blocks glycolysis, thereby interrupting flux over the sequence glucose-6-phosphate → pyruvate → acetyl-CoA → citrate → acetyl-CoA → malonyl-CoA. In ad-dition, glucagon and long-chain fatty acyl-CoA cause inhibition of acetyl-CoA carboxylase. The fall in malonyl-CoA thus produced disinhibits carnitine palmitoyl-transferase I (CPT I), the rate-limiting step in fatty acid oxidation, thereby activating the ketogenic pathway. Fatty acids delivered to the liver from adipose tissue are thus pref-erentially oxidized to acetoacetic and β-hydroxybutyric acids. The fall in malonyl-CoA also halts fatty acid synthesis.

genes for CPT I and CPT II have been cloned and sequenced in both rodent and human tissues. In liver, CPT I is distinct from CPT I in muscle, whereas CPT II appears to be the same in all tissues.

The activity of CPT I is regulated in large measure by the cytosolic concentration of malonyl-CoA. In the anabolic phase, malonyl-CoA concentrations in the liver, heart, and muscle are high and CPT I is inhibited. In tissues that synthesize fat, this assures that long-chain fatty acid synthesis and fatty acid oxidation do not occur simultaneously, thus avoiding a futile cycle. Under catabolic conditions, malonyl-CoA concentrations rapidly fall, thereby activating fatty acid oxidation, whereas lipogenesis simultaneously ceases as a result of a deficiency of substrate. The fall in malonyl-CoA is mediated in part by glucagon. One component of the mechanism is inhibition of glycolysis caused by the fall in fructose-2,6-bisphosphate previously described. The interruption of flux from glucose-6-phosphate to pyruvate reduces citrate production in the mitochondria, which in turn leads to failure of acetyl-CoA generation in the cytosol. Because malonyl-CoA is formed from the carboxylation of acetyl-CoA under the influence of the enzyme acetyl-CoA carboxylase, malonyl-CoA concentrations decrease, disinhibiting fatty acid oxidation. Glucagon also has the capacity to inhibit acetyl-CoA carboxylase (through cyclic AMP-mediated phosphorylation), as do long-chain fatty acyl-CoA concentrations, which also rise in liver during the catabolic adaptation (under some circumstances the carboxylase can also be inhibited by AMP-dependent protein kinase). These events are summarized in Figure 16-9. With refeeding, malonyl-CoA concentrations are restored to anabolic levels, thereby deactivating CPT I. The simultaneous rise in insulin, which inhibits lipolysis, normalizes the substrate wing of the process. Malonyl-CoA is also a regulatory molecule for fatty acid oxidation in nonhepatic tissues, and in the pancreatic β-cell it is thought to be instrumental in glucose-stimulated insulin secretion by causing elevation of the cytosolic long-chain acyl-CoA concentration.

DERANGEMENTS IN GLUCOSE, LIPID, AND PROTEIN METABOLISM

To illustrate the consequences of dysfunction in the anabolic–catabolic regulatory system, which normally is tightly controlled, some selected clinical disorders will be described briefly.

Obesity

Obesity, which has now reached epidemic proportions in developed countries, represents a serious breakdown of fuel homeostasis and is associated with a wide spectrum of co-morbidities including osteoarthritis, hypertension, and type 2 diabetes. Although excessive weight gain can only occur if there is an imbalance between calories consumed and calories expended, this simple logic belies the fact that there is genetically programmed variability among individuals in how they dispose of ingested calories (i.e., despite the same amount of food intake and physical activity, one person might maintain a stable body weight while another will lay down extra fat). From studies with normal and genetically obese rodents, early physiologists concluded that with expansion of fat mass a lipostatic factor is released from fat depots and, after transport through the blood, interacts with the hypothalamus to curtail food intake. It was further postulated that insufficient production of the putative material or a lower than normal ability of the hypothalamus to respond to it will lead to obesity.

This prophetic line of reasoning received major experimental support with the momentous discovery by Jeffrey Friedman and colleagues in 1994 of the hormone *leptin* (named after the Greek word "leptos," meaning "thin"). It was shown that leptin is a 16-kDa protein that is produced exclusively in fat cells and secreted into the blood. Moreover, it was found that the massive obesity of the *ob/ob* mouse stems from the complete absence of leptin production because of a mutation in the leptin gene. Not surprisingly, treatment of these animals with leptin corrected their hyperphagia, increased their metabolic rate, and restored them to a normal body weight.

There soon followed the cloning of the leptin receptor gene, which was found to encode both a long version and several truncated versions of the receptor. The long form, which contains a 303-amino acid cytoplasmic tail that confers signaling properties, is present in a variety of tissues but is particularly abundant in the hypothalamus. In keeping with earlier predictions, the *db/db* mouse (and also the Zucker *fa/fa* rat) was found to carry a mutation in the leptin receptor gene that results in failure to produce the long form of the receptor. As expected, leptin treatment of these animals is totally without effect on their hyperphagia, hypometabolism, or obesity.

Precisely how leptin's interaction with its hypothalamic (and possibly peripheral) receptor(s) influences feeding behavior and body habitus is not yet clear. With regard to its central effects, there is evidence that events downstream of the leptin–leptin receptor interaction include (a) a decreased synthesis of neuropeptide Y (NPY); (b) an increased synthesis of α-melanocyte-stimulating hormone (α-MSH); and (c) elevation in the ratio of sympathetic to parasympathetic signaling from the CNS to peripheral tissues. The NPY is known to be a powerful orexigenic substance (i.e., it drives food intake), whereas interaction of α-MSH with the melanocortin-4 receptor in the hypothalamus has the opposite effect. Thus, a leptin-induced decrease in NPY and increase in α-MSH levels would tend to suppress food intake. Enhanced sympathetic activity would be expected to accelerate adipose tissue lipolysis through catecholamine stimulation of β-adrenergic receptors, and to reduce malonyl-CoA levels both in fat and muscle cells. If, as is thought to be the case, there is a concomitant rise in uncoupling protein 2 or 3 activity in these tissues, conditions would be set for increased fat oxidation, elevation of the metabolic rate, and dissipation of fat stores. Whether leptin acts in this fashion, however, remains to be established.

Although the discovery of leptin and its receptor has electrified the field of obesity research, the initial hope that this hormone might provide a magic bullet for the treatment of human obesity has not materialized, for two reasons. First, although a few humans homozygous for serious mutations in the leptin gene have been found (one of whom weighed 94 kg at age 9 and is now losing weight rapidly with leptin treatment), these will probably be very rare. Second, most obese individuals have higher than normal circulating leptin levels, raising the possibility that leptin resistance might be a factor in the genesis of their condition. Because only a few hyperleptinemic obese individuals have proved to have a defect in their leptin receptor, it is likely that if leptin resistance turns out to be a common pathophysiogical entity, it will almost certainly be polygenic and heterogeneous in character. Accordingly, deciphering of the complex signaling pathways involved in leptin action is currently under intensive investigation and might well provide rational new approaches to the pharmaceutical treatment of obesity and its many complications.

Diabetes Mellitus

Diabetes mellitus is an extremely common metabolic disease affecting 1%–2% of the population in Western societies. The prevalence is much higher in certain groups such as the Hispanic and Native American subpopulations in the United States. There are two main types of diabetes, usually categorized as *insulin dependent* and *noninsulin dependent*. The former makes up about one-quarter of the total and is the more severe.

Current understanding of insulin-dependent diabetes (also known as *type 1 diabetes*) suggests that one inherits a genetic susceptibility to disease that is permissive but not causal. That multiple genes are involved has been suspected for some time and is reinforced by a recent search of the entire human genome, which revealed no less than 20 independent chromosomal regions with positive linkage to the disease. Of these, a particularly strong association was found with a gene located on the short arm of the sixth chromosome in the major histocompatibility complex. More than 90% of patients, when typed by a serologic test, exhibit human leukocyte antigen (HLA) DR3, DR4, or the combination DR3/DR4. It is currently thought that genes on the DQ β-chain may be more closely linked to diabetes susceptibility than those in the DR region. Some alleles appear to be susceptibility genes and others resistance genes, while still others are neutral. The HLA associations appear less informative in individuals developing diabetes after the age of 20.

The pathogenesis of autoimmune insulin-dependent diabetes is not precisely known. Leakage of cryptic antigens following a viral infection is one possibility. Alternatively, the mechanism of *molecular mimicry* may be involved. In molecular mimicry, homology between viral or food antigens and β-cell antigens fool the body's immune system into attacking itself. For example, a Coxsackie virus infection elicits an immune response. The cytotoxic T lymphocytes, armed against the viral antigens, cannot distinguish between the virus and the homologous amino acid segment in the β-cell, and thus attacks and destroys the latter.

Symptoms appear when 90% or more of the insulin-producing capacity of the islets of Langerhans is destroyed. Immune destruction is probably carried out both by humoral and cellular mechanisms, but the latter is considered dominant. Islet cell antibodies can be demonstrated in the plasma long before symptomatic diabetes appears. The most important predictive antibody recognizes glutamic acid decarboxylase (GAD) in the β-cell. The consequences of the immune attack are an absolute deficiency of insulin and a major overproduction of glucagon secondary to removal of the normal insulin restraint. The predictable metabolic consequences of a high [glucagon]:[insulin] ratio are overproduction of glucose by the liver, underutilization of glucose in nonhepatic tissues, and initiation of ketone body production in the liver, exactly as occurs in a normal fast. The only difference is that in normal individuals who do not eat, intact β-cells remain. Whereas a rising glucose concentration in plasma is the usual signal for insulin release, both ketone bodies and free fatty acids can also act in stimulatory fashion. Thus, in prolonged fasting, even though glucose concentrations are low, FFA and ketone bodies reach a threshold that stimulates insulin release, limiting lipolysis and thereby maintaining ketone production within the safe range. In uncontrolled diabetes, because insulin production is impossible, hyperglycemia steadily increases, adipose tissue lipolysis becomes excessive, and subsequent overproduction of ketone bodies by the liver leads to a life-threatening ketoacidosis.

The more common noninsulin-dependent diabetes mellitus (also called *type 2 diabetes*) is generally associated with obesity. Insulin resistance is a major problem, and insulin deficiency is relative rather than absolute. Obesity is a major cause of this resistance, but it can also be demonstrated in offspring of two parents with type 2 diabetes, even when they are not overweight or diabetic. The mechanism of the intrinsic insulin resistance has not been worked out, although there is growing evidence that fat accumulation in the muscle cell plays a role. Early in type 2 diabetes, insulin levels are high in absolute terms but are insufficient to overcome insulin resistance. Later, insulin levels fall as hyperglycemia worsens. The nature of the β-cell defect leading to diminished insulin reserve is not known, but here again an abnormal buildup of fat is thought to be one culprit. Because of the insulin resistance, glucagon levels are high and the [glucagon]:[insulin] ratio is elevated in terms of biological activity, even though the actual ratio may be near normal when assessed by radioimmunoassay. That is because the insulin present does not work well, leaving glucagon's actions unopposed. Once again the hormonal changes are those characteristic of the catabolic state and major hyperglycemia supervenes.

For reasons that are not yet clear, ketoacidosis does not develop in noninsulin-dependent diabetic subjects under most circumstances. Acetoacetic and β-hydroxy-butyric acid levels may rise after prolonged periods of poor medical control, but in general, they never exceed concentrations seen during the fasting state in normal people. Hyperglycemia may become extreme, reaching levels as high as 5000 mg/dl. It is not surprising that under these circumstances the blood has been described as "syrupy." Such profound elevations of the blood sugar result in severe body fluid losses through the kidney and ultimately lead to the syndrome called *hyperosmolar, nonketotic diabetic coma.* The former term refers to the fact that massive water deficits caused by glucose-driven urine production lead to increases in the plasma osmotic pressure from a normal of 280–300 mOsmol/liter to values as high as 400–500 mOsmol/liter. The term *nonketotic* does not mean that ketone bodies are not measurable in the urine or plasma, but simply that their production is not high enough to give ketoacidosis. Patients with hyperosmolar, nonketotic coma usually manifest altered consciousness or coma, convulsions, impaired kidney function, and sometimes pancreatitis and infections with gram-negative organisms. Mortality rates are very high.

The profound metabolic derangements of uncontrolled diabetes underline the importance of the control systems that normally govern fuel metabolism in the body. Although the metabolic disturbances of diabetes can usually be controlled well enough by dietary restriction and insulin therapy to prevent symptoms, it is almost impossible to maintain the plasma glucose within the normal range. Consequently, after many years of diabetes, patients become vulnerable to late degenerative complications involving the eyes, the nerves, the kidneys, and the blood vessels. Thus, diabetes is a leading cause of blindness, kidney failure, amputations, strokes, and heart attacks. It is these complications that make it such a devastating illness.

Hyperglycemia of Severe Injury

Nondiabetic subjects who sustain extreme injuries such as massive burns or major trauma may develop hyperglycemia even in the face of normal pancreatic function. The stress of such injuries leads to an outpouring of epinephrine and norepinephrine, which block insulin release from the β-cell, stimulate glucagon production, activate glycogenolysis, stimulate lipolysis, and induce proteolysis. In short, severe injury can quickly convert a normal state, even in a person who has just eaten, into the catabolic response. Stress overrides normal metabolism and does so by provoking sustained release of counterregulatory hormones.

Systemic Carnitine Deficiency

Systemic carnitine deficiency is a relatively rare syndrome in which carnitine concentrations are below the lower limits of normal in plasma and in multiple tissues, including muscle and liver. As noted above, protection against hypoglycemia requires the conversion of most tissues in the body from a carbohydrate to a lipid-utilizing state. This in turn requires that long-chain fatty acids be transported into the mitochondria for oxidation by the carnitine palmitoyltransferase system of enzymes. When carnitine is deficient, fatty acid oxidation is prevented, with the consequence that long-chain fatty acids cannot undergo terminal oxidation for energy generation or, in the liver, for the production of acetoacetic and β-hydroxybutyric acids. This means that all tissues remain dependent on glucose. Because the liver, even at maximal levels of gluconeogenesis, cannot deliver sufficient glucose in the plasma to meet body needs, profound hypoglycemia supervenes. Deficiencies of carnitine palmitoyltransferase or any of the enzymes of β-oxidation may lead to a similar syndrome. Children with systemic carnitine deficiency exhibit, in addition to hypoglycemia, massive storage of fat in all tissues of the body and also have the clinical picture of Reye's syndrome (hepatic encephalopathy, nausea, vomiting, increased arterial ammonia levels, and elevated liver enzymes in plasma).

Carnitine deficiency and related diseases of fatty acid oxidation illustrate the critical role of fat oxidation in protecting against hypoglycemia. Similar hypoglycemia can be seen in profound cachexia in the starvation belts of the world or in fat depletion consequent to cancer or other wasting illnesses.

Insulinoma

Insulin-producing tumors of the pancreas are not an uncommon medical problem and enter into the differential diagnosis of hypoglycemia. These tumors secrete insulin into the plasma in unregulated fashion. One might predict that counterregulatory hormones would protect against hypoglycemia under these circumstances, but persistent insulin secretion keeps glucagon suppressed to levels insufficient to overcome the actions of the β-cell hormone, with the result that blood sugar levels fall to concentrations that cause loss of consciousness, convulsions, or death. Just as severe injury can trigger sufficient release of counterregulatory hormones to overcome the capacity of the β-cell to respond, so can abnormal production of insulin abrogate the ability of counterregulatory hormones to respond. This emphasizes again how normal metabolism requires finely tuned and balanced interaction between the various components of the endocrine system.

Familial Hypercholesterolemia

Familial hypercholesterolemia (FH) is an autosomal dominant illness of humans that produces marked elevation of the plasma cholesterol. The latter, in turn, causes premature atherosclerosis with heart attacks occurring at an early age. In the more severe homozygous form of the disease (two abnormal genes for the LDL receptor), plasma cholesterol levels are in the range of 600–1200 mg/dl (normal, <200 mg/dl). In heterozygous patients (one mutant gene), levels are in the 300–550 mg/dl range. It is the LDL cholesterol fraction that is elevated. In homozygous familial hypercholesterolemia heart attacks commonly occur between the ages of 5 and 30 and have been reported as early as 18 months. In men with the heterozygous form of the illness there is a 5% chance of having a heart attack by the age of 30, 51% by the age of 50, and 85% by the age of 60. An interesting feature of the hypercholesterolemic states is the presence of cholesterol deposits in skin, tendons, and over bony prominences such as the elbows. These deposits, called *xanthomas,* are strong evidence of hypercholesterolemia. Careful palpation of the Achilles' tendon may reveal beaded xanthomas in patients who do not show typical deposits in the skin or over bony protuberances.

The elevation in plasma cholesterol is due in all cases to a genetic defect that produces an abnormal LDL receptor. Several types of defects are now known. Class 1 mutants synthesize no receptors. Class 2 mutants do not transfer LDL receptors efficiently from the endoplasmic reticulum to the Golgi apparatus so that the receptors are degraded in the cell before they can reach the cell surface. Class 3 mutants have LDL receptors that reach the cell surface but are unable to bind LDL. Class 4 mutants produce receptors that do not cluster in coated pits, thereby interrupting the normal metabolism of cholesterol.

It is possible to increase LDL receptors in heterozygous patients by giving bile-salt-binding resins. If endogenous cholesterol synthesis is then blocked by administering nicotinic acid or drugs that inhibit HMG-CoA reductase (e.g., lovastatin), substantial declines in plasma cholesterol can be obtained. Unfortunately, the drugs do not work in the homozygous form because no normal gene is available to stimulate.

Hypertriglyceridemia

Elevated plasma triglycerides may appear as primary genetic disease or secondary to other illnesses. The most common defect is a deficiency of lipoprotein lipase (LPL). Acquired deficiencies of LPL are seen in diabetes mellitus, hypothyroidism, alcoholism, lupus erythematosus (caused by antibodies against LPL or its co-factor, heparin), and uremia. Elevated triglycerides have two major detrimental effects. Acutely, they predispose to acute pancreatitis. Chronically, they lower HDL levels, predisposing to atherosclerosis.

SUGGESTED READING

Atkinson MA, and Maclaren NK: The pathogenesis of insulin dependent diabetes mellitus. N Engl J Med 331:1428–1436, 1994.

Bonnefont JP, Demaugre F, Tein I, Cepanec C, Brivet M, Rabier D, and Saudubray JM: Clinical deficiencies of carnitine palmitoyltransferase. In: *Current Concepts of Carnitine Research,* AL Carter, ed., CRC Press, New York, pp. 179–187, 1992.

Breslow JL: Genetic basis of lipoprotein disorders. J Clin Invest 84:373–380, 1989.

Brown MS, and Goldstein JL: A receptor-mediated pathway for cholesterol homeostasis. Science 232:34–47, 1986.

De Feo P, Perriello G, De Cosmo S, Ventura MM, Campbell PJ, Brunetti P, Gerich JE, and Bolli GB: Comparison of glucose counterregulation during short-term and prolonged hypoglycemia in normal humans. Diabetes 35:563–569, 1986.

Farooqi IS, Jebb SA, Langmack G, Lawrence E, Cheetham CH, Prentice AM,Hughes IA, McCamish MA, and O'Rahilly S: Effects of recombinant leptin therapy in a child with congenital leptin deficiency. N Engl J Med 341:879–884, 1999.

Friedman JM, and Halaas JL: Leptin and the regulation of body weight in mammals. Nature 395:763–770, 1998.

Gelfand RA, and Sherwin RS: Nitrogen conservation in starvation revisited: Protein sparing with intravenous fructose. Metabolism 35:37–44, 1986.

Havel RJ, and Rapaport E: Drug therapy: Management of primary hyperlipidemia. N Engl J Med 332:1491–1498, 1995.

Kahn CR: Banting lecture: Insulin action, diabetogenes, and the cause of type II diabetes. Diabetes 43:1066–1086, 1994.

Kather H, Bieger W, Michel G, Aktories K, and Jakobs KH: Human fat cell lipolysis is primarily regulated by inhibitory modulators acting through distinct mechanisms. J Clin Invest 76:1559–1565, 1985.

McGarry JD: What if Minkowski had been ageusic? An alternative angle on diabetes. Science 258:766–770, 1992.

McGarry JD, and Dobbins RL: Fatty acids and insulin secretion. Diabetologia 42:128–138, 1999.

McGarry JD, Kuwajima M, Newgard CB, Foster DW, and Katz J: From dietary glucose to liver glycogen: The full circle round. Annu Rev Nutr 7:51–73, 1987.

McGarry JD, Woeltje KF, Kuwajima M, and Foster DW: Regulation of ketogenesis and the renaissance of carnitine palmitoyltransferase. Diabetes Metab Rev 5:271–284, 1989.

Myers MG, and White MF: Insulin signal transduction and the IRS proteins. Annu Rev Pharmacol Toxicol 36:615–658, 1996.

Philipson LH, and Steiner DF: Perspectives. Pas de deux or more: The sulfonylurea receptor and K^+ channels. Science 268:372–373, 1995.

Pilkis SJ, and Granner DK: Molecular physiology of the regulation of hepatic gluconeogenesis and glycolysis. Annu Rev Physiol 54:885–909, 1992.

Ruderman NB, Saha AK, Vavvas D, and Witters LA: Malonyl-CoA, fuel sensing, and insulin resistance. Am J Physiol 276:E1–E18, 1999.

Schuit FC, and Pipeleers DG: Differences in adrenergic recognition by pancreatic A and B cells. Science 232:875–877, 1986.

Taylor SI, Accili D, and Imai Y: Insulin resistance or insulin deficiency—which is the primary cause of NIDDM? Diabetes 43:735–740, 1994.

Index